MEDICAL IMAGING IN CLINICAL PRACTICE

Edited by **Okechukwu Felix Erondu**

Medical Imaging in Clinical Practice
http://dx.doi.org/10.5772/45925
Edited by Okechukwu Felix Erondu

Contributors
Zongjin Li, Mojtaba Salouti, Akram Fazli, Marco Antonio Gutierrez, Francesco Alessandrino, Alfredo La Fianza, Giorgia Ricci, Esmeralda Eshja, Francesco Alfano, Carolina Della Fiore, Chiara Cassani, Carlos Costa, Frederico Valente, Augusto Silva, Patricia Carreño Moran, Julian Breeze, Michael Rees, Sonia Marta Moriguchi, Paulo Henrique Alves Togni, Katia Hiromoto Koga, Marcelo Santos, Tsuicheng D. Chiu, Takuya Osada, Laurence B Lovat, Rehan Haidry, Martín Gallegos-Duarte, Okechukwu Felix Erondu, Begona Garcia Zapirain, Maria Viqueira, Amaia Mendez Zorrilla

Published by InTech
Janeza Trdine 9, 51000 Rijeka, Croatia

Publishing Process Manager Danijela Duric
Technical Editor InTech DTP team
Cover InTech Design team

Additional hard copies can be obtained from orders@intechopen.com

Medical Imaging in Clinical Practice, Edited by Okechukwu Felix Erondu
p. cm.
ISBN 978-953-51-0986-0

For EU product safety concerns:
IN TECH d.o.o., Prolaz Marije Krucifikse Kozulić 3, 51000 Rijeka, Croatia,
info@intechopen.com or visit our website at intechopen.com.

Meet the editor

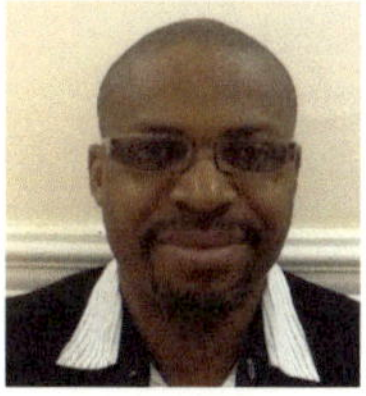

Dr. Felix Okechukwu Erondu is a practicing Medical imaging consultant and Cancer screening expert with clinical experience spanning over twenty years. He is an Adjunct senior lecturer in the Department of Medical Radiography and Radiological sciences in the University of Nigeria, Enugu campus and senior research fellow with over 40 scientific publications in renown international journals and three books to his credit. His research areas include ultrasound biophysics, radiation biology, diagnostic sonography, cross-sectional and breast imaging. He is actively involved in Group Cancer imaging and Advocacy work and chairs the Cancer Management Roundtable (CMRT), a private- public initiative. Dr Erondu is the Medical director of Image Diagnostics Ltd, Nigeria, a chain of ultramodern diagnostic facilities engaged in medical imaging and clinical support services. He has served as a board member of Nnamdi Azikiwe University Teaching Hospital and chairman of Radiographers Registration Board of Nigeria. He holds a masters degree in Medical Imaging and a doctorate in Medical Physics.

Contents

Preface

Everyday, millions of medical images are produced worldwide, to aid diagnosis and treatment of patients. A typical patient's diagnostic work-up is often incomplete without a medical imaging technique. The various techniques for achieving this have continued to evolve, from the basics through the sophisticated and now to the abstract. The concept of Medical imaging has therefore continued to widen, from the conventional like X-rays, ultrasound, CT, PET CT, MRI and nuclear Scintigraphy, to include various other recording and measurement techniques which may be documented by mapping or graphs.

This new book on 'Medical Imaging in Clinical practice' is another bold attempt to highlight the various research efforts and adaptations of newer and emerging techniques in the ever increasing world of medical Imaging. It seeks to explore the clinical applications of these newer techniques, while drawing parallels with the more conventional methods. It is by no means exhaustive, but achieves the overall purpose of widening the scope of knowledge and the readers' perception of the amazing world of medical Imaging.

I am sure, that most readers will not only be impressed, but encouraged to explore this ever evolving specialty of Medical Imaging and the bright hopes it offers in the future of clinical practice.

Dr. Okechukwu Felix Erondu
University of Nigeria Nsukka, Nigeria

Section 1

General Perspectives in Medical Imaging

Chapter 1

Content Based Retrieval Systems in a Clinical Context

Frederico Valente, Carlos Costa and Augusto Silva

Additional information is available at the end of the chapter

http://dx.doi.org/10.5772/53027

1. Introduction

Nowadays, digital images and protocols stand as a cornerstone of most modern health-care systems where they are used to provide important data and insights into the inner workings and ailments of the human body. The recent appearance of new modalities, the devices responsible for data acquisition, such as the fMRI[1] and the MDCT[2], produce copious amounts of data [1]. This, coupled with recent advances in storage technology has had as consequence an explosion in the amount of data produced at medical imaging institutions. For instance, the Geneva Hospital alone produced, in 2006, over 50000 images per day and such numbers are steadily rising [2]. Given the prevalence of digital images and protocols in the medical arena, we are, nonetheless, still a long way from fully taking advantage of the potential brought up by this digital revolution. The current data explosion makes it troublesome to a practitioner to sift through the imaging repositories while searching for data relevant for his context. This means we have the data, but not the information, which should be readily available to the experts in the area. In fact, data overload has been reported as a problem by practitioners from medium to large imaging institutions [3].

The current methods of data search, such as the ones provided by the standard query mechanisms present in Digital Imaging and Communication in Medicine (DICOM) are sub-optimal, relying on template matching over a limited number of textual fields [4] (which fields are available depend on the specific software backend), and can consequently be improved upon. It is expected that, by providing more refined and robust methods of searching the large image repositories that currently exist, diagnostic accuracy and efficiency can be improved and more accurate and useful Computer Aided Diagnosis (CAD) tools be devised.

1 Functional Magnetic Ressonance Imaging

2 Multi-detector computed tomography

A promising approach to solve the data explosion problem is to integrate computer-based assistance into the image querying and storage processes. This brings us into the topic of Content-Based Image Retrieval (CBIR). At its core, CBIR are a set of techniques to extract relevant pieces of information directly from an image or multimedia object itself with minimum (ideally none) intervention from a human.

The overarching goals are to improve the efficiency, accuracy, usability and reliability of medical imaging services within healthcare enterprises by analyzing content extracted directly from raw image data.

2. Picture archive and communication systems

In a medical imaging institution, such as a hospital or a clinic, the set of technologies employed through the processes of archiving, visualizing, acquiring and distributing medical images over a computer network (see Figure 1) is commonly referred to as a Picture Archive and Communication System (PACS). PACS have evolved tremendously since when, as early as 1972, Dr. Richard J. Steckel implemented a minimal imaging system, comprising not much more than a scanner next to a film developer for digitalization of radiographs, a communication protocol to transmit those images and a video monitor to receive and display them [5]. No more than a proof of concept back then, but fast forward to current days, however, and a properly integrated hospital, or an enterprise PACS implementation is now a major undertaking that requires careful planning and several million dollars of investment [6]. Such investment is often required since large PACS commonly have to handle more than 20000 radiological procedures per year each procedure comprising potentially hundreds of distinct images. This means around 10 Terabytes of imaging information are stored per year [7]. It is in such situations that Content Based Image Retrieval systems are expected to provide the largest benefits.

PACS are still a very active field of research where the ever-changing requirements and the desire to provide more efficient services coupled with new ideas. Figure 2 shows a chronological view of the different challenges that arose and of some of the problems in which the research community is currently focusing. The push for CBIR enabled PACS has gained momentum since the late 90's up to the present day, however, even nowadays there are very few such systems currently powering medical institutions.

2.1. Digital imaging and communication in medicine

A major step in the direction of modern PACS was given circa 1985 with the creation of an earlier form of what would become the current DICOM standard. This protocol stands as one of the key protocols involved in medical imaging systems. We can consider it as the glue that holds the equipment and software developed by multiple companies together. It is an expansible, object oriented protocol with support for multiple imaging modalities and respective structured reports that also allows for private data to be embedded in its objects. Of great importance is the fact that it defines how medical image data and correspondent metadata is to be stored, retrieved, and transmitted thus enabling communication between devices manufactured by distinct entities within a PACS.

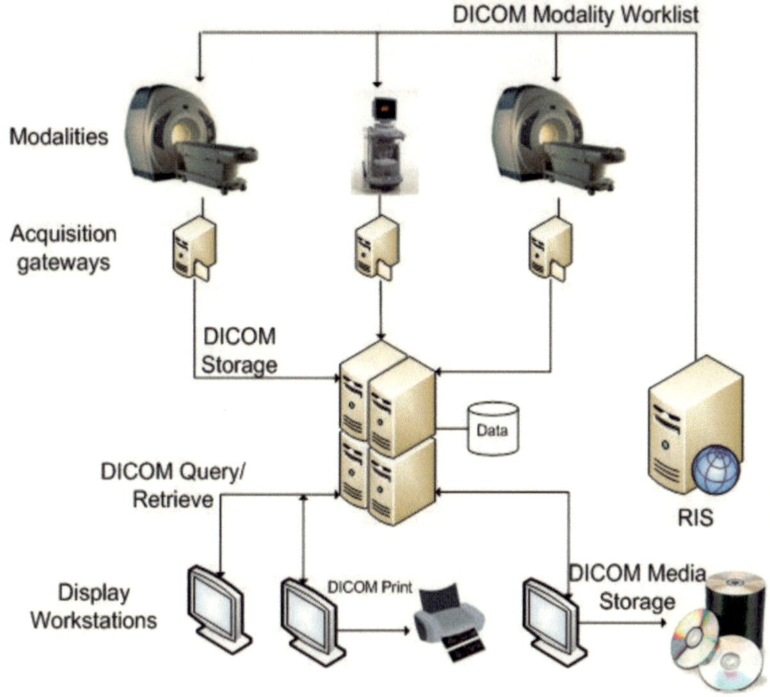

Figure 1. Outline of a PACS infrastructure comprising the most common components in an imaging institution

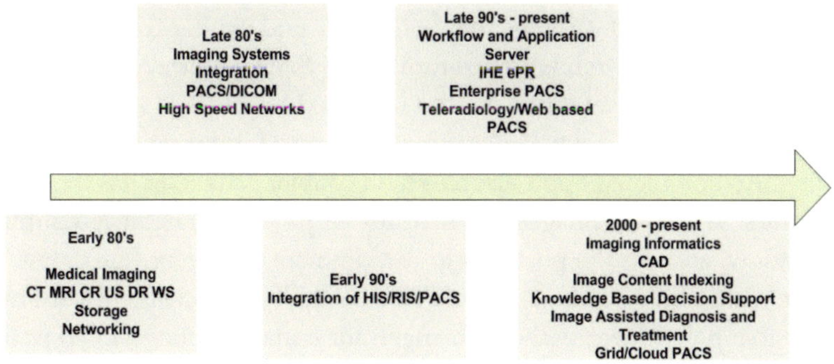

Figure 2. Evolution of PACS research and current trends

The protocol, first proposed by the National Electrical Manufacturers Association (NEMA), in 1983, and currently in its third version, was in itself a major contribution to the exchange of structured medical data [8]. With most available medical equipment providing embedded DICOM support, large sets of medical data have been produced in the DICOM file format. DICOM controls proper image display, it allows a large set of image post-processing from multi-planar reconstruction to the more advanced perfusion analysis, virtual colonoscopy and volume segmentation. This protocol can also be leveraged to enable a PACS-independent way of performing computer-aided diagnosis [9] and knowledge extraction [10]. In practice, much of the ease and flexibility radiologists enjoy today at work is due to this protocol.

However, while DICOM is an open standard, it was created with an eye on the future. As such, it is not set on stone and addends are continuously being added to support new services and modalities. DICOM uses an object oriented approach and its functionality can be extended. This is of great advantage since it allows bridging CBIR with PACS expanding on the DICOM protocol proving the extra functionality with minimal changes in infrastructure.

In DICOM, all data is organized in a patient, study, series and images hierarchy. These are viewed by DICOM as objects with a set of properties or attributes. The definitions for these objects and attributes are standardized according to predefined Information Object Definition (IOD). We can see IODs as templates for objects describing how each particular data object is constructed from attributes. It is then DICOM's group responsibility to maintain a list of all standard attributes and ensure consistency in their naming and composition [8]. The attributes comprise information regarding dates, radiation dosages or any other data of interest. Even image or video data are encoded within a DICOM object as a particular attribute (the attribute (0x7FE0, 0x0010) stands for the pixel data element).

3. Content based image retrieval systems

In its broadest sense, CBIR are systems that help users find similar content to a given image in large and potentially multi-modal repositories [11]. Even extremely large image archives, with often limited textual annotations, can be managed by CBIR as it allows navigation by visual content as opposed to keyword search or the more common form of direct patient/series searching. An automated approach based on content extraction has the advantage that it needs no manual tagging of images, the features employed are extracted automatically as part of the dataflow, and has the potential to discriminate even very fine details that escape the practitioner. Using information from DICOM Modality Worklists similar studies can be made available to a practitioner without the need for a manual query. Even in the presence of textual information (or rich enough DICOM metadata) content-based methods can potentially improve retrieval by offering additional insight into medical image collections [12]. It is important to note that, while striving to retrieve similar images, CBIR systems, unlike CAD systems, do not attempt to provide a diagnosis.

3.1. Searching information in content based image retrieval systems

Searching relevant data is a fundamental operation in CBIR. In relational databases the search procedure is applied to structured data, that is, numerical or alphabetical information that is searched for exactly. More sophisticated searches such as range queries on numerical keys or prefix searching on strings still rely on the concept that two keys are, or are not, equal. In order to guarantee query performance, traditional databases assume that there exists a total linear order on the keys which is used to establish indexes over the tables. That total order is something that does not arise naturally when dealing with unstructured high-dimensional spaces [13]. However, content-based retrieval relies heavily on similarity queries performed over them [14], hence a similarity function can be defined that establishes that ordering in relation to the source image.

When a query is performed with a source image, every element matches the input with a similarity value. If performed naively, without resorting to advanced indexing techniques, the outcome of similarity query is a permutation of all database content. That is, the elements are rearranged from the highest similarity value to the lowest [13]. This is a behavior that is not desirable. Assuming the similarity is properly defined there are two canonical types of queries that are of interest[3]:

- Range Query: Where we want to retrieve all elements that are closer than a given distance to the query content.
- Nearest Neighbor Query: Where we want to retrieve a certain number of the elements most similar to the query.

In order for a practitioner to perform a search he must provide input to the CBIR. Unlike in traditional query systems text is not used. Several approaches have been explored:

- Query by example – In this type of query a user merely provides a sample image and, relying on its analysis, the engine will provide the user with a set of similar images (see Figure 3).
- Query by region – From an image, the user selects a region of interest comprising the characteristics he is interested in. It is then up to the CBIR engine to retrieve images that share those same characteristics.
- Semantic query – A type of keyword query. However, it is not based on existent metadata but instead relies on mappings between the low level features extracted from an image and a high-level concept. An example would be a search for "micro-calcifications in a fatty tissue breast". Due to its complexity (it is still an unsolved problem) this types of query are only present in research systems.
- Query by sketch – Instead of using an image as source for a query, the user draws something alike what interests him. This methodology has been used to search for works of art in museums and images in the internet, but we know of no use-case in a clinical context.

---

3 Other, more complex types of query can be expressed over these.

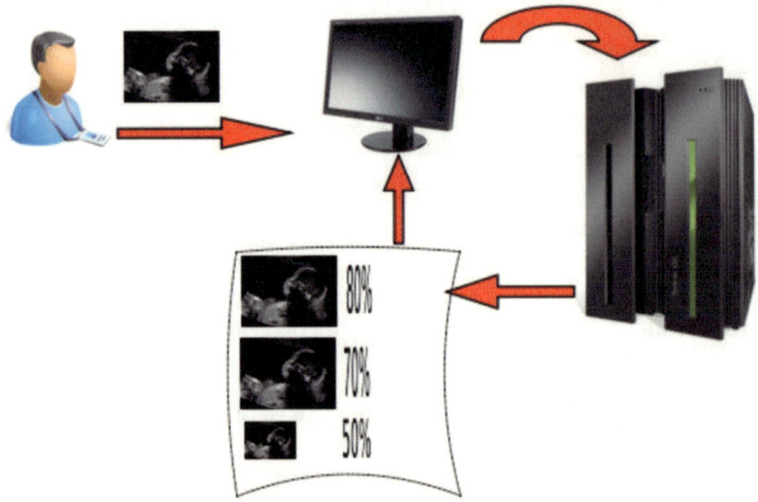

Figure 3. Query by example

3.2. Content based image retrieval systems in a clinical context

The push for the usage of CBIR of systems in a clinical context comes from their success in other areas where they have been successfully applied to handle large quantities of data. A recent example is Google's "search by image"[4] functionality that operates according to the query-by-example paradigm.

Several scenarios exist where medical practitioners can benefit from the use of these types of system. A key functionality that is of value to radiologists assessing medical images is the ability to provide them with a set of similar images, already diagnosed, thereby aiding them in their process of interpretation by quickly providing them with a second opinion. This proves to be orders of magnitude faster than the current mechanisms provided to manually browse the archives. The potential for this type of assisted interpretation is motivated not only by time constrains, but also by the recognition that variations in interpretation between practitioners, commonly based on perceptual errors, lack of training, or fatigue, do exist [11]. Significant inter-observer variation has been documented in numerous studies [15, 16]. Besides being a useful clinical tool, it is conceivable its use in an academic context where students can benefit from access to similar, diagnosed, data.

Selecting studies by similarity has another benefit. Considering a large repository, built over time, some of the retrieved images are bound to of some age. If a medical institution has kept track of a patient, performing more recent examinations, this data can be very useful to predict possible outcomes to an ailment's evolution. Furthermore, DICOM headers may contain a fairly high rate of errors, for example for the field anatomical region, error rates of 16% have been reported [17]. This hinders the correct retrieval of wanted images via textual search.

4 http://images.google.com/

http://dx.doi.org/10.5772/53027

Yet another important and useful outcome of CBIR is the possibility to bridge the semantic gap, allowing users to search an image repository for high-level image features. For instance a researcher may be interested in all studies containing a particular type or disposition of lymph nodes, or query only for images containing a particular feature. This concept expands on CBIR systems and requires that we establish a relation between the low level features employed and the high level concepts of a semantic interpretation.

3.3. Features and feature extraction

At the core of each CBIR there is a matching algorithm analyzing the similarity between the query content and the content stored in the database. However, except for the most trivial CBIR engines operating on simple content, it is not the actual content that is compared. As briefly mentioned, features extracted from the source content, are used instead. In the case of images, pixel by pixel comparisons are not commonly performed due to, not only to the computational effort involved, but also because such comparisons lacks any type of semantic meaning, are dependent on resolution and often are very sensitive to small changes. Furthermore, it is not clear which pixels from the one image correspond to pixels in another image. That said, a feature is simply a relevant piece of information, a synonym for an input variable or an attribute of an image [18], usually much smaller in size than the original data.

Thus, when there is a need to cope with large datasets, such as the ones present in medical repositories, or to deal with large inputs where most information is redundant or irrelevant, as is the case with some images, the analysis is commonly preceded by a pre-processing stage that provides a reduced representation of the original data. This step is called feature extraction and is of crucial importance for any CBIR currently deployed, as content matching operates by comparing features and only the features are indexed.

Using a feature based approach to image analysis brings several advantages to CBIR systems. Besides reducing the size of the input data, thus providing great performance improvements to the matching algorithms, its reduced representation also translates directly in a smaller storage footprint. Of great importance is that, by discarding redundant or useless information, some features can generalize a concept and allow predictive models to become both more general and accurate. Some features also map well into high level concepts (circles, nodes, shapes, nodes) and help bridge the semantic gap.

Generally a feature is represented by a set of values that can be organized into a vector. The global entropy of an image is a single real value but, on the other hand, a normalized intensity histogram or a texture descriptor can be understood as a n-dimensional vector where each index contains the probability of a pixel having an intensity value equal to that index.

In most CBIR systems, a single feature is very often not enough to fully represent the image in a way that makes possible to perform relevant queries. The usual approach is then to extract multiple features from the image and merge them into a single vector, canonically called the feature vector. The set of all possible feature vectors constitutes a feature space. Depending on the features, this can be a space with a very high dimensionality.

The types of features that can be used when designing a CBIR system are essentially limitless and new methods are continuously devised. However most features relate to the original image in a way that can be categorized as presented on table 1.

Criteria	Type	Description
Level of abstraction	Low level	Visual cues, such as color or texture extracted directly from the raw pixel data without any *a priori* information. Examples are edges, corners, contours, brightness histograms.
	Middle level	Regions or blobs obtained as result from image segmentation.
	High level	These types of features contain semantic information about the meaning of an image or the object represented. Usually require knowledge of contextual information and very often imply the use of a classification step. An example would be the number of cars present in an image or the location of nodes in a mammography.
Scope	Local	Features of this type describe a localized region of the image and are usually computed around interest points. A widely used method that uses these types of features is the scale-invariant feature transform.
	Global	Global features comprise information that somehow relates to the entire image. Image entropy is such a feature as is the color histogram.
Representation	Photometric	These are features that explore color and textural cues taken from raw pixel data. A relevant example is Gabor texture descriptors.
	Geometric	Instead of relying on color they employ shape-based cues, most features based on contours are of this type.
Domain	Binary	An on/off type of feature
	Categorical	Instead of having values in a numeric domain this features of this type are aggregated in categories. Usually high level features are also categorical.
	Continuous	Features of this type are represented by a continuous value or vector. Numerical features such as entropy are usually of this type.
	Structural	Where the feature is represented by a graph employed by structural descriptors based on segmentation.
	Vectorial	Sets of continuous values that are related amongst themselves such as histograms, space-based shape descriptors or centers of mass of clusters.

Table 1. Feature taxonomy

The relevancy of a feature is, however, highly dependent on the domain of the problem. This brings the problem of what features should be selected or are relevant in a given context. Namely, what features should be used to perform efficient CBIR in a medical environment where multiple modalities are in place? This is a topic of great interest nowadays and the subject of intensive research.

3.4. Similarity

Due to the unstructured nature of content in images, CBIR systems eschew exact matching and rely instead in nearest neighbor or range queries based on a similarity function. Hence, one of the most important tasks in both the research and development of CBIR systems is to properly define that similarity. Implicitly, one person has a clear notion of whether any two objects or images are similar. Even so, humans are also very much subject to subjective opinions and those can vary wildly. Nonetheless, when searching for reasonable similarity measures, the most obvious place to look is at the human similarity assessment. After all, when a user searches for something similar, he already has in mind his own concept of similarity, whose form is doubtlessly quite different from the metric spaces (such as the Euclidean) typically used for feature vector comparison. The similarity used by the CBIR systems should then be as similar as possible to the human concept of similarity if the results of the search are to be satisfactory [19]. Algorithmically modeling that behavior thus requires that the internal image representations closely reflect the ways in which users interpret, understand, and encode visual data. Finding suitable image representations, based on the types of features described previously is an important step towards the development of effective similarity models [14]. However, creating such algorithmic functions is complicated due to the fact that there is no single model of human similarity. Furthermore a user may have in mind a very specific type of similarity or criteria he is interested in. For instance, in a radiology setting, a practitioner may wish to place more emphasis in finding mammographs sharing a certain disposition of micro-calcifications rather than those containing the same tissue type or having a similar breast size.

Combining multiple representation models can partially resolve this problem. If a retrieval system allows parameterized or multiple similarity functions, the user should be able to select those that most closely model his or her perception [14]. This is not a trivial problem to solve by any means and similarity selection functionality is hardly present in current medical CBIR. In fact such feature is lacking in even most CBIR systems. However, within a medical institution often exist multiple modalities and the DICOM protocol offers support for all those types of distinct imagery.

3.4.1. Similarity measures

Of crucial importance in a CBIR system is the design of the similarity metrics used to match a query to the database feature vectors. Mathematically we can define these metrics as a function $f(x,x')$ that takes as arguments the set of features belonging to two distinct images and returns a value from an ordered set (such as the set of real numbers). This sorting embodies the idea that some images look more like the query than others and allow a content engine to return, not only the closest match, but a bundle of images arranged by similarity thus increasing the probability that the user has of finding what he is looking for. Typically, smaller values correspond to higher similarity although that depends, of course, on the specific function being used. The similarity measures employed in CBIR systems are deeply tied with the representation of the features extracted by the system. We now present some of the most applied functions.

- **Vector distance –** One of the most common similarity measures. A function of two feature vectors is defined over the feature space. These are often applied due to their conceptual simplicity. Simpler distances, such as the Euclidean, are also quick to compute, however, that is not always the case, other measures such as the EMD[5] or statistical distances can have significant complexity.
- **Shape based –** These are used when features consist of points delineating a shape boundary. The similarity between shapes is defined in terms of the transformations required to transform a shape into another.
- **Structural/Graph matching -** A class of similarity measurements that apply when the extracted features are represented by a graph. The similarity can be computed by an attributed graph-matching scheme such as relaxation schemes or combinatorial algorithms.
- **Classifier-based -** These classifiers employ machine learning techniques to classify the image as pertaining to a set of predetermined labels. This scheme does not follow the concept of a similarity function, however, in most systems the label obtained is merged with the existing feature set and a vector distance metric is subsequently applied.

In table 2 we find a list containing some of the methodologies employed for similarity measurements in various CBIR projects.

3.4.2. Relevance feedback

While CBIR systems should operate in a transparent manner, in order to increase their overall accuracy it can be desirable to allow a user to relate back to the system which results are actually relevant. Relevance feedback is the process of automatically adjusting an image query using the information provided from the expert on previously executed queries [20]. A way to achieve this goal is to expose to the user an interface that allows him to provide feedback on the relevancy of the results on a per-image basis. A new query can then be executed in order to replace non-relevant results and the feedback loop is repeated many times until the user is satisfied. A key issue is in how to effectively utilize the feedback information to improve the retrieval performance. This aspect depends on the particular implementation of the CBIR given it modifies the way the similarity computation is performed and several methodologies have been explored. An overview of these mechanisms can be found in [21].

5 Earth Mover's Distance

http://dx.doi.org/10.5772/53027

3.5. Indexing and performance

When the number of images in the database is small, as is often the case with research systems, a sequential linear search across all elements can provide an acceptable performance. However, with large-scale image databases, such as the ones present in medical systems, more efficient query mechanisms become a necessity. The search task can be significantly improved by relying on multidimensional indexing structures. Like traditional databases, the indexing of an image database should support an efficient search based on the extracted features.

The basic idea behind any indexing procedure (figure 4) is a hierarchical division of space that increases the lookup speed by removing the need to sift the entire feature space o obtain the desired resuls. Due to the nature of CBIR queries, which require quick lookup of the nearest neighbors to a data point in the feature space, the indexing structure must preserve locality.

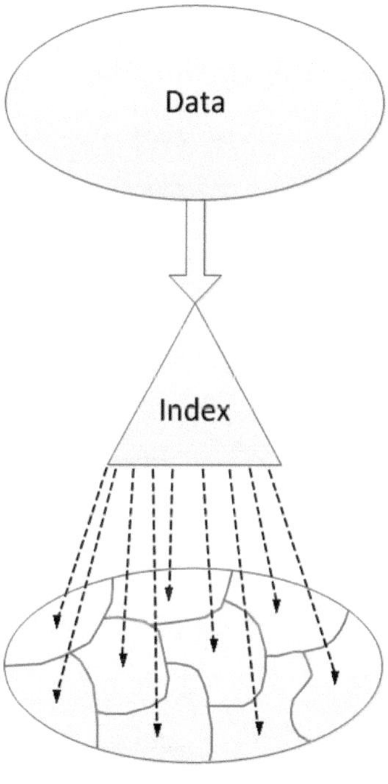

Figure 4. Indexing a feature space

The most popular class of indexing techniques in traditional databases is the B-tree family which provides very efficient searches when the key is a scalar. However, they are not suitable to index the content of images represented by high-dimensional features. Nonetheless, multidimensional indexing techniques exist. There are a large variety of multidimensional indexing methods, which differ in the type of queries they support and the dimensionality of the space where they are advantageous. The R-tree [22] and its variations are probably the best-known multidimensional indexing techniques in general purpose content retrieval engines. Other approaches are the k-d tree and variants such as the R+-tree and the R*-tree [23].

If a similarity function is at the same time a distance, and thereby a metric to the feature space, a distinct set of methods that operate in a metric space are available. These methods rely only on the definition of the distance function and make no other assumptions. Hence they prove to be very general indexing structures. A study on such methods is available in [13] and [24]. One reason these types of data-structures are not more pervasive in medical CBIR is that research is still being conducted on how to provide mechanisms in Database Management System (DBMS) that allow users to easily incorporate them into search engines.

3.6. Architectural overview of content based retrieval engines

Taking into account the presented requirements and operations for CBIR systems, in figure 5 we show how a generic architecture to a PACS-aware CBIR architecture can be designed. In this architecture the CBIR engine operates outside the PACS repository. This guarantees the integrity of the imaging repository and allows clinical operations to proceed should the CBIR engine fail.

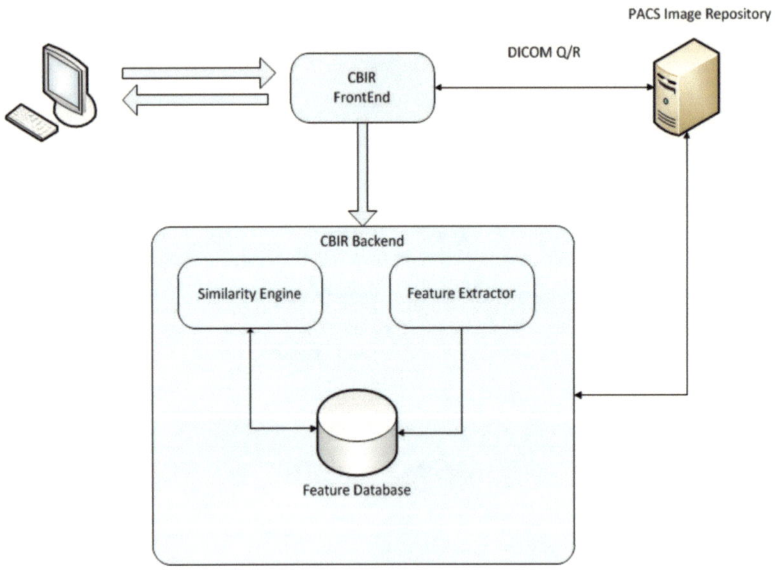

Figure 5. General architecture of a PACS enabled CBIR system

The frontend is the component in charge of receiving similarity requests. Such requests can be triggered manually, by a practitioner, or by analyzing DICOM's Modality Worklist. It replies to the requests with a list of DICOM files to be retrieved which are similar to the source image of the request.

The Feature Extractor component's, main responsibility is, like the name indicates, to extract the relevant features from an image. This behavior is triggered during an initialization procedure, when analyzing images from the PACS repository, or upon the creation of new images by the modalities. The extracted features are then passed to the Feature Database which indexes them and allows for fast nearest neighbor queries. The last major component, the similarity engine comprises the set of metrics and similarities that can be applied.

3.7. Review of CBIR applications

Most radiological CBIR applications are still in a conceptual or research stage. In table 2 we present a brief listing of such systems together with the most important aspects present in a CBIR. This table is based on a similar, more complete table presented in [11].

The features column is arranged in three categories: General, Mixed and Specialized. General features are low and middle level features, extracted from the image with no *a priori* domain specific knowledge and typically extracted with no user input. Mixed features comprise both general features and extra annotations, whether provided from a practitioner or extracted from other sources. Specialized features rely on specific knowledge about the nature and type of the dataset and are typically not automated requiring an expert to provide extra information such as regions of interest.

Ref	Features	Similarity measures	Relevance feedback	PACS Integration
[25]	General	Classifier-based	Yes	No
[26]	General	Classifier	No	No
[27]	Mixed	Classifier	No	No
[28]	Mixed	Vector distance	No	No
[29]	Specialized	Classifier	No	No
[30]	Specialized	Structural	No	No
[31]	General	Vector distance	No	No
[32]	General	Classifier	No	No
[33]	Mixed	Vector distance	No	No
[34]	Mixed	-	No	Yes

Table 2. Overview of medical CBIR systems

Of the presented systems, only [34] focuses specifically on PACS level integration, however, only the concepts and methodology are discussed.

4. Dicoogle

We have developed Dicoogle[6], an open-source PACS with support for data indexing, peer-to-peer communication and CBIR functionality. This tool complements, and may even replace a traditional PACS server and enhance it with a more agile indexing and retrieval mechanism [35]. Besides providing basic DICOM services such as Storage and Query/ Retrieval, Dicoogle can automatically extract, index and store all metadata present in a DICOM header (including data present in private data elements). The indexed data can then be queried using free text. A more advanced search mechanism is also provided using a rich query language based on Lucene's syntax. This syntax has support for element selection, numerical and range-based search, wildcard expansion and Boolean operators such as AND, OR and NOT. As a data-extraction tool, Dicoogle has been used in several small to medium imaging institutions. For instance, in [36] Dicoogle was used to demonstrate several inconsistencies in the handling of some DICOM attributes by the modalities and to perform a study on the radiation dosage of the patients handled at the site.

Recently, Dicoogle was extended to support CBIR over a DICOM image repository using a query-by-example paradigm (see figure 6) and following the architectural considerations exposed on the previous sections.

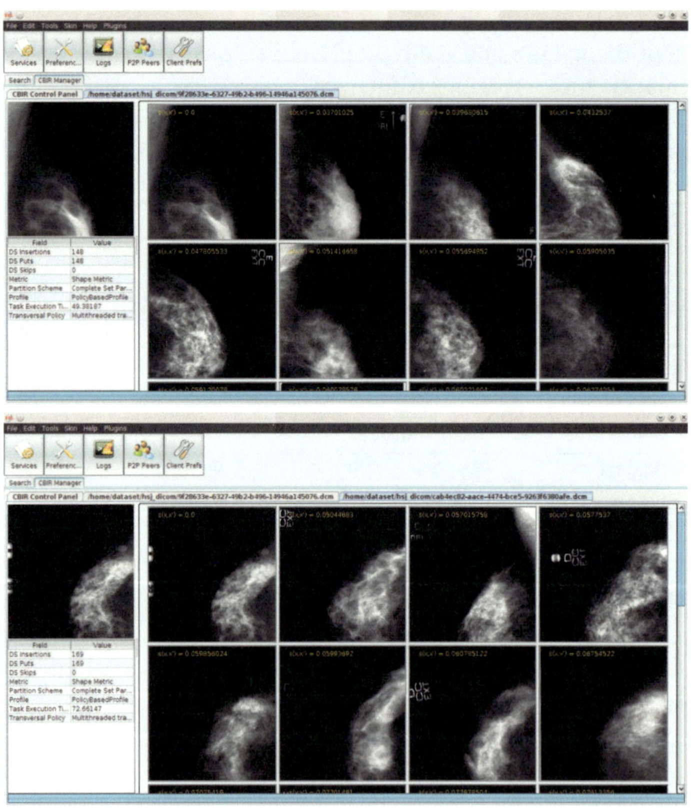

Figure 6. Dicoogle's Query by example results

6 http://www.dicoogle.com

4.1. A profile-based approach to CBIR in a medical context

In the context of multi-modality institutions each modality has distinct criteria to evaluate similarity. Structures identifiable in CT scan images likely have no meaning in the context of mammograms. Similarly, a feature set apt to describe an image within a context of a modality can be entirely useless in another. Likewise for the functions that express the similarity from those features. In a multi-modal environment it seems a needless imposition to use a single set of features and a single measure for similarity, independent of context. Particularly since feature sets coupled with similarity functions can be used to highlight different aspects of an image. In the context of mammographies there is a tendency to focus on microcalcifications to provide the relevant similarity rather, than, for instance, tissue type or size of breast.

Therefore we've separated the similarity metric from the feature extraction process and provided the user with the concept of "CBIR profiles". A profile contains information on the metric to be used and which features are required to apply it. A profile also contains hints to the indexing mechanism to limit the search space and on which modalities it can be applied. Profiles can be automatically selected using data provided by the DICOM header. Using profiles our CBIR engine allows a practitioner to specify what is of interest to him and fine tune the query if required. In figure 7 we show the dataflow of Dicoogle's CBIR engine.

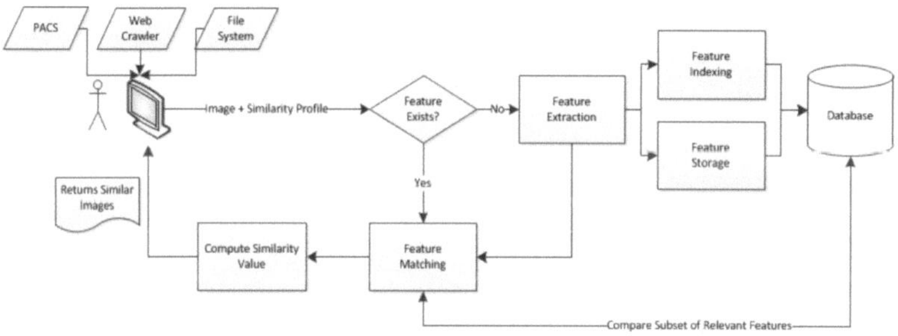

Figure 7. Flow diagram of the interactions between the distinct components of Dicoogle CBIR

5. Challenges and opportunities

In spite of its success in other areas, CBIR is still not a widely deployed technology as a decision support tool. It is the author's opinion that this is currently due to both a lack of integration with the standards that operate through medical institutions, as well as from the stringent requirements that must be fulfilled when operating in an area as critical as the health-care industry. Nonetheless, these types of systems provide enough benefits to the practitioner fully justifying the effort and research applied towards their implementation. Moving towards a clinically useful CBIR in radiology will, however, require a concertated and multi-disciplinary approach. We now point out some challenges that arise from both the general topic of CBIR and its integration with the medical imaging infrastructures.

- **PACS and DICOM integration.** We proposed an approach that complements a PACS by externalizing the CBIR and interacting through the DICOM protocol. However, in this approach, third party tools are limited to images pushed to them through the DICOM C-Move operation. This needlessly hampers the possibility of cooperation between applications as third party tools are either passive, must conform to a private API or must implement themselves an indexing and similarity mechanism.

- **Enabling multi-dimensional database systems.** Several studies exist on how to perform multi-dimensional indexing. However, databases that natively provide support for indexing multi-dimensional data-points according to an arbitrary similarity function and able to cope with large, dynamic volumes of information are, to the best of our knowledge, inexistent. This leads researchers and application developers resorting to either implement indexing mechanisms atop relational databases or to completely ignore the problem and focusing on the other aspects of a CBIR.

- **Multi-modal data integration.** To rely exclusively in pixel data imposes some limits to CBIR systems, not only in the medical arena. Gathering information from multiple sources, such as demography data of a patient from the Radiology Information System, and combining it with the extracted data has the potential to further improve clinical CBIR. A further step forward will be to move from single image analysis and retrieval and merge information from the multitudes of sources that may be present in a DICOM study. Combining this information is not trivial due to missing information, the heterogenetic nature of the data and the problems involved in relating a set of images to another in a meaningful way. This will allow CBIR engines to move to a study-based paradigm, the most common unit of search for practitioners in most modalities. Tackling this problem is likely to have the biggest impact in a clinical environment [37].

- **Lack of a Gold Standard for CBIR.** It is currently not possible to compare the performance across different medical CBIR systems. Not only their respective application domain and specific goals differ, but there is a lack of a common Gold Standard. The ImageCLEFmed[7] is one of the few platforms to evaluate and compare different systems. Other public datasets exist with annotated data, however, the fact they are scattered and the annotations provided do not follow any particular structure makes them cumbersome to use. To access the research effectively, task-related standardized databases on which distinct groups can apply their algorithms are needed. Cooperation with clinical experts is a necessity to provide the necessary relevancy assessments.

- **Towards semantic search.** Much emphasis is being placed on automatic and assisted concept extraction. This effort is directed towards bridging the semantic gap and further increase the accuracy of CBIR systems [38]. An advantage of a CBIR operating in the medical field is that semantics in the medical domain are much better defined and there is a vast accumulation of formal knowledge representations that could be exploited to support semantic search for any specialty areas in medicine [39].

---

7 http://www.imageclef.org/

http://dx.doi.org/10.5772/53027

This idea expands on CBIR systems and requires that we establish a relation between the low level features employed and the high level concepts of a semantic interpretation. Several strategies currently under study are the following [38]:

- Usage of object ontologies to define high-level concepts
- Employ machine learning concepts to perform the association between features and concepts
- Rely on users and perform relevance feedback for continuous learning
- Generate semantic templates (profiles) to support the association
- Rely on the meta-data or other textual information provided by the user

The major functionality enabled by semantic search is the advanced textual queries that can be provided to a practitioner. For example, queries such as *"show me blood smears that include polymorphonuclear neutrophils"*[8] should become a possibility.

6. Conclusion

In this chapter we've exposed the some of the most common methodologies employed in Content-based Image Retrieval and provided an overview of the state of such systems in a clinical context. We pointed out how CBIR, being a query mechanism more adapted to the workflow of a radiologist than the traditional string matching present in DICOM, can help improve diagnosis speed and accuracy in a clinical context.

It was shown how the creation of accurate and performing CBIR systems in a clinical context is a task hard to tackle, ripe with non-trivial challenges that arise from a multitude of factors such as the need for integration with currently deployed PACS, the need to handle multiple modalities and cope with stringent performance requirements.

Furthermore, we presented Dicoogle, our approach to bring CBIR to DICOM enabled PACS systems relying on a profile-based approach.

The goal of CBIR systems is not to replace the practitioner or, unlike CAD tools, provide automated diagnosis, but to empower the expert with tools that allow for faster and more accurate diagnosis in a workflow adapted to his needs.

Acknowledgements

This work has received funding from "Fundação para a Ciência e Tecnologia" (FCT) under grant agreement PTDC/EIA-EIA/104428/2008

8 An example from the ImageCLEFmed competition as shown in [2]

Author details

Frederico Valente, Carlos Costa and Augusto Silva

Universidade de Aveiro, IEETA, Portugal

References

[1] Rubin GD. Data explosion: the challenge of multidetector-row. European Journal of Radiology. 2000;: p. 74-80.

[2] Henning Muller XZADMPJsIaAG. Medical Visual Information Retrieval: State of the Art and Challenges Ahead. 2007 IEEE International Conference on Multimedia and Expo. 2007;: p. 683-686.

[3] Andriole K. Addressing the coming radiology crisis - the society for computer applications in radiology transforming the radiological interpretation process (trip) initiative. Journal of Digital Imaging. 2004;(17): p. 235-243.

[4] National Electrical Manufacturers Association. DICOM Part 4: Service Class Specifications. 2009..

[5] Steckel J. Daily x-ray rounds in a large teaching hospital using high-resolution closed-circuit television. Radiology. 1972; 105(2).

[6] Huang HK. PACS and Imaging Informatics: Basic Principles and Applications: John Wiley & Sons; 2010.

[7] Oliveira MC, Cirne W, Marques PM. Towards applying content-based image retrieval in the clinical routine. Future Generation Computer Systems. 2007 March; 23(3): p. 466-474.

[8] Oosterwijk H, Gihring P. DICOM basics.: Tech; 2002.

[9] CAD–PACS integration tool kit based on DICOM secondary capture, structured report and IHE workflow profiles. Computerized medical imaging and graphics : the official journal of the Computerized Medical Imaging Society. 2007 June; 31(4).

[10] Lehmann TM, Güld O, Deselaers , Keysers , Schubert , Spitzer , et al. Automatic categorization of medical images for content-based retrieval and data mining. Computerized Medical Imaging and Graphics. 2005 March; 29(2).

[11] Akgül B, Rubin DL, Napel , Beaulieu CF, Greenspan , Acar. Content-Based Image Retrieval in Radiology: Current Status and Future Directions. Journal of Digital Imaging. 2011 April; 24(2).

[12] Lew MS, Sebe , Djeraba , Jain. Content-based multimedia information retrieval: State of the art and challenges. ACM Transactions on Multimedia Computing, Communications, and Applications. 2006 February; 2(1).

[13] Chavez E, Navarro , Baeza-Yate , Marroquin JL. Searching in metric spaces. ACM Computer Survey. 2001; 33.

[14] Castelli V, Bergman LD. Image databases: search and retrieval of digital imagery: Wiley; 2002.

[15] Siegle RL, Baram EM, Reut SR. Rates of disagreement in imaging interpretation in a group of community hospitals. Academic Radiology. 1998; 5(3).

[16] Soffa D, Lewis R, Sunshine J, Bhargavan M. Disagreement in interpretation: a method for the development of benchmarks for quality assurance in imaging. Journal of the American College of Radiology. 2004; 1(3).

[17] Guld MO, Kohnen , Keysers , Schubert. Quality of dicom header information for image categorization. 2002..

[18] Guyon I. Feature extraction: foundations and applications (Studies in fuzziness and soft computing): Springer-Verlag; 2006.

[19] Santini , Jain. Similarity queries in image databases. In IEEE Computer Society Conference on Computer Vision and Pattern Recognition; 1996.

[20] Pinjarkar L, Sharma , Mehta. Comparative Evaluation of Image Retrieval Algorithms using Relevance Feedback and it's Applications. International Journal of Computer Applications. 2012 June; 48(18).

[21] Pinjarkar , Sharma , Mehta. Comparison and Analysis of Content Based Image Retrieval Systems Based On Relevance Feedback. Journal of Emerging Trends in Computing and Information Sciences. 2012 July; 3(6).

[22] Qian , Tagare. Optimal embedding for shape indexing in medical image databases. In Medical Image Computing and Computer-Assisted Intervention - MICCAI 2005; 2005.

[23] Beckmann , Kriege HP, Schneid. The r*-tree: an efficient and robust access method for points and rectangles. In SIGMOD; 1990. p. 322-331.

[24] Zezula , Amato , Dohnal , Batko. Similarity Search: The Metric Space Approach: Springer; 2006.

[25] Bhattacharya M, Desai B. A framework for medical image retrieval using machine learning and statistical similarity matching techniques with relevance feedback. IEEE Transactions in Information Technologie in Biomedicine. 2007; 11(1).

[26] Greenspan H, Pinhas A. Medical image categorization and retrieval for PACS using the GMM-KL framework. IEEE Transaction in Information Technologies in Biomedicine. 2007; 11(2).

[27] Lim J, Chevallet J. Vismed: A visual vocabulary approach for medical image indexing and retrieval. In Second Asia Information Retrieval Symposium; 2005; Jeju Island.

[28] Müller H ea. The Use of MedGIFT and EasyIR forImageCLEF 2005. in Accessing Multilingual Information Repositories. In Accessing Multilingual Information Repositories.: Springer p. 724-732.

[29] Petrakis E, Faloutsos C, Lin K. ImageMap: an image indexing method based on spatial similarity. IEEE Transactions in Knowledge Data Engineering. 2002; 15(5).

[30] Amores J, Radeva P. Registration and retrieval of highly elastic bodies using contextual information. Pattern Recognition Letters. 2005; 26(11).

[31] Mohammad-Reza et al. Content-based image database system for epilepsy. Computer Methods and Programs in Biomedicine. 2005; 79(3).

[32] Alto H, Rangayyan R, Desautels J. Content-based retrieval and analysis of mammographic masses. Journal of Electronic Imaging. 2005; 14(2).

[33] Kim J et al. A new way for multidimensional medical data management: Volume of interest (VOI)-based retrieval of medical images with visual and functional features. IEEE Transactions in Information Technologies in Biomedicine. 2006; 10(3).

[34] Benedikt Fischer et al. Integration of a Research CBIR System with RIS and PACS for Radiological Routine. In Proceedings of the SPIE; 2008.

[35] Costa CaFCaBLaRLaSAaOJ. Dicoogle - an Open Source Peer-to-Peer PACS. Journal of Digital Imaging. 2011; 24(5): p. 848-856.

[36] Santos , Bastião L, Costa C, Silva A, Rocha N. DICOM and Clinical Data Mining in a Small Hospital PACS: A Pilot Study. In Communications in Computer and Information Science; 2011: Springer Berlin Heidelberg. p. 254-263.

[37] Medical Visual Information Retrieval: State of the Art and Challenges Ahead. In IEEE International Conference on Multimedia and Expo; 2007; Geneva. p. 683 - 686.

[38] Ying , Zhang , Lu , Ma WY. A survey of content-based image retrieval with high level semantics. Pattern Recognition. 2007 January; 40(1).

[39] Zhou XS, Zillner S, Moeller M, Sintek M, Zhan Y, Krishnan A, et al. Semantics and CBIR: a medical imaging perspective. In CIVR '08 Proceedings of the 2008 international conference on Content-based image and video retrieval; 2008. p. 571-580.

Chapter 2

Challenges and Peculiarities of Paediatric Imaging

Okechukwu Felix Erondu

Additional information is available at the end of the chapter

http://dx.doi.org/10.5772/51611

1. Introduction

Although some, diseases seen among children and infants are similar to those in adults, diagnostic imaging of these category of patients can both be interesting and challenging.

Paediatric imaging therefore requires specific training and certification that gua rantees application of thorough knowledge, expertise and a variety of dedicated or adaptable equipment. This is hardly the case in many countries; where there may not be sub specialty training in paediatric imaging and practice may not have specific requirement except interest in children. Historically, there are few recruitment training centers for paediatric imaging specialists, and this area appear to be one of the least subscribed of all radiology sub specialities. It is also difficult, to establish quality imaging service for children defined as ' A service where the child is examined and diagnosis made by specialists with appropriate expertise, is imaged using dedicated facilities and equipment and where the child is at the center of all decisions made' (Report of National Imaging Board, NHS).

It is important to recognise that children are increasingly irritable and unusually aware of strangers and unfamiliar environments. This presents a huge challenge for the radiographer or the clinical care personnel who must try to gain the child's trust and co-operation before and throughout the duration of an examination. This can be a daunting task in children who may both be ill as well as experiencing pain. Coercion and support from parents is usually enough to achieve this, but in some extreme cases (such as MRI and CT), it may be necessary to sedate the child. Even with a quality examination, the accurate interpretation of diagnostic images, also requires a deep knowledge of the intricate and dynamic face of anatomy and some peculiarity in pathological presentations.

This paper seeks to draw attention to the peculiarities of Paediatric Imaging and the need to encourage expertise in this area.

Challenges of paediatric imaging can be discussed as follows:

This chapter will be divided into 3 Major Areas namely service delivery, technical peculiarities and Clinical Applications.

2. Service Delivery

2.1. Lack of Specialist Training

Inspite of the vulnerability of this category of patients and obvious need for specialized diagnostic services, there are few training centers or programs dedicated to Paediatric imaging. In Nigeria, there is no specialist training for would be paediatric radiologist, outside the regular fellowship. In some countries like Switzerland, a two year sub specialty Fellowship and certification is available for Radiologist, but nothing specific for Radiographers and Imaging Technologists. There is evidence that enrollment and popularity of paediatric imaging as a speciality is low in United States and Europe. In the United Kingdom, all radiology trainings programs include core paediatric experience, and full adaptation can be achieved after a 6 months of pediatric focused training. Alternatively, a paediatric consultant may need up to 1 year training in radiology, but the short period of rotations during residency is usually not enough to provoke sufficient interest in this category of practitioners.

Among Radiographers, there is no recognition of Pediatrics as an area of specialty or professional registration for pediatric Radiographers. There is no formal training programs dedicated to this area, or career pathways or incentives for Specialist paediatric radiographers. The picture appears to be replicated in most African and SubSaharan countries where lack of manpower may further inhibit the development of this potentially important specialty.

2.2. Lack of Dedicated Children Imaging Centers

This challenge is almost similar to the one earlier described. In practice, there is a wide variation in the provision of specialist imaging centers with services tailored specifically for the children. According to an NHS report, majority of routine, emergency and trauma imaging takes place in district hospitals, equipped with variable degree of local expertise.

2.3. Specialized Equipment

Imaging equipment and facilities suitable for use by children and toddlers require some specialized features. Sometimes, these equipment may differ from the premature to the adult sized teenager. Equipments that are easy to manipulate, while allowing fast acquisition of diagnostic information is the gold standard.Where necessary, image viewing and workflow stations allow fast transfer of images to PACS, for easy reporting and audits by radiologists.

2.4. Environment

Children require stimulating environments that easily catch their attention and make them less suspicious of strangers and their intentions. The environment should usually be friendly and tailored to make the child patient feel relaxed. For instance, the walls should have bright colors, with paintings and designs as well as images with toys, play characters, cartoons and toys.

http://dx.doi.org/10.5772/51611

Provision to allow children run around, play and use murals and stencils can be of immense use.

The designs can also be such that allows a lot of natural lighting into the room. This can be achieved with glass panels and windows and special lightings.

2.5. Safety and Radiation protection

With the advent of CT and fluoroscopy, the amount of radiation doses available to paediatric patients has become increasingly significant. Consequently, issues of radiation protection are more stringent in paediatric imaging and both local rules and international standard must be maintained.

It is recommended that low dose imaging systems be deployed using digital detection components, optimized for paediatric use to ensure dose reduction.

Imaging systems that are ultra fast are often needed to reduce the time of investigation while optimizing image quality, and this comes with a huge financial burden to hospital authority, since they cost higher. It is also important to ensure the physical safety of the child while in the department.

2.6. Extended Work Hours

The need to have immediate intervention in children especially following trauma and emergencies, may necessitate the extension of working hours and off peak availability of personnel. This means placing Radiographers and Radiologists with pediatric experience on call, to handle such cases. This obviously places most departments under work pressure to keep this category of workers.

2.7. Quality Assurance

The need to obtain images of optimum quality requires that the imaging equipment function to their maximal capacity. Diagnosis of many paediatric ailments depend on exquisite demonstration of anatomical detail, and subtle changes. Quality assurance programs are tailored towards ensuring optimum performance, often requiring constant calibration of these equipment.

Double check protocols are necessary to ensure there is no missed diagnosis, through proper clinical audits.

2.8. General Guidelines for Paediatric Imaging Departments

The standard protocols should be adopted as a general rule:

1. There must be a clinical justification for any imaging procedure

2. The clinical benefits should outweigh any potential risk

3. When possible, children should not be examined with facilities dedicated to adults

4. The protocols for each investigation must be specific and tailored to meet individual patient situations.

5. Service hours and sessions must be sufficient to cover both booked and emergency cases.

6. Radiation protection services must be available and optimization principles such as ALARP (As Low As Reasonably Practical) should be applied.

7. There should be care providers with sound understanding of the anatomical and pathological processes in the paediatric age group.

8. A thorough knowledge of various diagnostic and imaging techniques by practitioners, including indications, contraindications and complications.

9. Knowledge of the advantage as well as limitations of each imaging modality, is necessary to make informed choice and guide clinical management.

10. Good communication and interpersonal skills are needed to deal with children.

11. Access to interventional and emergency care must be ensured at all times.

12. All protocols must take into consideration, the personal or physical safety of the children while in the imaging department.

3. Technical Peculiarities

Conventional X-ray

There are existing policy guidelines regarding acceptable quality and criteria for diagnostic radiography in the pediatric population. Such guidelines like that of the European Commission, sets out to ensure the triple objectives of producing adequate and uniformly acceptable image quality, providing accurate radiological interpretation of the image and using a reasonably low radiation dose per radiograph. A typical guideline will take into account a specific image criteria, taking into consideration anatomical, patho-physiological, size and degree of cooperation expected of a child. It will emphasize good Radiographic technique and patient dose limitations. The general requirements include but not limited to the list below

1. High quality images produced by computed or digital radiography is recommended, so that exposure factors can be optimized and repeats are avoided.

2. Films of high contrast and capable of yielding high resolution images are recommended.

3. Low absorption cassette or image plates, grids, tabletops should be used. While the use of grids may often be unnnecessary, the introduction of digital or computed Radiography has reduced the use and importance of some of these accesories)

http://dx.doi.org/10.5772/51611

4. Exposure Parameters should be stringent, with appropriate combination of KV, MA and Time. Due to a likelihood of motional blur, short exposure times is compensated for by slight increase in KV and MA.

5. The technique with positioning, centering, collimation, side markers, image identification, restraining methods are carefully chosen.

6. There should be proper collimation devices with fine focus techniques necessary to reduce radiation dose without loss of detail. Protective radiation shields should be used whenever necessary.

7. Radiographs should show both soft tissue and bony detail.

8. Comparison films are often necessary to make accurate diagnosis.

9. Where possible, effort should be made to produce the area of interest with minimal projections. For example, A single projection showing chest and abdomen would be preferable in an eight month old baby, rather than two view of the chest and abdomen respectively.

10. In acute injury, two projections (Ap and Lateral) should be done as an emergency.

When necessary, radiographs may be obtained under mild sedation especially in the very uncooperative patient.

Due to the increasing radiation sensitivity of children compared with adults, balancing radiation protection with image quality is of utmost importance. The dynamic face of the immature growing and partially ossified skeleton, requires experience and good knowledge of the radiological image and developmental variants. Radiation protection should also follow already made guidelines like the ICRP draft report consultation on ' Radiological Protection in Pediatric diagnostic and interventional Radiology' published in the Annals of the ICRP ref 4839-3982-4649 of May 2011 (readers are encourage to view this document for further details).

Paediatric MRI

MRI in children is performed under a variety of settings including neurological, cardiac, musculoskeletal as well as for diagnosis and follow up of malignant disease. The major challenges in imaging children with MRI stem from the following

A. Peculiarity of anatomy

The relatively smaller anatomic structures in children create a challenge in terms of available signal as well as limit of resolution.

These anatomical structures which are smaller than the adult such as inner ear, cranial nerves, brachial plexus, biliary tree, peripheral joints and blood vessels require high resolution. In other words, imaging these structures require high signal to noise ratio. This scenerio becomes even more significant in the presence of anomalies or congenital defects, as well as the changing face of structural developments.

This can be achieved with high field strengths, acquisition of thinner slices and improved spatial resolution.

B. Evolving development.

The anatomy in children appear to be evolving as they develop and mature. This is true with cerebral imaging where the corticosulcations, patterns of myelination change rapidly as the child matures. At birth, the water content of brain tissue is significantly higher than that of adults. The abundance of Hydrogen molecules from water and the lack of commensurate fatty signals requires an increase in TE on T2- weighted imaging to achieve good contrast. Also visualization of joints should take into consideration changes in the growth of the epiphyses and and apophyseal cartilage.

C. Patho- Physiological challenges.

The rates of acquisition of images, contrast injection rates may be influenced by physiological changes. For instance, the heart rate, pulse rate, breathing and blood flow rates are different in neonates, necessitating shorter times for image acquisition. Children may also find it difficult to hold their breaths and this may introduce artefacts during the image acquisition process.

It is often difficult to perform an exhaustive clinical examination in children and symptoms may be vague and non- specific. Consequently, MRI request can frequently be non- specific, making the choice of protocols and modification in techniques more cumbersome.

D. Behavioral challenges

Children are increasingly aware of changes in their environment and less likely to co-operate with strangers. Some MRI studies require a reasonable period of cooperation and calm. This poses more difficulties on the time and energy of the staff. To achieve cooperation, the child may be sedated or given general anaesthesia, thereby increasing the inherent risk and often requiring staff with requisite skills.

E. Safety

The thermoregulatory mechanisms in children are poorly developed and children have high basal temperatures, thereby exposing them to higher risk of radiofrequency heating effects. This becomes magnified by the relatively higher surface area to weight ratio in children, increasing the area exposed to RF heating with a concurrent reduction in heat dissipation. The implications of the high specific absorption ratio (SAR) from MRI in children is unclear, but the need for close monitoring in the critically ill child cannot be over emphasised. Further safety concerns stem from possible side effects of anaesthesia like nausea, vomiting, drowsiness, agitation which are exaggerated in the pediatric population.

Generally speaking several issues come to mind

1. Improving signal to noise ratio requires higher field strengths (up to 3T)
2. Achieving the above also means more expensive hardware and sophistication in techniques

3. The use of greater field strength means better spatial and temporal resolution with altered T1 contrast (longer T1 and T2 relaxation times).
4. The likelihood of artifacts are higher especially for cardiac and abdominal imaging.
5. The SAR ultimately increases due to higher fields strengths in addition to introductio of B- field inhomogeneities.
6. Chemical shift, motion and susceptibility artefacts are increased.
7. Safety issues become more stringent as the field strength increases.

Due to the absence of radiation exposure, whole body MRI is considered a useful sequence in the evaluation of children with systemic abnormality or bone metastases.

Some general rules to achieving a successful MRI in children would include engaging them to become aware and participate in the procedure, allowing considerable distractions with audiovisual aids, puzzle tasks and relaxation breathing techniques. In addition to this, conscious effort to separate intravenous cannulations from the main MRI exam as well as carefully planning the sequences and protocols to include only the necessary ones are techniques that ultimately help.

3.1. Paediatric CT

There are general concerns about the amount of radiation exposure from paediatric CT due to the radio sensitivity of developing and immature tissues in children. Evidence abound to prove that pediatric CT will result in significantly increased lifetime radiation risk for cancer over adult CT, due to increased dose per milliamperes second and the increased lifetime risk per dose. There are also issues with who makes appropriate decisions for the referral of children, clinical benefit of the procedure, dose information and poor knowledge and compliance to laid down guidelines.

In a particular survey, there is poor compliance to guidelines in imaging children with torticollis, ventriculoperitoneal shunt and sinusitis. Sometimes, unnecessary examinations may be seen in cases of uncomplicated headache, suspected Pulmonary embolism, pre- op chest survey, and in the evaluation of appendicitis.

The use of Helical CT techniques for volume acquisition during CTA (CT Angiography), also has several challenges in children. To perform successful CTA's in children, factors like reduced contrast volume, injection rates, timing of scans, radiation dose minimization and breath holding abilities must be considered. For most indications, helical CT of the chest using low dose techniques provides adequate image quality without a significant loss of diagnostic information. Modifications in equipment design has allowed optimization of scan parameters to achieve desired results. These include reduction in the rotation time (0.4 to 0.5seconds), reduced detector coverage commensurate to body size, reduced slice thickness and pitch especially with multiple slice facility. Others are reduced field of view (FOV), KV and use of smart MA/ auto MA options to optimize exposure levels.

When used, CT facilities should be equipped to accommodate ventilated neonates and appropriately trained medical and nursing staff must accompany such patients.

3.2. Paediatric Ultrasound

The procedure for paediatric ultrasound does not differ significantly from that of children. Equipment and facilities may not differ significantly except for the choice of transducers. Most ultrasound machines come with options for paediatric probes. This is especially true for transcranial and cardiac work. Most paediatric probes would be relatively smaller than adult probes and may have adjustable usually higher frequencies to cope with various depths and patient needs. The compromise is usually between the degree of penetration and resolution required for each case.

Patients may either be awake or sleeping, but there is usually no need for sedation in most circumstances.

Ultrasound is relatively safe with no risks of radiation, cheap and readily available. Ultrasound scans may be repeated over and over again, without any significant risks. The challenges for the care giver is similar to that in most other modalities; getting the cooperation of the child.

A warm friendly environment, good interpersonal skills will help the sonographer perform the investigation with ease. The practice of warming the gel and towels is often desirable for the child patient. The cooperation of the parents or guardian is usually solicited as this helps the child to remain calm during the investigation. As a general rule, most pediatric ultrasound scans are performed in the presence of accompanying adult.

For neonates in intensive care units, portable scanners may be used, equipped with transducers with various frequencies, and Doppler to perform the investigation at the bedside. Special care and aseptic procedures must be maintained to prevent risk of infection to infants.

The general rule is to get an ultrasound whenever possible, as it can be repeated over and over again.

4. Clinical Applications

The clinical implications of the above challenges are highlighted below for the various regions.

Pediatric chest: The chest radiograph is the most common imaging technique employed for pediatric thoracic abnormalities. Pediatric chest radiography presents peculiar challenges due to the wide range of tissue densities present in the thorax. This is complicated by the need to minimise radiation dose, the varying thoracic sizes, difficulty in achieving inspiration and likelihood of motional blurr. The continous improvement in screen- film technology and development of digital systems produce a wider dynamic range and linear response to xray exposure. This ensure that useful images can be obtained in a wide latitude of expo-

http://dx.doi.org/10.5772/51611

sures and digital processing allows adequate contrast and detail to be achieved. This means a better control of radiation exposure as repeats are almost eliminated. The neonatal chest radiograph will most undoubtedly include portions of the abdomen and appendicular skeleton. The ABC approach typically is to examine the whole radiograph and not just the chest. This can be put in this simplified format

A- Abdomen region is examined for abnormal gas patterns, calcification and situs

B- Bone to exclude fractures, metabolic diseases eg rickets or definite bone lesions

C- Chest for position of the mediastinum, cardiac size and contours, vascular markings, abnormal air spaces, pneumothorax or atelectasis, determine positions of central venous line, umbilical venous catheter and endotracheal tube, pleural effusions.

In addition, soft tissue appearance to exclude abnormal swellings, or loss of body mass like in malnutrition and wasting states. Rapid advancement in imaging technologies has widened the opportunities provided to more specifically explore pathologies of the chest by the introduction of CT, MRI, PET CT. In conjunction with tremendous input of digital techniques has improved acquisition of morphological and functional information regarding the chest. Helical CT scans allow short acquisition times, reduce motion artefacts and with dynamic contrast injection can produce remarkable information of the thoracic bony cage as well as vascular and pulmonary architexture, simultaneously.

MRI holds a high promise in the evaluation of thoracic disease. It has ability to clearly distinguish between mediastinal fat, blood vessels and soft tissues. Cardiac anomalies, mediastinal masses, and chest wall lesions can be delineated with MRI. The emphasis on the possibility of acquiring dynamic and functional information of the lungs has led to introduction of many techniques such as Functional MR, He- enhanced MR, and Fluorodeoxyglucose (FDG)PET studies. MR techniques hold much promise in the examination of obstructive airways disease including cystic fibrosis, by allowing excellent delineation of lung parenchyma and patterns of ventilation.

PET studies appear to be increasingly useful in lymphoma imaging in children.

Pediatric Abdomen

The plain abdominal radiograph can provide variable degree of information allowing initial assesment of disease processes. Similar to the approach adopted for chest interpretation, plain films of the abdomen require specific methodology.

The plain abdomen radiograph typically includes the lower chest and thus the bases of the lungs and diaghragm are examiaimed for pneumonia and abnormal gas appearance beneath the dome respectively. The erect abdomen radiograph appears to be the most vital single projection, allowing tremdous insight into chest and abdominal changes.

Bones are examined to exclude fractures, osteomyelitis and abnormal changes due to metabolic or neoplastic disease.

The psoas muscles, retro-peritoneal fat lines, calcification or abnormal gas patterns are visualized within the abdominal cavity. This can be interpreted as CBA (chest, bone, abdomen), a reversal of the pattern described earlier.

In suspected intestinal obstruction, a plain radiograph may be sufficient to differentiate low from high obstruction, by providing information on the presence, extent and level of gas in the bowel. A water soluble contrast examination of the upper gastrointestinal tract will help to determine cause, for example pyloric stenosis and gastric outlet obstrauction. Barium enema may be necessary to differentiate the possible causes of low intestinal obstruction especially in equivocal cases of ileal atresia, meconium plug or ileus.

Ultrasound is both safe and reliable to assess intrabdominal organs and to determine origin and perhaps vascular extension of a potential abdominal mass. Initial assessment of the liver, spleen, kidneys are best performed with ultrasound. Ultrasound would equally be useful to differentiate medical from obstructive jaundice and initial suggestion of biliary atresia. In an experienced hand, abdominal ultrasound can provide a tremendous amount of information in cases of suspected intestinal obstruction. Diagnosis of pyloric stenosis and gastric outlet obstruction, hiatus hernia, intussusception can comfortably be made with ultrasound.

Computed tomography or MRI is usually necessary to determine the exact extent of a mass and to exclude spread, especially when the need to have a sectional information arises. CT has its use in the determination of injuries to organs following trauma, perforated viscus, abscesses, appendicitis. The use of spiral CT techniques encourages better evaluation of the liver for acquired vascular abnormalities, vascular masses, pre operative evaluation of renal tumors. The advances in MR techniques have significantly altered the investigation of abdominal and pelvic disease in children. MRI will profoundly help in the visualization of the biliary tract, pancreas as well as intra and extra- luminal bowel disease. MR urography is especially useful for anatomical and functional assesment of the urinary system.

Pediatric Brain

The use of ultrasound in the imaging of neonatal brain has tremendous advantages. Ultrasound is safe, cheap and available and therefore is the preferred modality at this stage. In older children, ultrasound is no longer useful once the fontanels are closed.

Brain CT is usually recommended for children with traumatic brain injury, which is relatively common. The recommendation takes into account traditional clinical guidelines for determining the at risk patient and the risk of radiation and possible sedation for the critically ill. Such a guideline would ultimately depend on the clinical scenario and age of the patient. The problem typically lies in the ability to determine this category of patients who clinically qualify for the procedure and to differentiate them from those at low risk for serious treatable head injury for whom cranial CT would be unnecessary.

Structural and functional MR techniques are invaluable in investigating brain tissue development. Practical and technical constraints exist in MR imaging in children and have been discussed in the technical section. Some peculiar techniques employed in Paediatric MRI include susceptibility-weighted Imaging (SWI) which is useful in imaging trauma, vascular

http://dx.doi.org/10.5772/51611

disease, telengiactasia, cavernous and venous angiomas, tumors and epilepsy and Diffusion Tensor Imaging allowing changes in the developing brain, trauma, and white matter disease. Other techniques include arterial spin labeling useful in identifying perfusion changes in the brain.

Paediatric Skeleton

Hussain et al (2007) noted that the unique features of children's growing skeletons create challenges in imaging and specifically result in injuries and fractures. The imaging of skeletal structures following trauma in children typically start with plain film radiography. Additional modalities include MRI and CT which are used as Adjunct procedures. MR imaging has evolved as the most important diagnostic tool for the local staging of primary bone and soft tissue rumors, for monitoring response to chemotherapy and also in the detection of postoperative tumor recurrence. MR imaging provides accurate postoperative staging of local tumor extension and helps to obtain adequate safety margins and planning of successful limb- salvage surgery.

Bone scintigraphy with 99mTc-polyphosphate or 99mTc-pyrophosphate can be carried out in children with suspected bone disease. Scintigraphy is effective to demonstrate skeletal metastases, primary osteosarcoma, fibrous dysplasia, and osteomyelitis. Abnormal accumulation of radioactivity in soft tissue lesions can also be demonstrated in primary adrenal neuroblastoma, Hodgkin's granuloma, and metastatic Burkitt's lymphoma.

Radionuclide bone scintigraphy is also highly sensitive and specific for diagnosing the musculoskeletal disorders of childhood. Conditions such as neonatal osteomyelitis, septic arthritis, diskitis of childhood, Legg-Calve-Perthes disease, the osteochondroses, the toddler's fracture, sports injuries, spondylolysis, myositis ossificians, and reflex sympathetic dystro phy can easily be made. Risks may include allergic reactions and exposure to radiation.

5. Conclusion

The challenges and pecularities discussed so far underscores the need for expertise and care during paediatric imaging procedures.

This expertise can be acquired through structured training as well as experience.

There is need to encourage Pediatric radiology as a sub specialty, as well as the training of Radiographers specifically for this purpose. There is need to encourage separate registration and licensing with career pathways and incentives to would be pediatric Radiographers. This may involve a review of the current training curriculum for Radiographers and radiologists.

There is need to have a joint commitment and responsibility towards achieving quality service delivery to the pediatric patient population.

Author details

Okechukwu Felix Erondu[1,2]

Address all correspondence to: okerons@yahoo.com

1 Department of Clinical Imaging, Image Diagnostics, Image Place, Port Harcourt, Nigeria

2 Department of Medical Radiography and Radiological sciences, College of Medicine, University of Nigeria, Enugu Campus, Nigeria

References

[1] Bisset, G. S. (1989). Pediatric thoracic applications of MRI. *J Thoravic Imaging* , 1989 April, 4(2), 51-7, Pubmed.

[2] Brenner, D. J., Elliston, C. D., Hall, E. J., & Berdon, W. E. (2001). Estimated Risks of Radiation- induced Fatal cancer from Pediatric CT. *AJR*, 176, 289-29.

[3] Dagla, Charuta, & Ditchfield, Michael. (2008). T MRI in paediatrics. Challenges and clinical applications. *Eur. J. Radio*, 68(2), 309-319.

[4] Conway, J. J. (1986). Radionuclide bone scintigraphy in pediatric orthopedics Pediatr. *Clin. North Am.J.* , Dec 1986, 6, 1313-1334.

[5] Cohen, R. S., Trush, D. P., & Donnelly, L. F. (2000). Data acquisition for paediatric CT angiography Problems and solutions. *Pediatr Radiol*, 30, 813-822.

[6] Cohen, M. M., Cameron, C. B., & Duncan, P. G. (1990). Pediatric Anaesthesia morbidity and mortality in the peri operative period. *Anaesthesia and Analgesia*, 70, 160-7 (cross-ref).

[7] Coren, M. E., Ng, V., Reubens, M., Rosenthal, M., et al. (1998). The value of ultra fast computed Tomography in the investigation of pediatric chest disease. *Pediatr Pulmonol*, 26, 389-395.

[8] D'Alessandro, M. P., & D'Alessandro, M. D. (2012). Virtual Pediatric Hospital. http://www.vitualpediatrichospital.org, Accessed 29 th May 2012.

[9] Crush, D. P., Siegel, M. J., & Bisset, G. S. (1997). Challenges of pediatric spiral CT. *Radiographics July*, 17, 939-959.

[10] Dagia, C., & Ditchfield, M. (2008). T MRI in paediatrics: Challenges and clinical applications. *Eur. J. Radiol.*, doi:10.1016/j-ejrad.2008.05.019.

[11] Darge, K., Anupindi, S. A., & Jaramillo, D. (2001). MR imaging of the abdomen and pelvis in infants, children and adolescents. *Radiology*, 261(1), 12-29.

[12] Diederich, S., Leutschig, M. G., Winter, F., Roos, N., & Bongartz, G. (1999). Detection of pulmonary nodules vs non-overlapping image reconstruction at spiral CT. *Eur Radiol*, 9, 281-286.

[13] Edeling, C. J. (1976). Bone scintigraphy in children. *Nuklearmedizin*, 1976 Oct, 15(5), 228-32, pubmed.

[14] Frush, D. P., Donnelly, L. F., & Chotas, H. G. (2000). Contemporary Pediatric Thoracic Imaging. *AJR*, sep 2000, 175, 3, 841-851.

[15] Partan, Gerald, Pamberger, Petra, Blab, Edmund, & Hruby, Walter. (2003). Common tasks and problems in paediatric radiology. *Eur. J. Of Radiol*, 48(1), 103-124.

[16] Cahoon, Glenn. (2011). Techniques in Pediatric MRI- Tips for Imaging children. *Magnetom Flash*, www.siemens.com/Magnetom-world.

[17] Hearty, M. P., & Krammer, S. S. (1998). Recent advances in pediatric pulmonary imaging. *Curr opin Pediatr*, 10, 227-235.

[18] Hussain, H. M., & Barnes, C. E. Pediatric skeletal trauma Plain film to MRI. *Applied Radiology*, 36(8), 24-33.

[19] ICRP draft report. (2011). Consultation on 'Radiological Protection in Pediatric diagnostic and interventional Radiology'. *Annals of the ICRP*, No. 4839-3982-4649 of May 2011.

[20] Kirks, D. R., et al. (1991). *Practical Pediatric Imaging*, (2nd Ed) Boston: Little, Brown and Co.

[21] Kohn, M. M., Moores, B. M., Schibilla, H., Schneider, K., Stender, H., Stieve, F. E., Teunen, D., & Wall, B. European Guidelines on Quality criteria for Fiagnostic Radiographic Images in Paediatrics. *European Commission. Directorate-General XII:science, Research and Development*.

[22] Lang, P., Johnston, J. O., Arena-Romero, F., & Gooding, C. A. (1998). Advances in MR imaging of pediatric musculoskeletal neoplasms. *Magn Reson Imaging Clin N Am.*, 1998 Aug, 6(3), 579-604.

[23] Machata, A. M., Willshike, H., Kaban, B., Prayer, D., et al. (2009). Effect of Brain MRI on body core temperature in sedated infants and children. *Brit J. Anesthesia*, 102(3), 385-9, cross-ref.

[24] Michael, R. (2008). Potential of MR-imaging in the paediatric abdomen. *Eur J Radiol*, 2008 Nov, 68(2), 235-44, Pubmed.

[25] NHS- National Imaging Board. (2010). Delivering quality Imaging services for Children. 30th March 2010 (www.dh.gov.uk).

[26] Raschle, N., Sliva, D. D., Franceschi, A., Grant, P. E., Benasich, A. A., et al. (2012). Pediatric neuroimaging in early childhood and infancy: challenges and practical guidelines. *Annals of the New York Academy of sciences*, April 2012, 1252, 43-50.

[27] Ravin, C. E. (1998). Future directions in pulmonary imaging. *Radiology*, 206, 9-10.

[28] Riccabona, M., Avni, F. E., Blickman, J. G., et al. (2008). Imaging recommendations in paediatric uroradiology. *Paediatric. Radiol*, 38, 138-145.

[29] Singh, S., Kalra, M. K., Moore, M. A., Shailam, R., Liu, B., Toth, B. S., et al. (2009). Dose Reduction and Compliance with Pediatruc CT protocols adapted to patient size, clinical indication and number of prior studies. *Radiology*, July 2009, 252, 200-208.

Chapter 3

Clinical Applications of Nuclear Medicine

Sonia Marta Moriguchi, Kátia Hiromoto Koga,
Paulo Henrique Alves Togni and
Marcelo José dos Santos

Additional information is available at the end of the chapter

http://dx.doi.org/10.5772/53029

1. Introduction

Nuclear Medicine is a medical specialty in which radioactive substances are used for diagnostic and therapeutic purposes. Historically, its major development occurred after the Second World War. After the attack on Pearl Harbor, the United States developed nuclear reactors to produce atomic bombs, which were subsequently dropped on the Japanese cities of Hiroshima and Nagasaki. After the end of the war, the United States was involved in the campaign for application of *Atomic Energy for Peace*, which stimulated implementation of knowledge of nuclear energy for medical applications, among other beneficial actions. There is no doubt that this was the greatest advance in the production and distribution of radionuclides for medical purposes. The first radionuclide for medical applications was iodine-131, and this was followed by several others. Artificial production of technetium for diagnostic purposes was a milestone in the history of nuclear medicine. Today, this radioisotope is used the one most for producing imaging.

In the beginning, the images were documented using rectilinear scanner and subsequently using scintillation cameras or so-called gamma cameras, with images of poor definition. With technological development, improvements to gamma cameras became possible. The acquisition of functional images, which had previously only been done on a two-dimensional plane, became tomographic with three-dimensional reconstruction. This was named Single-Photon Emission Computed Tomography (known as SPECT), and it increased the sensitivity of detecting abnormalities or lesions. More recently, gamma cameras have been coupled with computed tomography (CT) or magnetic resonance imaging (MRI), thereby forming hybrid machines and increasing the effectiveness of identifying lesions or functionally abnormal tissues, at their sites. Technological advances have also been important for

Positron Emission Tomography (known as PET), thereby massively increasing the applicability of this method, especially related to oncologic processes, with molecular imaging.

The diagnostic and therapeutic applications are based on the kind of radiation used. In general, gamma emitters are used for diagnosis, and technetium-99m is the most common agent for this purpose. For therapy, beta radiation emitters such as iodine-131 are the agents most used.

Scintigraphy is a noninvasive imaging diagnosis method using low doses of radiation, it is painless, has reasonable cost and availability, and enables functional or metabolic assessment of organs or structures. Its advantage is clear, especially when the possibility of analysis using other methods is limited. It is based on administration of radiation-emitting substances to patients, with detection by scanning using a scintillation camera. These radioactive substances may migrate to the organs themselves or, when that does not happen, they may bind to other substances, thus forming complexes called radiopharmaceuticals that are taken up by the target organ. There are specific pharmaceuticals for each organ, e.g. MDP, DTPA, sestamibi, etc., thus making it possible to perform bone, renal or cardiac scintigraphy, respectively. The great majority of radiotracers represent the physiology or metabolic activity of some part of the body, but without altering the function of these structures or forming part of the metabolism.

The main characteristic of scintigrams is that they provide information on the functioning and metabolism of organs and structures. Hence, they differ from other imaging methods such as ultrasound, CT scans or MRI, which are anatomical, and thus complement the diagnostic investigation.

From this perspective, it is important to distinguish between the diagnostic approaches for benign or malignant diseases. In benign lesions, the most important information comes from functional assessment of each organ. This may show that the organ function is normal or is deviating from normal, and this is assessed together with the evolution of the disease or the post-intervention changes. Malignancies are assessed based on metabolic activity and findings of active primary or metastatic tumors. Details relating to residual tumors, viable tumors, recurrence, or disease progression are important and can be differentiated. Based on this information, the clinical application of nuclear medicine is to highlight the physiological or metabolic structures or organs involved.

This chapter does not aim to teach the methodology for performing scintigraphy, but to provide some knowledge for professionals who are not specialists in this field, so that the usefulness of this method in relation to various diseases can be seen.

This chapter is divided into applications and therapy using conventional scintigraphy with single-photon emitters.

The radionuclide most used for performing single-photon scintigraphy is technetium 99m, which is a pure gamma radiation emitter, with energy of 140 keV. This is considered to be a low energy level with ideal characteristics for producing images. It can be administered alone or coupled with pharmaceuticals to form complexes with specific characteristics relating to the preferential uptake for various human organs or structures. For each type of scintigraphy,

http://dx.doi.org/10.5772/53029

there is a specific radiotracer uptake mechanism that interfaces with the metabolism or excretion of the organ. In the following, most of the applications of diagnostic nuclear medicine in different systems of the human body are presented. The general precautions to be taken in cases of pregnancy, breastfeeding, breastfed infants and young children, for all the procedures in nuclear medicine, are indicated. This should be discussed on a case-by-case basis.

2. Gastrointestinal system

Application of nuclear medicine to the gastrointestinal (GI) system is very useful for investigating many diseases. This is a noninvasive and painless examination, with administration of low doses of radiation to patients. It is easy to perform and is indicated for diagnosing and following up gastrointestinal diseases. The long acquisition time for most examinations increases the sensitivity for detecting gastrointestinal abnormalities. Scintigraphy is generally of use for assessing organ function and the kinetics of gastrointestinal transit or excretion.

2.1. Salivary gland imaging

This assesses the function and excretion of the salivary glands, both in the initial diagnosis and in post-treatment follow-up. The main indications include: tumors, cysts, inflammatory or infectious diseases, calculosis and Sjögren's syndrome.

The radioisotope used is pertechnetate, an anion that is concentrated and secreted by the epithelial cells of the salivary glands in the same way as seen with the anions that make up the saliva. Thus, this substance reflects the production and physiological secretion of the saliva. This radiotracer is administered intravenously, and sequential images of the head are acquired for 30 minutes. Over the first ten minutes, increasing concentration of radiotracer in the salivary glands is observed, which represents the function. After administration of citric stimulus, generally using lemon, the excretion phase begins. The uptake peak usually occurs five to ten minutes after starting to administer the radiotracer, and complete excretion begins immediately after the stimulation with lemon (Figure 1).

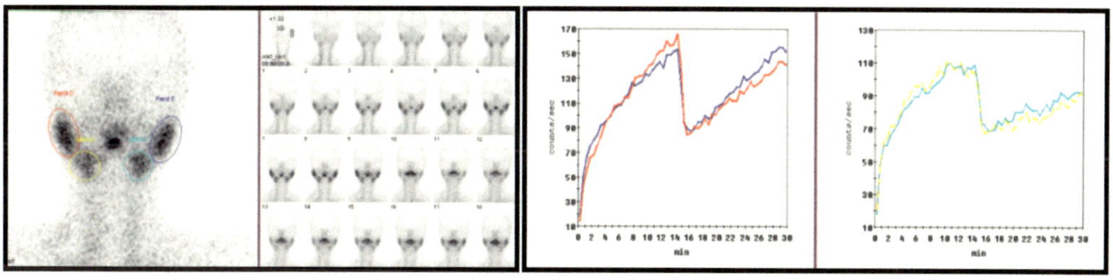

Figure 1. Normal salivary gland imaging. Dynamic images are performed during 30 minutes and citric stimulus is on first fifteen minutes. Region of interest are placed on right and left parotid (red and dark blue) and submandibulary (yellow and light blue) glands and time activity curves are created showing quantitative uptake and excretion analyses.

The scintigraphic abnormalities depend on the type and severity of disease. Most tumors present diminished or absence of uptake radiotracer, except for Warthin's tumor. Acute inflammatory and infectious diseases present uptake increased because of the increased vascularization and diminished secretion. Abscesses and cysts do not show any uptake. Patients with Sjögren's syndrome either do not concentrate radioactive material or concentrate very little of it (Figure 2).

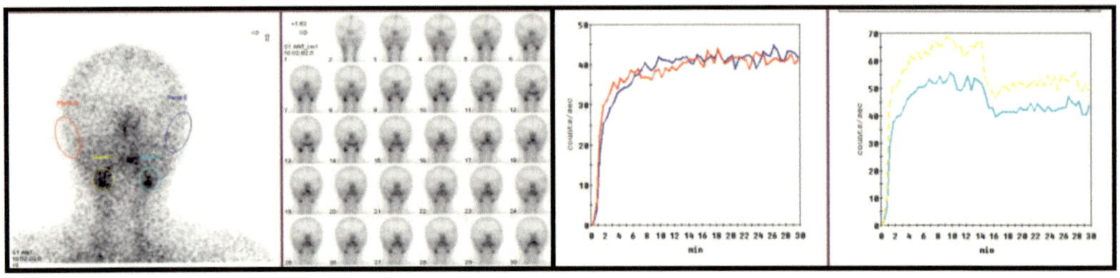

Figure 2. Anormal salivary gland imaging. Absence uptake and non excretion in parotid glands confirmed by quantitative curves by region of interest (red and dark blue).

Other agents that are used to assess the salivary glands include gallium-67 and 111 In/ 99mTc-labeled white blood cells, in cases of inflammatory or infectious diseases.

2.2. Scintigraphy on esophageal transit and emptying

Scintigraphy on the esophageal transit is a noninvasive examination with oral administration of radiotracer that supplies information on esophageal motility, in relation to the duration of esophageal transit and segmental motor abnormalities such as adynamia and lack of coordination. It is indicated for patients with suspected primary or secondary motor disorders, both for diagnosis and for follow-up of therapeutic interventions, in conditions such as achalasia, scleroderma, diffuse esophageal spasm, nutcracker esophagus, diabetic enteropathy, nonspecific motor disorders, Chagas' disease, neoplasm, systemic lupus erythematosus, polymyositis, myasthenia gravis, myotonic dystrophy, esophagitis, alcoholism and others. The radiopharmaceuticals indicated for these assessments are those that are not absorbed by the esophageal mucosa, such as colloids and chelates: technetium-^{99m}Tc-sulfur colloid and diethylenetriamine pentaacetic acid (DPTA). The radiopharmaceuticals are administered orally, diluted in 10 ml of water, and deglutition is stimulated every 20 seconds with the patient in either a supine or an upright position. The transit time for the entire esophagus and in its three segments (upper, middle and lower) is quantified and the motor abnormality pattern (adynamia or lack of coordination) is determined (Figure 3).

http://dx.doi.org/10.5772/53029

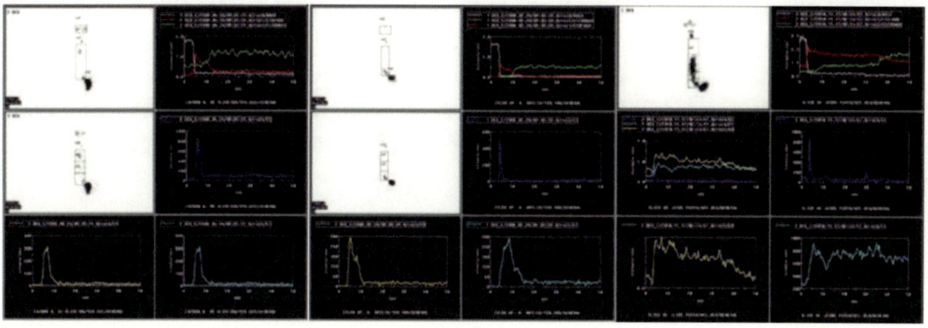

Figure 3. Scintigraphy on esophageal transit. Normal, adynamia and adynamia with incordination patterns, respectivelly.

2.3. Investigation of gastroesophageal reflux

Scintigraphy is the most sensitive noninvasive method for detecting gastroesophageal reflux, especially in children. Colloids with low absorption rates in the esophageal and gastric mucosa are used, thereby reflecting the kinetics of the tracer within the digestive system. After oral administration of ^{99m}Tc colloid, and with a field of view covering the stomach and esophagus, episodes of gastroesophageal reflux are identified and information on the quantity and duration of the reflux and the point that it reaches are obtained (Figure 4). It has the advantage of continuous and more prolonged acquisition, which increases the sensitivity of the method. Other additional information obtained includes assessment of pulmonary aspiration, in the event that the reflux of the ingested material reaches the pulmonary tree.

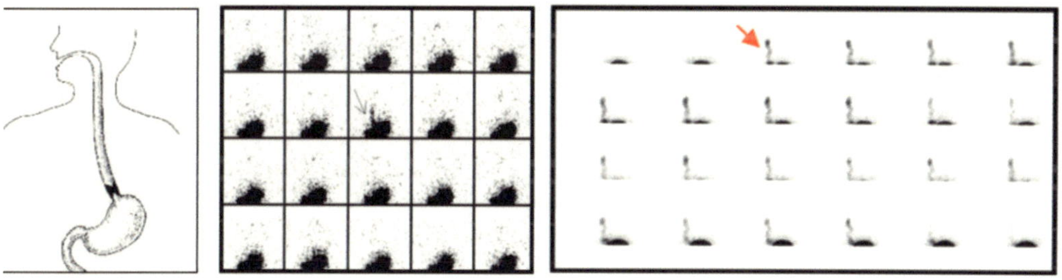

Figure 4. Gastroesophageal reflux scintigraphy. A single episode with a short time, reaching the upper esophageal segment (black arrow) and during a long time (red arrow).

2.4. Gastric emptying

This is a noninvasive examination performed after intake of solid foods, liquids or a mixture of these. The emptying time and kinetics of the radiotracer in the stomach depend on the composition of the food ingested. Several pharmacological materials can be labeled with the radioactive substance, and the composition of both the food and the radiotracer depends on the standard adopted by each laboratory as the reference value. Computer acquisition is required to determine the half-time of emptying and/or percent of emptying and to generate gastric emptying time-activity curves. The main indications include diabetic gastroparesis, anorexia nervosa, gastroesophageal reflux, gastritis, gastric ulcer, duodenal ulcer, Zollinger-Ellison disease, connective tissue disorders and others, along with postsurgical evaluations, vagotomy and gastrectomy.

2.5. Liver-spleen imaging

Other imaging methods such as MRI, CT and ultrasound offers better information about the anatomic display of liver and spleen than does this exam. The radionuclide colloid imaging is capitalized by phagocitosis by Kupffer cells of liver and spleen. The uptake and distribution of ^{99m}Tc-colloid in liver and spleen reflects perfusion and the distribution of functioning reticulendothelial cells. Usually, the information of liver-spleen scan include the size, shape and position, the distribution aspect of activity within the organs, as homogeneity or non-homogeneity, presence of any or many focal defects in activity and relative distribution of colloid among the liver, spleen and bone marrow. Most of the masses seen on MRI, CT or US, which take up ^{99m}Tc colloid contain Kupffer cells, and are benign. These present with increased hepatic uptake and include: focal nodular hyperplasia (Figure 5), cirrhosis with regenerating nodule, Budd-Chiari syndrome and Superior vena caval obstruction. Masses with decreased hepatic uptake can be benign or malignant. These include: hepatoma, metastasis, cyst, adenoma, hemangioma, abcess, and pseudotumor. The most common causes of focal defects in the spleen include: abcess, cyst, infarct, lymphoma, and hematoma.

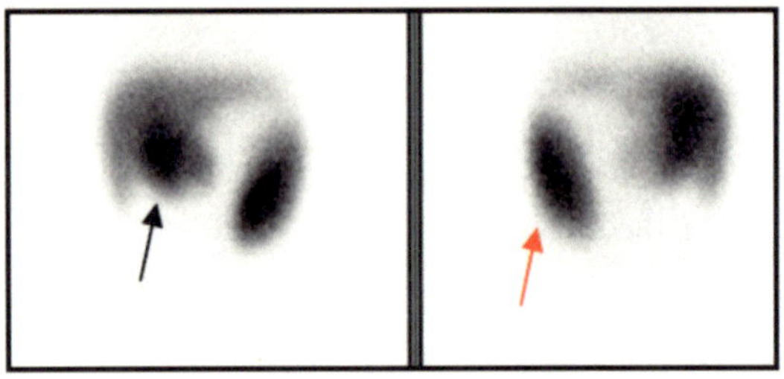

Figure 5. Liver-spleen scintigraphy. Focal nodular hyperplasia. Anterior and posterior images. Focal uptake increased in liver (black arrow). Spleen increased too (red arrow).

2.6. Hepatic blood pool imaging

This exam is indicated for evaluating hemangiomas. These lesions are clusters or large blood filled sinuses. They are usually asymptomatic, and are found as incidental findings during MRI, CT or US performed for others indications. The radiotracer used is ^{99m}Tc-red blood cells (RBC), injected intravenously. The typical appearance of ^{99m}Tc-RBC scan is a focal area of decreased perfusion on the first study (flow phase), and in the immediate images because the flow with ^{99m}Tc-RBC is relatively low compared to the hemangioma. About 1 or 2 hours later, the radiolabelled cells reach the hemangioma vessels, and then these lesions present as a focal hot spot, with intensity similar to the heart. This method is highly specific to confirm hemangioma.

2.7. Gastrointestinal bleeding imaging

The common causes of lower GI bleeding in adults include neoplasms, inflammatory bowel disease, diverticular disease and angiodysplasia. The GI Imaging is a noninvasive method that provides information especially of lower GI bleeding. The effective therapy for acute GI bleeding depends on accurate localization of the site of bleeding. There are two radiotracer that localize the GI bleeding; ^{99m}Tc-RBC and ^{99m}Tc-colloid. The first one is preferred in the investigation of GI hemorrhage, especially in cases of intermittent or slow bleeding, because the radiotracer remains in the intravascular space. Imaging may be performed over a period of 24 hours. The second one is high, specifically to identify the bleeding site, but the sensitivity is low, because it is performed for a short time and the bleeding needs to be present at the moment of scintigraphy.

3. Cardiovascular system

Nuclear medicine examinations play an important role in the noninvasive evaluation of cardiac physiology.

3.1. Myocardial perfusion imaging

Myocardial perfusion imaging (MPI) has high sensitivity to evaluate perfusion in the left ventricular wall and thus indirectly assess coronary flow. The ischemic cascade is the basis and the best justification for the use of nuclear medicine examinations in the evaluation of coronary artery disease.

Myocardial perfusion imaging can be performed with thallium-201 chloride and Pharmaceuticals labelled with 99mTc (sestamibi, tetrofosmim and teboroxime). To use thallium-201 chloride it is necessary to fast for at least 4 hours. Radiopharmaceuticals labelled with 99mTc have advantages and disadvantages when compared to thallium-201 chloride, as best rate of counts and less sensitivity to assess viability, respectively.

The stress phase can be accomplished by exercise or by the use of drugs such as dipyridamole, adenosine, and dobutamine. The sensitivity and specificity of these types of stress are similiar.

Clinical applications of the study with thallium-201 chloride are: diagnosis of coronary artery disease, assessing the extent and severity of coronary stenosis, myocardial viability assessment and therapeutic efficacy (CABG and angioplasty).

Radiopharmaceutical labelled with 99mTc are usually associated with cardiac monitoring during image acquisition, thus allowing quantitative analysis with motility evaluation of the left ventricular wall and ejection fraction.

Clinical applications of the study using radiopharmaceuticals labelled with 99mTc are: a diagnosis of coronary artery disease, risk stratification post-myocardial infarction and therapeutic efficacy (Figure 6).

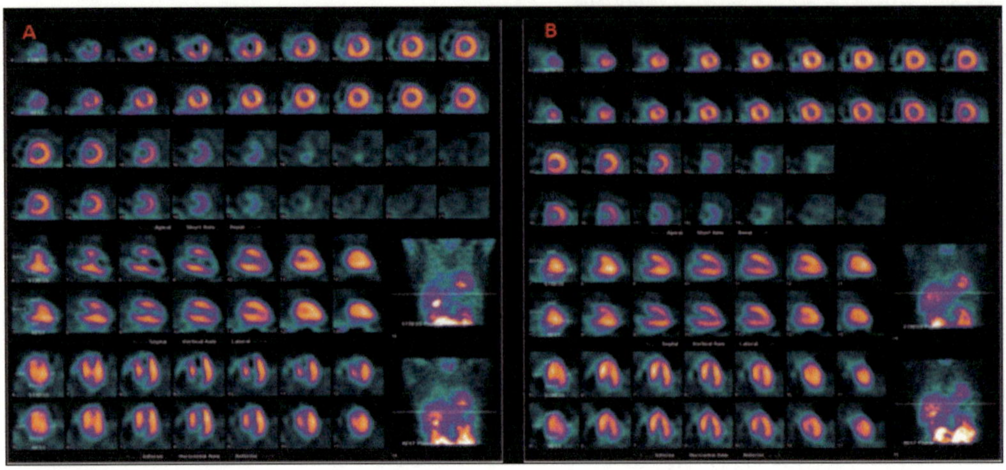

Figure 6. Myocardial perfusion scintigraphy with 99mTc-sestamibi. A: Pre-angioplasty: ischemia of the apex and the middle and apical regions of the anteroseptal wall of the left ventricle. B: Post-angioplasty: a study without evidence of myocardial ischemia.

3.2. Myocardial viability imaging

The principle objective of myocardial viability assessment is to identify patients eligible for coronary artery bypass grafting (CABG). Several criteria were used to determine the clinical impact of CABG: improvement in regional left ventricular function, in global left ventricular function (ejection fraction), symptoms, functional capacity, in cardiac remodeling and long term prognosis [1].

Imaging with thallium-201 chloride and home-redistribution protocol can be used to assess the presence of viable myocardium. Using the protocol stress-rest-reinjection, in addition to similar information, the presence of ischemia can be evaluated.

3.3. Myocardial infarction imaging

Currently this study has been little used, due to advances in methods of enzymatic detection of acute myocardial infarction. Radiopharmaceuticals used can be 99mTc-pyrophosphate and Antimyosin-Fab-DTPA-In-111.

The maximum uptake of 99mTc-pyrophosphate occurs 24 to 72 hours after the event. Planar imaging with 99mTc pyrophosphate detect acute transmural with a sensitivity of at least 90% and a specificity of 70% (Figure 7). Tomographic imaging (SPECT) can improve the specificity to around 80%.

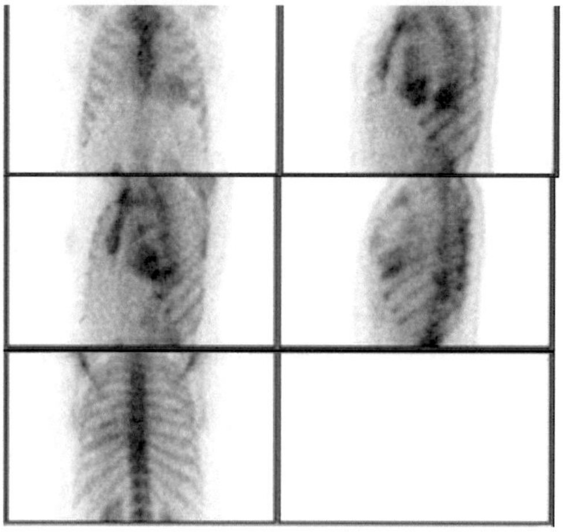

Figure 7. Imaging of myocardial infarction with 99mTc-pyrophosphate. 99mTc: trasmural infarction in the anterolateral wall of the left ventricle.

Antimyosin has an overall sensitivity of 92% for the detection of acute MI [2].

3.4. Multi Gated Acquisition (MUGA)

The objective is to assess the global and regional ventricular function. The radiopharmaceutical used is ^{99m}Tc-red blood cells (RBC), erythrocytes labeled with 99mTc. The parameters evaluated in this study are: motility of the ventricular wall, left ventricular ejection fraction, analysis of phase and amplitude. The clinical indications are: acute myocardial infarction, coronary artery disease, cardiomyopathy, valvular disease, congenital heart disease, therapeutic efficacy assessment and evaluation of cardiotoxic drugs.

3.5. Cardiac adrenergic imaging

The sympathetic and parasympathetic innervation of the heart plays an important role in regulating the cardiac function [3]. The activation of sympathetic innervation causes increased heart rate (chronotropic effect), contractility (inotropic effect) and conduction atrioventricular [4]. Norepinephrine is produced and stored in presynaptic vesicles in sympathetic nerve terminals [5]. Thus, the radionuclide used for cardiac adrenergic imaging is 123I-MIBG (metaiodobenzylguanidine) that is an guanethidine analogue which mimics norepinefrina [6]. The clinical indications are: heart failure, cardiomyopathy, cardiac transplantation, ischemia and myocardial infarction and ventricular tachyarrhythmias.

4. Pulmonary system

Pulmonary embolism (PE) is an important and treatable illness caused by migration of thrombus to the pulmonary circulation, commonly from the veins of the lower extremities.

Untreated, PE can cause death [7]. The treatment includes oral anticoagulants, heparin and thrombolytic agents. The clinical presentation of PE is variable, from asymptomatic to sudden death, including cough, hemoptysis, chest pain, breathlessness, syncope, palpitations, tachypnoea, cyanosis, tachycardia, pulmonary hypertension and right heart failure. But, these symptoms are not specific of PE, needing more tests to confirm or refuse the PE diagnostic. Recently, Bajc et al, purposed a clinical algorithm for the investigation of patients with suspected PE. If the clinical likelihood of PE is low and the quantitative D-dimer is negative, a diagnosis of PE is unlikely and further investigations are not required. If the clinical likelihood of PE is low and the quantitative D-dimer is positive, further investigations for a range of diagnoses including PE may be required, particularly if the D-dimer level is markedly elevated. If the clinical probability is other than low, it seems more appropriate to skip the D-dimer test and refer the patient directly to the appropriate imaging technique. This may be Ventilation (V) and perfusion (P) imaging (V/P_{SCAN}) or multidetector computed tomography of the pulmonary arteries (MDCT) depending on the local availability, medical expertise, and the patient's clinical condition. V/PS_{CAN} has virtually no contraindications and yields a substantially lower radiation burden than MDCT [8].

A combined ventilation and perfusion study increases the specificity for PE diagnosis. A combined 1-day protocol is preferred. The scan can be with planar lung imaging (anterior, posterior, left and right lateral and left and right posterior oblique) or Spect imaging. In pregnancy only a perfusion scan is recommended.

4.1. Ventilation lung scintigraphy (V)

Ventilation studies, in general, are performed after inhalation of inert gases ^{133}Xe and ^{81m}Kr, radiolabelled aerosols ^{99m}Tc-DTPA and ^{99m}Tc-labelled Technegas. It is performed for mapping regional ventilation.

4.2. Perfusion lung scintigraphy (P)

Perfusion scintigraphy is accomplished by microembolization with radiolabelled particles injected into a peripheral vein. The commercially used particles are MAA, which are labelled with ^{99m}Tc. The particle distribution accurately defines regional lung perfusion.

V/P_{SCAN} exploits the unique pulmonary arterial segmental anatomy. Each bronchopulmonary segment is supplied by a single end-artery. In principle, conical bronchopulmonary segments have their apex towards the hilum and base projecting onto the pleural surface. Occlusive thrombi, affecting individual pulmonary arteries, therefore produce characteristic lobar, segmental or subsegmental peripheral wedge-shaped defects with the base projecting to the lung periphery. V/P mismatch within bronchopulmonary segment(s) defected by PE, ventilation is usually preserved. This pattern of preserved ventilation and absent perfusion within a lung segment gives rise to the fundamental signiture for PE diagnosis using V/$P_{SCAN,}$ known as V/P mismatch.

Follow-up of PE using imaging is essential to assess the effect of therapy, differentiate between new and old PE on suspicion of PE recurrence and investigate physical incapacity after PE [9].

http://dx.doi.org/10.5772/53029

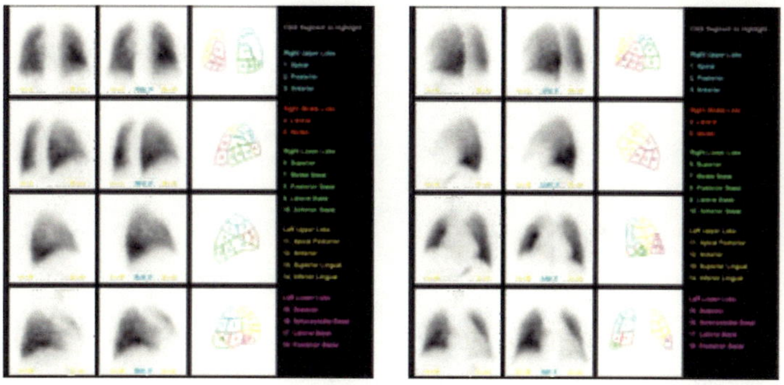

Figure 8. Normal pulmonary scintigraphy.Inhalation and perfusion images are compared. Homogeneous uptake in lungs. Matched findings.

5. Genitourinary tract imaging

In nuclear medicine the studies of genitourinary system can be divided into superior and inferior genitourinary tract. Studies evaluating the superior genitourinary tract include the kidneys, allowing evaluation of several characteristics such as blood flow, function, anatomy and integrity of the collection system, aiding in the diagnosis of different pathologies. For the lower genitourinary tract studies are represented by radionuclide cystography and testicular scintigraphy.

Renal radiopharmaceuticals commonly used to meet the various pathologies are 99mTc-MAG3, 99mTc-DTPA, 99mTc-GHA and 99mTc-DMSA, being dependent on the indication of particular characteristics. 99mTc-MAG3 has as a main uptake mechanism tubular secretion (98% tubular secretion, 2% of glomerular filtration and extraction fraction of 40-50%). the 99mTc-DTPA has as a main uptake mechanism glomerular filtration (100% filtration and extraction fraction of 20%). 99mTc-GHA has a mixed uptake mechanism, being, glomerulo-tubular (10-20% tubular secretion and 80-90% glomerular filtration). The 99mTc-DMSA is attached to the renal cortical (40-50% cortical binding in 2 hours).

5.1. Clinical applications in the superior genitourinary tract

Dynamic renal scintigraphy renogram represents the study commonly used to evaluate the various pathologies associated with superior genitourinary tract.

5.1.1. Obstruction of the genitourinary tract

It is the main indication of renal dynamic studies. The exam is simple, painless, easy to perform and only prior hydration is necessary. It lasts 30 to 50 minutes, and such variation is associated with the use of diuretics (Figures 9 and 10).

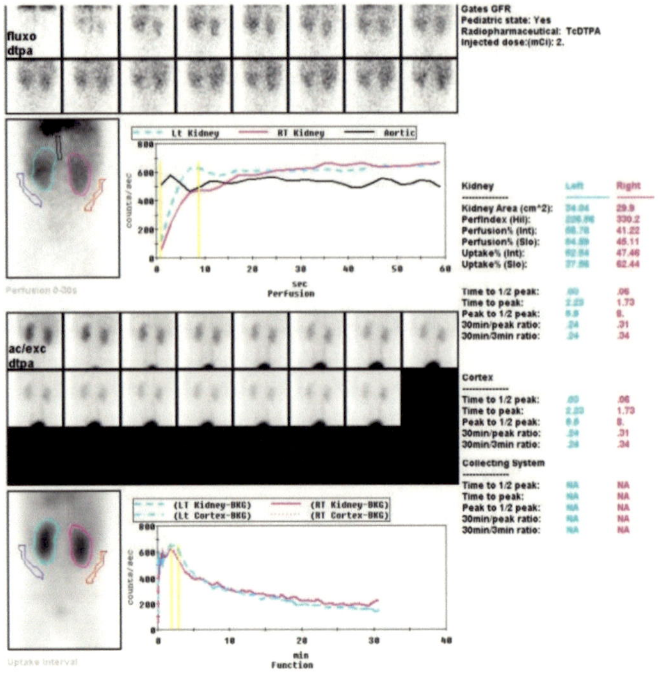

Figure 9. Dynamic renal scintigraphy with 99mTc-DTPA: flow, normal function and nonobstructive excretory pathways.

5.1.2. Hypertension of renovascular origin

For this condition, the renal dynamic study is done in two phases: one utilizing a stimulus by angiotensin converting enzyme inhibitor, one hour before administration of the radiopharmaceutical and the other from the merely studying renal dynamic without stimulus considered study baseline.

According to the pathophysiology of renovascular disease, the standard pattern of diagnosis is an abnormal study with stimulation of the angiotensin converting enzyme inhibitorassociated with a normal baseline study.

5.1.3. Renal transplant

In renal transplant, renal dynamic study is mainly used for evaluation of its most common complications such as acute tubular necrosis and rejection. The scintigraphic pattern of acute tubular necrosis and acute rejection are very similar, with preserved or slightly reduced flow and reduced glomerular filtration rate. The time and symptoms are the key to diagnosis. In serial renal studies, the renal graft dysfunction secondary to acute tubular necrosis should improve or remain unchanged, while the rejection demonstrates progressive deterioration. Currently, ultrasound is the method of choice for renal transplant dysfunction [10].

http://dx.doi.org/10.5772/53029

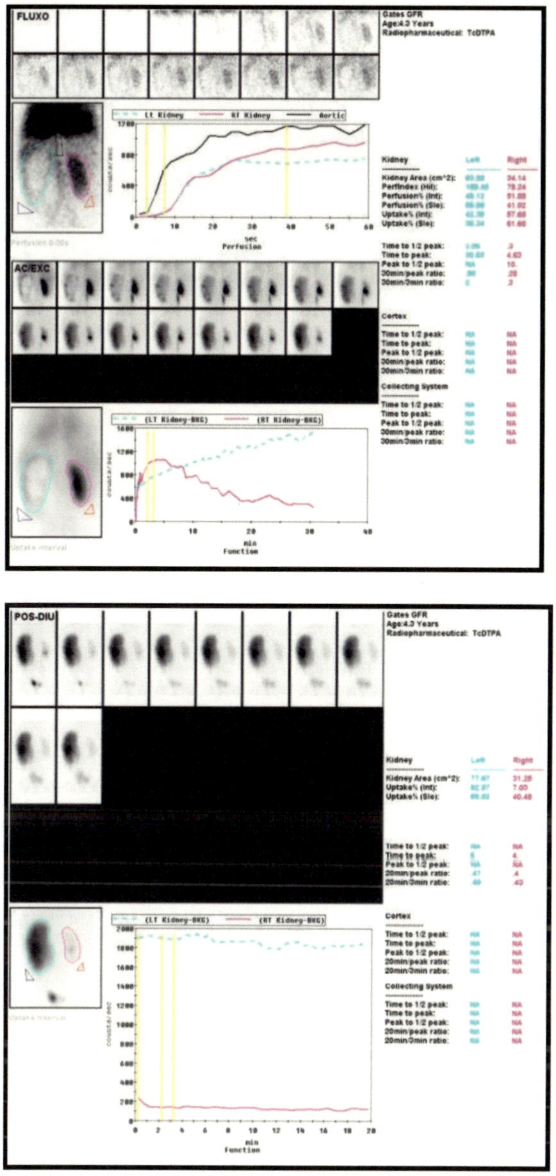

Figure 10. Dynamic renal scintigraphy with 99mTc-DTPA and use of diuretic: Deficit of flow and left renal function associated with obstructive hydronephrosis.

5.1.4. Acute pyelonephritis and renal scarring

The renal cortical scintigraphy with 99mTc-DMSA is the procedure of choice for evaluating acute pyelonephritis and renal scarring. The image acquisition takes place 2 to 3 hours after intravenous administration of the radiopharmaceutical so that attachment occurs at the same cortical. The scintigraphic patterns in acute pyelonephritis are focal involvement of a single area or multiple areas and diffuse involvement of the kidney. It has 100% sensitivity and specificity above 87% [11].

Renal scarring is a consequence of acute pyelonephritis, which may develop in 37% to 80% of children after an episode of infection [11,12] (Figures 11 and 12).

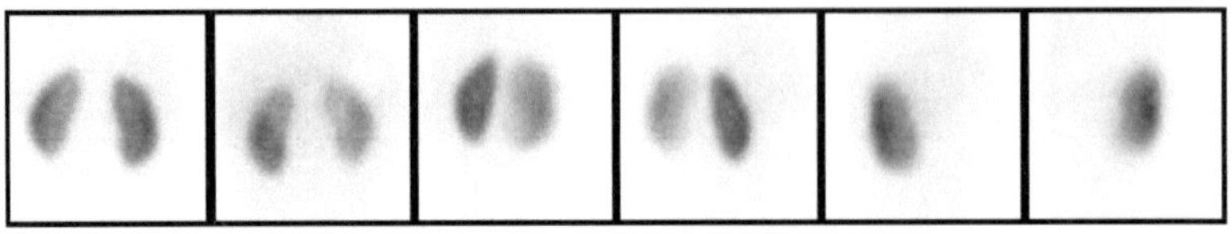

Figure 11. Normal renal scintigraphy with 99mTc-DMSA.

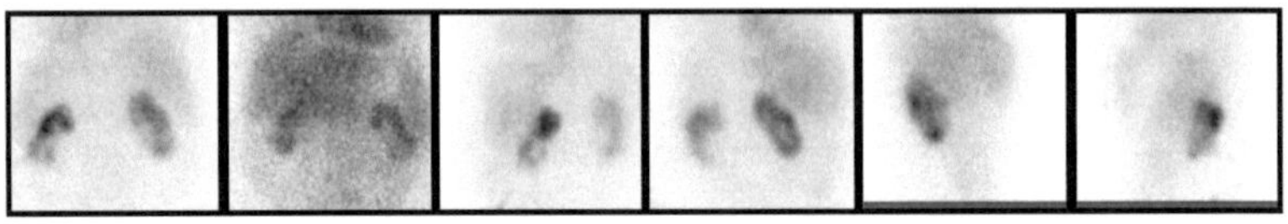

Figure 12. Renal scintigraphy with 99mTc-DMSA, renal scars.

5.2. Clinical applications in the lower genitourinary tract

5.2.1. Assessment of vesicoureteral reflux

Radionuclide cystography permits visualization of very small volumes of reflux, and is probably more sensitive than contrast cystography [13]. The procedure is performed by infusion of saline and radiopharmaceuticals within the bladder through the catheter, thereby evaluating the presence of reflux (Figure 13).

5.2.2. Testicular torsion

Testicular torsion is considered a surgical emergency and the availability of this tissue is mainly related to ischemic time. The testicular ultrasound is a simple method and easily performed for evaluation of this condition, however, in children evaluating the flow can be difficult, testicular scintigraphy is indicated.

The scintigraphic findings depend on the stage of testicular torsion, in the early phase there is a normal flow, reduced or absent and the still image is a slight reduction in uptake of the radiotracer within the testicle, followed by an increase in flow and static image appearance of halo of mildly increased activity around a centrally cold testicle, ending with testicular infarction, in which there is an increased flow rate and persistent halo of increased activity around a cold center.

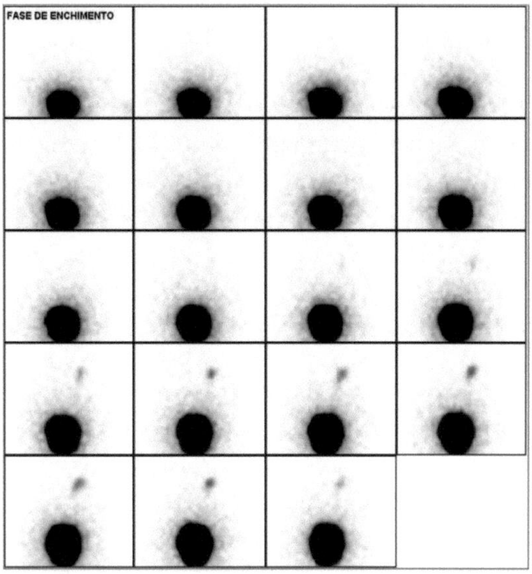

Figure 13. Radionuclide cystography: right vesicoureteral reflux.

6. Musculoskeletal system

6.1. Bone scintigraphy

Bone scintigraphy identifies single or multiple focal or diffuse areas with increased osteoblastic activity, which reflects local bone remodeling. It is a highly sensitive examination for detecting such abnormalities, but its specificity is limited. It needs to be analyzed in conjunction with other imaging examinations. It is indicated for both adults and children, but should be interpreted differently for these two groups, given that the normal distribution of radiopharmaceutical in the skeleton differs between adults and children, particularly because of the presence of physiological osteoblastic activity in the growth cartilage of children. These bone scans are based on the principle of phosphonate uptake in bone tissue, especially in blastic lesions. For example, from this principle, the presence of osteoblastic metastases from breast tumors or prostate tumors can be seen, among others. Likewise, changes typical of benign diseases such as bone infections, inflammatory activity of rheumatic diseases, and prosthesis complications like loosening, infection, etc., can be seen.

The radiopharmaceutical used most, which is called ^{99m}Tc-methylene diphosphonate (^{99m}Tc-MDP), binds to the amorphous phase of hydroxyapatite crystals by means of chemoadsorption. It is administered intravenously as a bolus. Images can be acquired immediately afterwards when information on the blood supply and vascular permeability is important, like in cases of infectious or tumor growth processes. They may also only be acquired later on, after 2-3 hours of injection, with acquisition of whole-body images in the anterior and posterior projections, in order to acquire information on osteoblastic activity. It is worth emphasizing that this examination shows low sensitivity to predominantly lytic pathological conditions or to conditions with low bone remodeling, except in cases associated with significant osteoblastic abnormalities, such as in investigations of associated fractures, for example, in patients with multiple myeloma. The great advantage of this method is that it assesses the whole body in a single examination with high sensitivity, and it guides other examinations that are more specific.

6.1.1. Clinical applications for children

Based on informations above, the mean indications of bone scan include: primary benign or malignant bone tumors and bone metastases; acute osteomyelitis versus soft-tissue inflammation; subacute and chronic osteomyelitis; septic arthritis as a complication of osteomyelitis; and aseptic arthritis; aseptic necrosis (Legg-Calvé-Perthes disease) and sickle cell disease; equivocal radiographic findings after trauma; stress fractures; occult fractures; child abuse; multiple trauma; complications of fractures and therapy; and Sudeck's atrophy; surgery-guided by bone scintigraphy, like as osteoid osteoma; bone dysplasia; Camurati-Engelmann disease; evaluations on skeletal involvement (brown tumors); and hyperparathyroidism; arthritis and bone pain [14]. Scintigraphies in children are showed in figure 14.

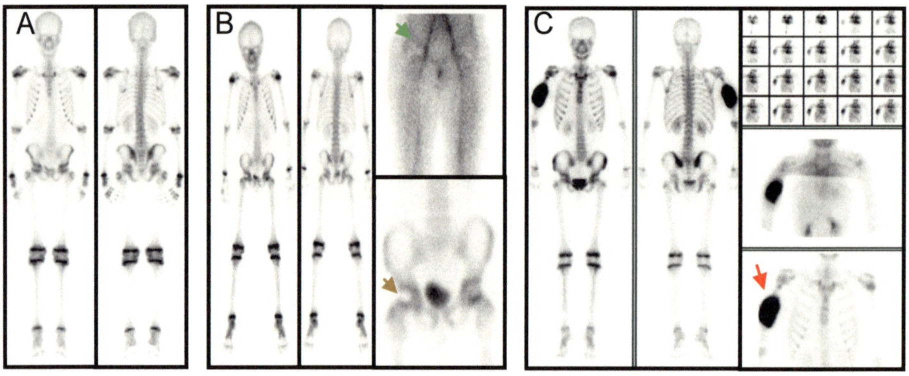

Figure 14. Bone scintigraphy in children. A. normal scan: Symmetric uptake on the skeletal and presence of physiological osteoblastic activity in the growth cartilage. B. Acute phase of avascular necrosis in right femoral head. Vascular permeability decreased (green arrow) and photopenic area (brown arrow) in right femoral head. C. Three phase bone scan. Osteosarcoma in the right humerus. Flow, vascular permeability and osteoblastic activity increased in right humerus (red arrows).

6.1.2. Clinical applications for adults

A little difference is observed between the chindren`s and adults`indications of bone scan. In this last group, the pathologies include: primary and metastatic bone tumors: staging, follow-up and post-therapy evaluation; distribution of osteoblastic activity prior to radiometabolic therapy (89Sr, 153Sm-EDTMP and 186Re-HEDP); osteomyelitis; Paget's disease, osteoporosis and hyperparathyroidism; arthropathy, low back pain and sacroiliitis; fibrous

http://dx.doi.org/10.5772/53029

dysplasia and other rare congenital conditions; stress fractures, shin splints, occult fractures; avascular necrosis and loose or infected joint prosthesis [15] (Figure 15).

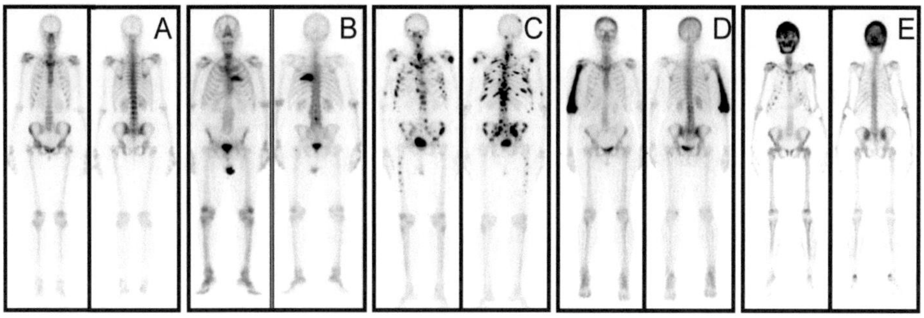

Figure 15. Bone scintigraphies in adults. A. Normal scan: symmetric uptake on the sckeletal. B. Single bone metastasis on left rib. C. Multiple bone metastasis. Multiple focal uptake on skull, scapulas, ribs, spine, pelvis and right femur. D. Monostotic Paget Disease on right humerus. Intense uptake on right humerus. E. Hyperparathyroidism. Intense uptake on skull and focal uptake on ribs.

7. Scintigraphy with gallium-67 citrate

Because of the characteristics of gallium-67 uptake in tissues, this radiotracer can be used in relation to neoplastic diseases, especially lymphomas, and in cases of chronic inflammatory or infectious processes, such as those in fever of unknown origin or in patients with acquired immunodeficiency.

The radiotracer is administered intravenously 48 hours before producing whole-body initial images in the supine position, in the anterior and posterior projections. Delayed images, produced at least from 72 hours and up to 5 days after injection, may be needed to differentiate normal colonic activity from lesions in the abdomen. This allows clearance of nonspecific activity from the body, and enhancement of the target in relation to the background in the images. The technologist or physician should give the patient a thorough explanation about the examination. Food and liquid restrictions are not mandatory. Bowel preparation is optional. In patients with constipation, oral laxatives prior to imaging may decrease the activity in the bowel. In this case, laxatives should be given on the day before gallium-67 scintigraphy (at least 18 hours prior to scanning). Gallium-67 scanning should be avoided within 24 hours of blood transfusion or gadolinium-enhanced MRI, which could interfere with gallium-67 biodistribution. It is also advisable to wait 3-4 weeks after chemotherapy before performing follow-up imaging.

Management of patients with lymphoma is very useful, especially in intermediate or high-grade tumors. Low-grade lymphomas may not uptake gallium-67 and therefore may not benefit from this method. Although anatomical diagnostic methods such as CT and MRI are superior to gallium-67 for initially staging the patients, an initial examination using gallium-67 is important because it serves as the basis for post-therapy monitoring of patients and indicates which patients may benefit from this method. If the tumor does not concentrate gallium-67 in the first examination, this radiotracer should not be used for the follow-up. For lymphomas that concentrate gallium-67, this tool becomes very useful for assessing the response to the treatment, since gallium accurately assesses tumor viability and the extent of the disease, indicates the prognosis and, especially, is important for restaging, given that the anatomical changes that occur after the treatment make it difficult to interpret anatomical images. Other tumors that may benefit from this method are lung cancer, head and neck tumors, hepatocellular carcinoma, germ cell tumors, neuroblastomas, sarcomas, multiple myelomas and melanomas. These tumors present avidity for gallium-67, but the use of this imaging method in these tumors is not well defined (Figure 16).

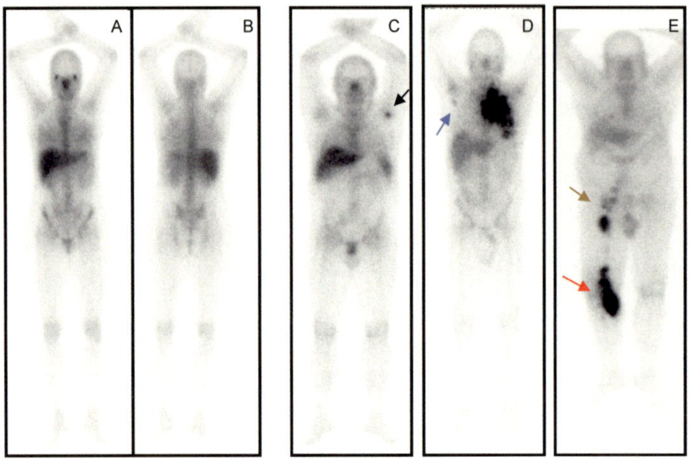

Figure 16. Whole body scan with gallium 67. A. normal scintigraphy. B. Lymphoma with lymphonodopathy. Uptake in left axillary lymphonode. C. Lymphoma with lymphonodapathy in right axillary, supravicular and mediastinal chain and left lung. D. Lymphoma in inguinopelvic lymphonode and soft tissue in right leg.

In addition, gallium-67 has been used to detect infections or inflammations such as osteomyelitis, sarcoidosis and myocarditis, and to evaluate interstitial lung disease and examine patients with acquired immunodeficiency syndrome (AIDS). It has been suggested that gallium-67 may be clinically useful for assessing adults presenting fever of unknown origin because of the possibility of locating pathological uptake (both malignant and benign).

Precautions need to be taken in relation to cases of suspected or confirmed pregnancy. If diagnostic procedures are performed on such patients, a clinical decision weighing the benefits against the possible harm from carrying out the procedure is necessary. Moreover, if diagnostic procedures are performed on breastfeeding mothers, the breastfeeding should be discontinued.

Because of the high radiation exposure, children aged less than 14 years should not undergo gallium-67 scintigraphy, except when there is clear evidence of malignancy.

http://dx.doi.org/10.5772/53029

In laboratories with PET/CT the gallium scintigraphy was replaced by ^{18}F-FDG in the pathologies described above, because of the best accuracy of the PET.

8. Scintimammography

Scintimammography was approved by the FDA in 1987 as a complementary examination for use when mammography is indeterminate in investigating malignant breast tumors. It is not used for screening, although new technologies for the equipment have improved the accuracy of this method. On the other hand, it is now indicated when mammography presents limitations in investigating tumor processes, such as in cases of dense breasts, asymmetrical density, architectural distortion acquired after the procedures or belonging to the breast, detection of tumor viability or recurrence, and very small breasts, particularly in men when breast compression cannot be performed. Lymph node status is also assessed, although with low sensitivity. ^{99m}Tc-Sestamibi (a cation with affinity for malignant tumor processes) is used, with summing of factors such as negative transmembrane potential, activity, mitochondrial density, cell count and cell mitotic activity.

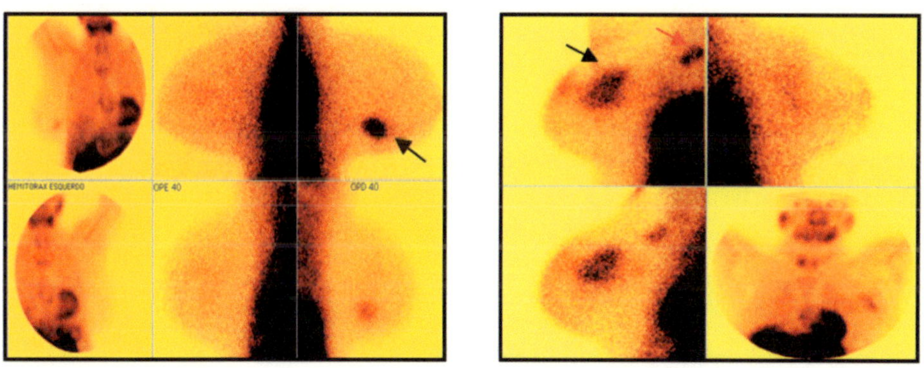

Figure 17. Scintimammgraphy. Breast carcinoma in right and left side (black arrows) and lymphonodal metastase (red arrow).

9. Dacryoscintigraphy

This examination is indicated for cases of epiphora. It is a simple and easy-to-perform examination, with administration of microdrops of pertechnetate in the epicanthus of the eyes. In a normal examination, the radiotracer is expected to progressively pass through the palpebral fissure, lacrimal canaliculi, lacrimal sac, nasolacrimal ducts and nasal cavity. The retention or obstruction patterns do not show progression of the radiotracer.

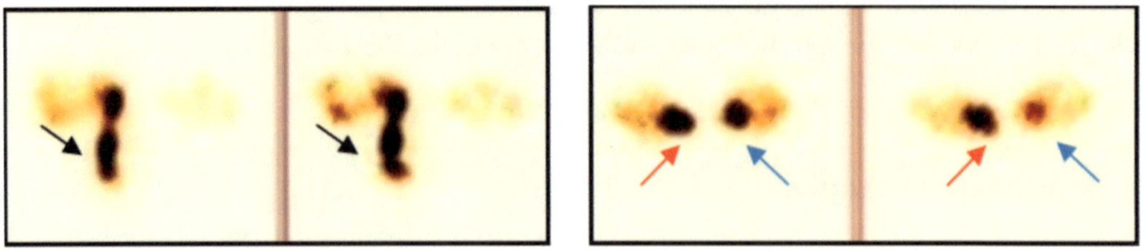

Figure 18. Dacrioscintigraphy. Normal exam. Radiotracer reachs right nasal cavity (black arrows). Total retention in billateral lacrimal sacs. Right lacrimal sac (red arrows) and left lacrimal sac (light blue arrows).

10. Radioguided procedures

Radioguided procedures were introduced in the 80s, and are based on the search of concentrated lesions of radioactive material guided by a small detector. There are three types of procedures: the search for occult and/or radioguided lesion (ROLL), the search of sentinel lymph node (SLN), and the association of the two methods (SNOLL).

ROLL are lesions with difficult to be found when is necessary to be located for biopsy. The mean indications are: nonpalpable breast lesions, like a small lesions, deep lesions or microcalcifications; for biopsy of parathyroid, osteoma, bone metastasis and so on.

SNL is the first lymph node to be reached by neoplasms cells from the primary tumor. When the lymph node was not metastatic, the second lymph nodes are not. Then, the total lymphadenectomy can be avoided (Figure 19 and figure 20).

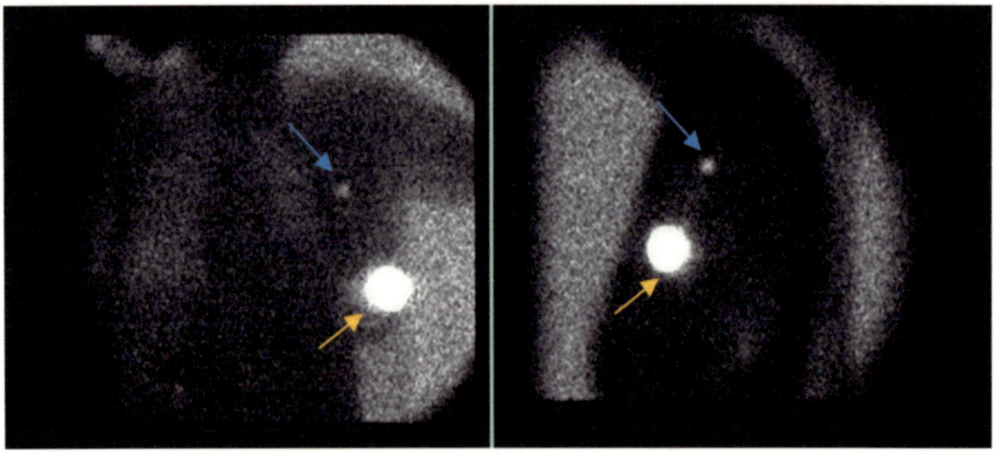

Figure 19. Breast lymphoscintigraphy. Anterior and left lateral images. After injection of radiopharmaceutical substance in left breast (yellow arrows) and SLN in left axillary lymphatic chair (light blue arrows).

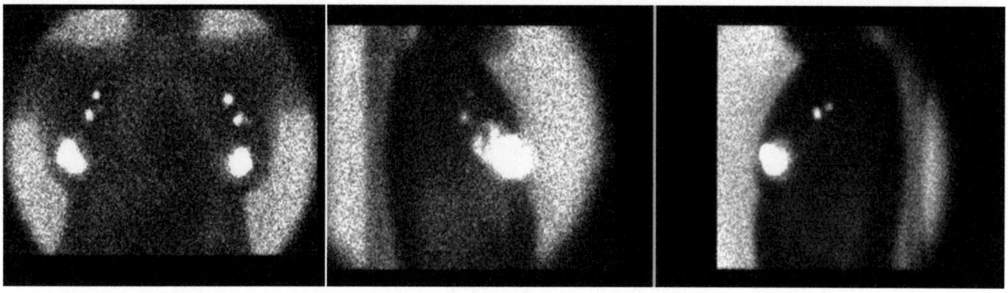

Figure 20. Billateral breast lymphoscintigraphy. Two sentinel lymph nodes are identified in left and in right axillary lymphatic chain.

11. Therapy

11.1. Therapy with radioiodine

Radioiodine therapy consists of oral administration of iodine-131 to treat benign and malignant diseases of the thyroid. Iodine-131 is a beta-emitting radionuclide with a physical half-life of 8.1 days. The main gamma rays have energy of 364 keV and the beta radiation has maximum energy of 0.61 MeV, mean energy of 0.192 MeV and tissue reach of 0.8 mm. Because of cellular damage it is necessary to have some precautions.

Mean absolute contraindications include: Pregnancy: Female patients of fertile age should ideally undergo a pregnancy test 72 hours or less before radioiodine therapy. Occasionally, when the patient's history clearly demonstrates that there is no possibility of pregnancy, the test may not have to be done; Breastfeeding: Patients who are breastfeeding have to be advised to postpone radioiodine therapy until lactation ceases. This has the aim of minimizing the radiation absorbed by the breast. Lactation ceases between four and six weeks after delivery when there is no breastfeeding, and four to six weeks after the end of breastfeeding. This milk should not be stored.

Mean relative contraindications are: Urinary incontinence that is difficult to manage: The physician should obtain confirmation of the patient's urinary incontinence in order to take the necessary measures to avoid contamination through the urine; uncontrollable hyperthyroidism; active exophthalmia.

The clinical indications for benign disease of thyroid including: hyperthyroidism: Graves' disease, toxic multinodular goiter and autonomous nodules; non-toxic multinodular goiter: therapy with iodine-131 has been successfully used to reduce non-toxic multinodular goiter [15,16](Figure 21).

And for malignant thyroid diseases, specially for: well-differentiated neoplasms of the thyroid that synthesize thyroglobulin. In these cases, iodine-131 has been used to ablate the remains of the thyroid after total thyroidectomy, and to treat residual cancer and metastatic disease after total thyroidectomy. Cerebral metastases have to be assessed carefully, since there is a risk of bleeding and cerebral edema. In general, the more invasive the cancer is, the bigger the dose will be.

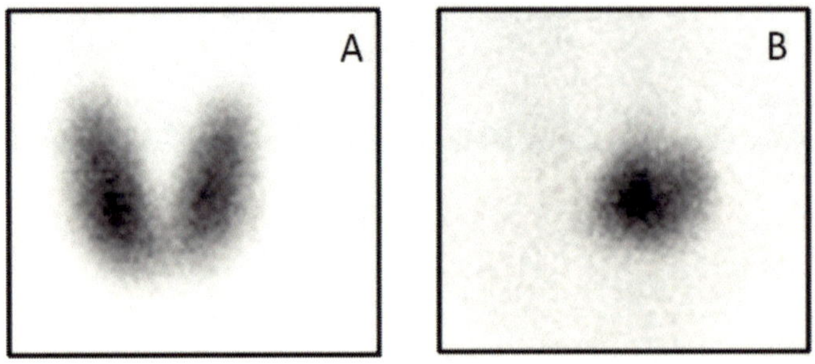

Figure 21. Thyroid scintigraphies. A. Graves' Disease. Diffuse thyroid uptake. B. Plummer's Disease. Nodular uptake on left thyoid lobe with suppression of the gland.

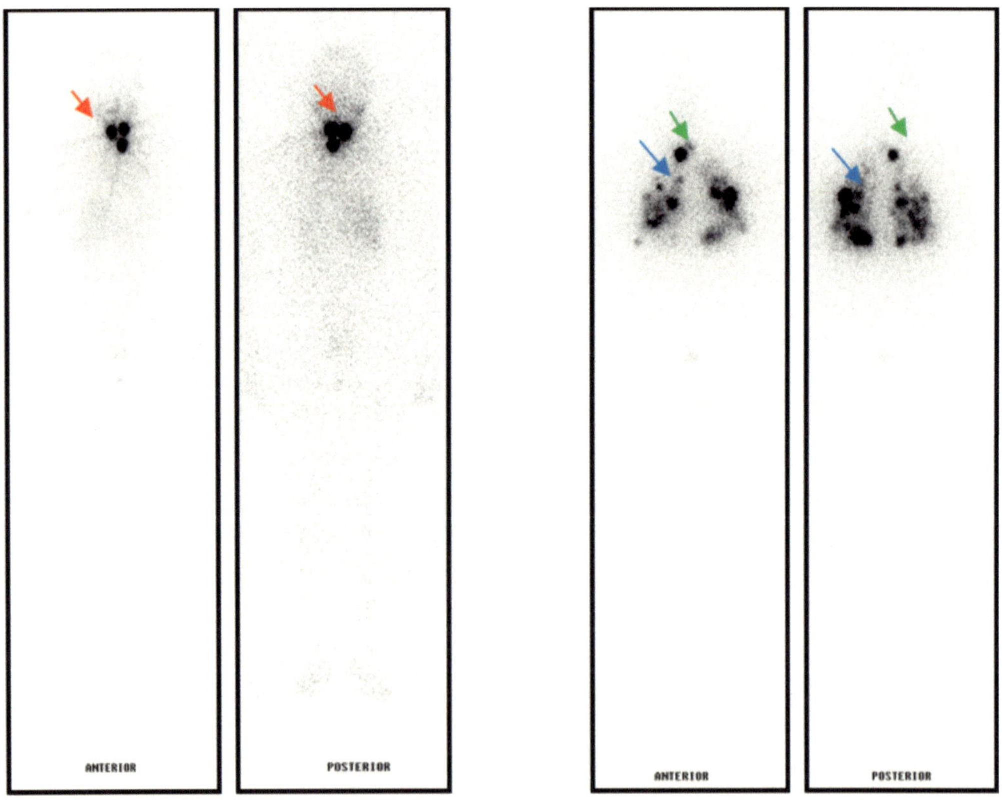

Figure 22. Whole body scan post radioiodine therapy. Radioidine on thyroid tissue and on cervical lymphodes (red arrows). In another patient, notice lymphonode (green arrows and lung (light blue arrows) metastasis.

http://dx.doi.org/10.5772/53029

11.2. ^{131}I-meta-iodobenzylguanidine therapy (^{131}I-mIBG)

This consists of 131I-mIBG intravenous infusion, selectively accumulated by neuroectodermal tissue, including tumours of neuroectodermal origin. Uptake occurs by active via and passive diffusion. mIBG is a meta isomer of the guanethidine derivative iodobenzylguanidine, stored within cytoplasmic storage granules and 131I.

Common indications include: neuroectodermal tumours derived from the primitive neural crest, and showing uptake and retention of labeled mIBG, especially in inoperable or malignant phaeochromocytoma (Figure 23), inoperable or malignant paraganglioma, inoperable or malignant carcinoid tumour Stage III or IV neuroblastoma, inoperable, malignant medullary thyroid cancer.

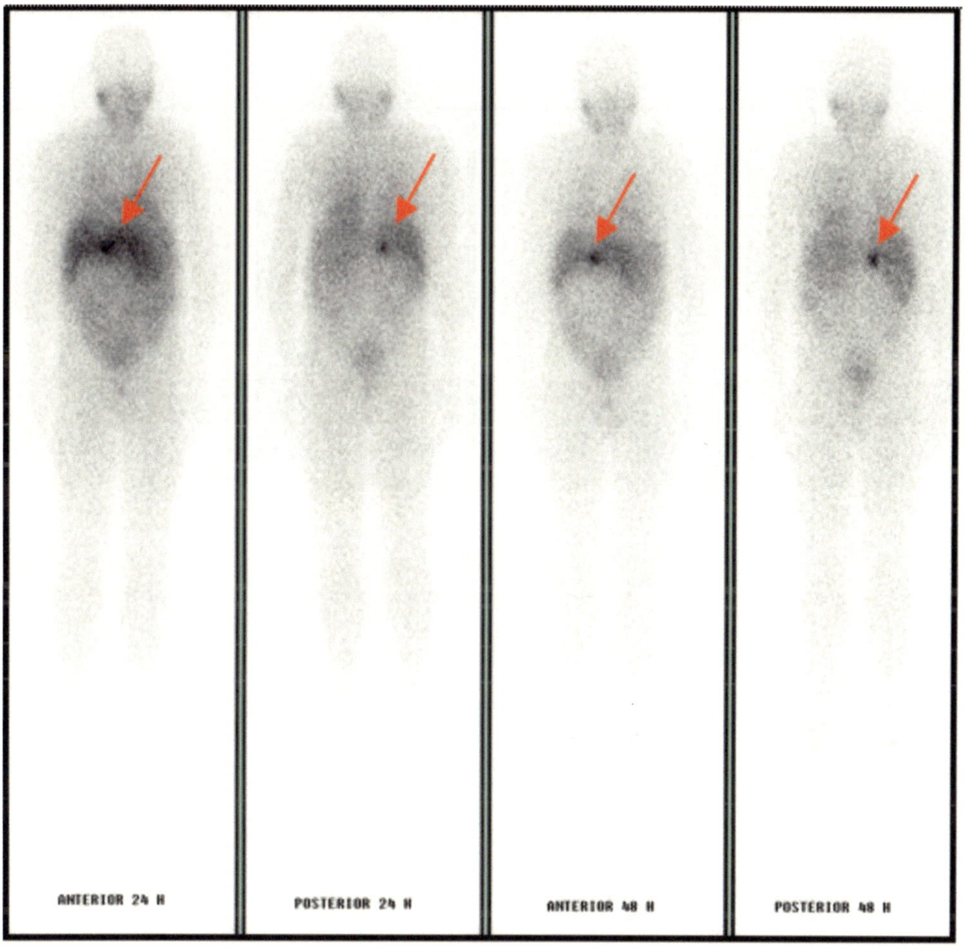

Figure 23. Phaeochromocytoma. Focal uptake in posterior abdomen aspect (red arrows). Late images are better to identify the lesion.

11.3.Treatment of refractory metastatic bone pain

Bone pain is a common symptom of metastatic disease in cancer, experienced with various intensities during the development of their disease, generally in the terminal phases. In addition to other therapies, such as analgesics, bisphosphonates, chemotherapy, hormonal therapy and external beam radiotherapy, bone-seeking radiopharmaceuticals are also used for the palliation of pain from bone metastases (Figure 24). Substantial advantages of bone palliation radionuclide therapy include the ability to simultaneously treat multiple sites of disease with a more probable effect in earlier phases of metastatic disease. The tissue destruction is also based on beta-emitting radionuclide. This therapy consists of intravenous administration of ^{89}Sr-chloride in aqueous solution, ^{153}Sm-EDTMP or ^{186}Re-HEDP that reaches the osteoblastic or mixed metastasis from prostate, breast, lung or any other tumor with osteoblastic presentation. Caution is necessary because this therapy develops myelotoxicity. Usually the bone pain decreased after two weeks depending on the radionuclide administered [17].

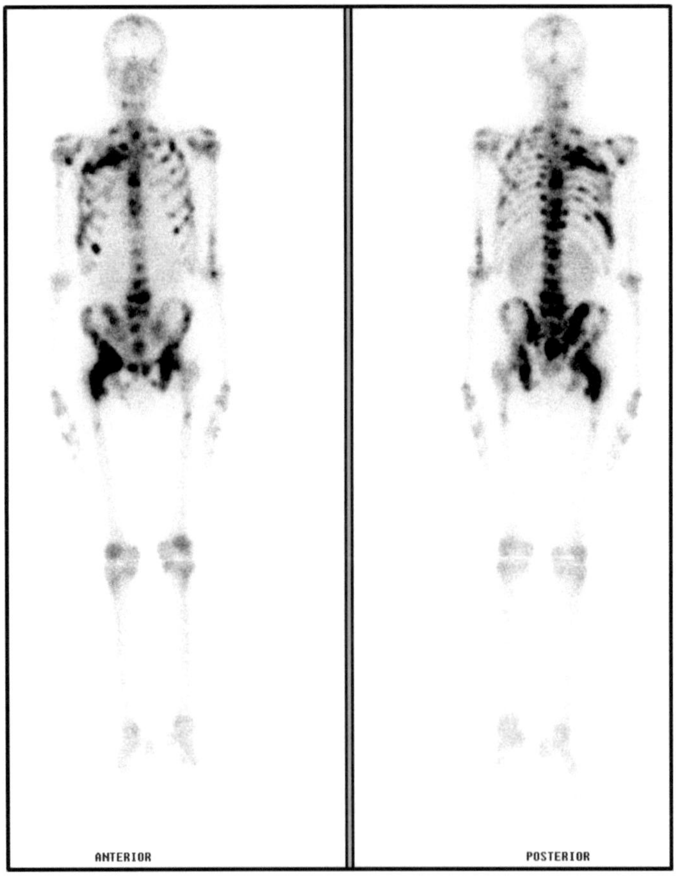

Figure 24. Bone scan. Bone metastasis.Multiple focal uptake on skeletal,

http://dx.doi.org/10.5772/53029

12. Conclusion

In conclusion, the information about the nuclear medicine applications, based on metabolic and functional evaluations, make this method a co-adjuvant of the others anatomic exams on investigation of many pathologies, without competition with them and being preferred on the functional lesion follow up, metastasis screening and viable tumor issue.

Author details

Sonia Marta Moriguchi[1,2*], Kátia Hiromoto Koga[2], Paulo Henrique Alves Togni[1,3] and Marcelo José dos Santos[4]

*Address all correspondence to: soniamoriguchi@gmail.com

1 Togni Nuclear Medicine, Sao Jose do Rio Preto, Brazil

2 Nuclear Medicine Department, Botucatu Medical School, Sao Paulo State University Botucatu, Brazil

3 Catanduva Medical School, Catanduva, Brazil

4 Nuclear Medicine Department, Barretos Cancer Hospital, Barretos, Brazil

References

[1] Schinkel, AFL, Poldermans D, Elhendy A, Bax JJ. Assessment of myocardial viability in patients with heart failure. J Nucl Med 2007; 48: 1135-1146.

[2] Manspeaker P, Weisman HF, Schaible TF. Cardiovascular applications: Current status of immunoscintigraphy in the detection of myocardial necrosis using antimyosin (R11D10) and deep venous thrombosis using antifibrin (T2G1s). Semin Nucl Med 1993; 23: 133-47.

[3] Patel AD, Iskandrian AE. MIBG imaging. J Nucl Cardiol 2002; 9: 75-94.

[4] Carrio I. Cardiac neurotransmission imaging. J Nucl Med 2001; 42: 1062-1076.

[5] Kelesidis I, Travin MI. Use of cardiac radionuclide imaging to identify patients at risk for arrhythmic sudden cardiac death. J Nucl Cardiol 2012; 19: 142-52.

[6] 6. Chen W, Botvinick EH, Alavi A, Zhang Y, Yang S, Perini R, et al. Age-related decrease in cardiopulmonary adrenergic neuronal function in children as assessed by the I-123 metaiodobenzylguanidine imaging. Nucl J Cardiol 2008; 15: 73-79.

[7] Barritt, D.W. & Jordan, S.C. Anticoagulant drugs in the treatment of pulmonary embolism. A controlled trial. Lancet. 1960; 1:1309–12. ISSN: 0140-6736.

[8] Bajc, M., Neilly, J.B., Miniati, M., Schuemichen, C., Meignan, M. & B. Jonson, B. EANM guidelines for ventilation/perfusion scintigraphy. Part 1. Pulmonary imaging with ventilation/perfusion single photon emission tomography. Eur J Nucl Med Mol Imaging. 2009; 6(36):1356–70. E ISSN: 1619-7089. (a)

[9] Bajc, M., Neilly, J.B., Miniati, M., Schuemichen, C., Meignan, M. & B. Jonson, B. EANM guidelines for ventilation/perfusion scintigraphy. Part 2. Eur J Nucl Med Mol Imaging. 2009; 6(36):1528–38. E ISSN: 1619-7089.(b)

[10] Boubaker A, Prior JO, Meuwly JY, Delaloye AB. Radionuclide investigations of the urinary tract in the era of multimodality imaging. J Nucl Med 2006; 47: 1819-1836.

[11] Chiou YY, Wang ST, Tang MJ, Lee BF, Chiu NT. Renal fibrosis: prediction from acute pyelonephritis focus volume measured at ^{99m}Tc dimercaptosuccinic acid SPECT. Radiology 2001; 221: 366-370.

[12] Hitzel A, Liard A, Véra P, Manrique A, Ménard JF, Dacher JN. Color and power Doppler sonography versus DMSA scintigraphy in acute pyelonephritis and in prediction of renal scarring. J Nucl Med 2002; 43: 27-32.

[13] Eggli DF, Tulchinski M. Scintigraphic evaluation of pediatric urinary tract infection. Semin Nucl Med 1993; 23(3): 199-218.

[14] Stauss J, Hahn K, Mann M, Palma D. Guidelines for paediatric bone scanning with 99mTc-labeled radiopharmaceuticals and 18F-fluoride. Eur J Nucl Med Mol Imaging. 2010; 37: 1621-28.

[15] EANM procedures guidelines for therapy benign thyroid disease, 2010; 37:2218-28.

[16] EANM procedures guidelines for therapy with iodine 131. Eur J Nucl Med Mol Imaging. 2003; 30: BP27-BP31.

[17] Bodei, L., Marnix Lam, M., Chiesa, C., Flux, G., Brans, B., Chiti, A. & Giammarile, F. (2008). EANM procedure guideline for treatment of refractory metastatic bone pain. Eur J Nucl Med Mol Imaging. 2008, 35:1934–40. Eletronic ISSN: 1619-7089.

Chapter 4

Current Perspectives on Molecular Imaging for Tracking Stem Cell Therapy

Lingling Tong, Hui Zhao, Zuoxiang He and Zongjin Li

Additional information is available at the end of the chapter

http://dx.doi.org/10.5772/53028

1. Introduction

The main objective of stem cell therapy is to repair the tissue with functional cells differentiated from stem cells, and contribute to the lost organ function together with the remaining functional native cells. Nevertheless, there also remain important questions unanswered, regarding the engraftment, viability, biology and safety of transplanted stem cells, as well as interaction with the environment. Consequently, novel molecular imaging techniques are necessary for investigating the behaviors and the ultimate feasibility of cell transplantation therapy of stem cell.

Along with the rapid development of sensitive, noninvasive technologies, several molecular imaging approaches have been implicated to track the fate of stem cells *in vivo* [1-4]. Continuously observing the process of tissue regeneration after stem cell transplantation would markedly improve knowledge about the underlying cellular mechanisms and analysis of the molecular pathways that control this process. Although, this is inconsistent with the most current studies, in which the cells are observed in hours or days time point without definite cell population. So far, there is no single imaging modality that is ideal to observe all the relevant aspects of stem cell therapy with a continuous manner [5]. The new development of molecular imaging technology push the researches of stem cell therapy much closer to the single-cell level, and make the observation of different types of stem cells more continuous and comprehensive.

2. Promises, challenges, and needs for molecular imaging of stem cell therapy

Molecular imaging is a rapidly emerging biomedical research discipline that provides integrated information on specific molecules of interest within the cells of *living* subjects and thus holds great promise as an effective way to track certain cellular and subcellular events of the transplanted cells [2, 6-8]. The visual representation, characterization, and quantification of biological processes within intact *living* organisms obtained from molecular imaging techniques is particularly helpful in evaluations of the functional outcomes of cell engraftment and may shed light on the mixed findings regarding stem cell therapy. In recent years, a variety of imaging technologies is being investigated as tools for evaluating stem cell therapy in living subjects. Molecular imaging modalities include optical bioluminescence, optical fluorescence, targeted ultrasound, molecular magnetic resonance imaging (MRI), magnetic resonance spectroscopy (MRS), single-photon-emission computed tomography (SPECT), and positron emission tomography (PET) [9]. Moreover, many hybrid systems that combine two or more of these modalities are already commercially available [9]. The use of noninvasive, longitudinal, and quantitative imaging of the fate of stem cells can facilitate preclinical experimental studies in animal models and can help in human stem cell therapy trials as well.

A wide variety of stem or progenitor cells, including adult bone marrow stem cells, endothelial progenitor cells, mesenchymal stem cells (MSCs), resident cardiac stem cells, and embryonic stem cells, have been shown to have positive effects in preclinical studies and therefore hold promise for treating and curing debilitating and deadly diseases. Several of these types of stem cells have been tested in early-stage clinical trials, such as MSCs [10], human embryonic stem (hES) cells [11]. However, to realize the full therapeutic potential of stem cell technology, it will be necessary to develop novel and improved quality assessments that can be used readily to determine the exact cellular state of the transplanted cells.

After the systemic or local administrating, stem cells may be able to proliferate, migrate and repopulate in pathologic sites to bring tremendous therapeutic effect. However, the transplantation success is companied with risks of the stem cell misbehavior after delivered, especially embryonic stem cells [6, 12]. Consequently, real-time visualization of the fate of the transplanted cells over time *in vivo* is a vital step to determine the efficiency of the implantation. By tracking the optimal number of transplanted cells, researchers can define therapeutic windows and monitor cells growth and possible side effects for regenerative therapies [13].

The ability to label and track stem cells in humans would provide a method to answer some of the ongoing, unsolved issues in the field. The most efficacious route of delivery, the appropriate choice of stem cell type(s), the optimal cell population for treatment in a chronic setting and the favorable time-point of cell delivery, however, is still unknown and requires further study. A safe, noninvasive, and repeatable imaging modality that could identify injected stem cells would be able to answer questions about cell viability and retention in future clinical trials of stem cell therapies, as well as provide the ability to adjust the assessment of bioactivity on the basis of actual delivered doses of cells. With the desire to monitor stem cells long-term continuously with high temporal resolution and good biocompatibility, which have the properties of differentiation and self-renew over long periods of time, stem-cell-derived regeneration still faces in its efforts to improve.

http://dx.doi.org/10.5772/53028

Despite significant progress in molecular imaging, no single technique meets all the stem cell tracking criteria. Combined imaging modalities, such as PET-CT, are already well accepted and offer high sensitivity and anatomical detail [14]. Multimodality imaging approaches are likely to play an important role in illuminating different aspects of stem cell biology *in vivo* and elucidating the mechanisms of tissue repair and regeneration. In brief, noninvasive imaging stem cell therapy could provide greater insight into not only the therapeutic benefit, but also the fundamental mechanisms underlying stem cell fate, migration, survival and engraftment *in vivo*.

3. Approaches and implications of stem cell imaging

A number of methods are available to track stem cells by molecular imaging. In general, there are two methods to label the cells: [1] direct labeling method, which physically introduce marker(s) into the cells before transplant; [2] indirect labeling method, which genetically introduce reporter gene(s) into the cells before transplant. The current noninvasive imaging approaches for tracking stem cells *in vivo* include imaging with magnetic particles, radionuclides, quantum dots (QDs) and reporter genes (Figure 1).

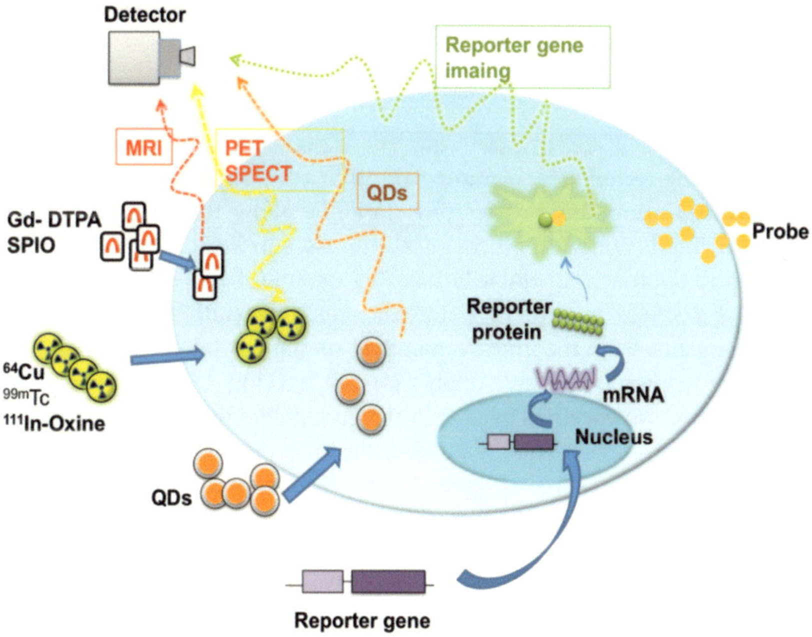

Figure 1. Conceptual basis for noninvasive imaging of transplanted stem cells in living animals. It shows imaging techniques including magnetic resonance imaging, radionuclide imaging, quantum dots imaging and reporter gene imaging. Abbreviations: Gd-DTPA, gadolinium-diethylenetriamine penta-acetic acid; SPIO, superparamagnetic iron oxide; ^{99}mTc, ^{99}mTc-hexamethylpropylene amine oxime; ^{111}In-Oxine, ^{111}In-oxyquinoline.

Imaging of stem cell therapy requires the selection of a molecular target, an imaging probe, and an imaging system. Specific molecular targets along with advances in imaging modalities increase the sensitivity and specificity of stem cell imaging. The commonly used labeling methods are discussed below.

3.1. Magnetic particle labeling

Possessing the advantages of high spatial resolution (ranging from 50μm in animal and up to 300μm in whole body clinical scanners) and high temporal resolution, magnetic resonance imaging (MRI) is widely used for *in vivo* cell tracking in preclinical and clinical studies. The fundamental principle underlying MRI is magnetic dipoles (such as hydrogen atoms in water and organic compounds), which align themselves when placed into a magnetic field. To be tracked in ischemic tissues, stem cells need to be enriched with a contrast agent that produces a sufficient positive or negative signal to distinguish them from the background. One type of contrast agents is the agent containing gadolinium-diethylenetriamine penta-acetic acid (Gd-DTPA), and the other type is the agent containing super paramagnetic iron oxide (SPIO). At present, SPIO are the preferred agent for short-term stem cell tracking. With the high spatial and temporal resolution, MRI allows the location of iron-labeled donor cells to be monitored noninvasive over several weeks *in vivo* [3, 15]. However, it is difficult to distinguish iron-labeled cells from the surrounding air, hemorrhage, necrosis, and macrophages. To address these problems, off-resonance (OR) MRI has been developed for imaging iron-labeled hES cells to generate positive contrasts through enhancement of signal and suppression of background tissue [3].

3.2. Radionuclide labeling

Radionuclide imaging techniques, including positron emission tomography (PET) and single-photon emission computed tomography (SPECT), allow the imaging of radiolabeled makers and their interaction with biochemical processes in *living* subjects. Current clinical molecular imaging approaches primarily use PET or SPECT-based techniques. Compared with MRI, PET and SPECT provide high intrinsic sensitivity ($<10^{-11}$M) and can use a variety kind of imaging agents. With the improvements in spatial resolution (1-2mm), radionuclide imaging has been made particularly suitable for cell tracking. Direct labeling of cells with radiometals in clinical practice has used ^{111}In-oxyquinoline and ^{99m}Tc-hexamethylpropylene amine oxime. Imaging plays a role in monitoring short-term cell tracking, long-term cell survival and function, and as a surrogate marker of implant efficacy. Labeling implanted cells with relatively long-lived isotopes, such as ^{111}In-Oxine for SPECT and ^{64}Cu for PET, allows shorten, real-time cell tracking, to determine biodistribution and availability in the target organ [16].

However, these cell-labeling techniques have some significant disadvantages. They are limited by concerns such as the potential transfer of radiotracer to nontargeted cells and potential adverse effects of the radiotracer on stem cell viability, function, and differentiation capacity. Thus, the effects of labeling on the capacity to differentiate stem cells of various origins are needed to be studied.

http://dx.doi.org/10.5772/53028

3.3. Nanoparticle labeling

QDs are emerging as an important class of fluorescent agents. Luminescent colloidal QDs are inorganic semiconductor particles with physical properties that enable them to emit fluorescent light from 525 to 800 nm. The nanoparticles are consisting of an inorganic core, a shell of metal and an outer organic coating. The total diameter of quantum dots is 2–10 nm [17], depending on the physical properties of the material due to the quantum nature of QDs. With the capability of being excited by one single wavelength and emission light of different wavelengths, QDs are ideal probes for multiplex imaging. By contrast, conventional organic labeling agent cannot be easily synthesized to emit different colors and have narrow excitation spectra and broad emission spectra, making it difficult to use these dyes for multiplexing. Due to their extreme brightness and resistance to photobleaching [18], QDs are appropriate for live stem cells imaging, which requires long-term observation under the excitation light source. The approaches of QDs entering stem cells include passive loading, receptor-mediated endocytosis or transfection. Passive loading has been found to be the most effective method owning to the high label efficient and limited damage to surrounding cells. QDs are capable of single quantum dot tracking, multiplex imaging, and 3-D imaging reconstruction.

Unquestionable, quantum dots represent a novel strategy to tracking stem cells *in vivo*. However, the effects of QDs on stem cell biology remain unclear because mixed results have been reported using different stem cells or experimental protocols [19, 20]. Moreover, light scattering limits the applicability of this approach, especially to the brain in humans, making it difficult to use in 3D localization or quantitative estimation of cell survival. Last, several other obstacles, including nonspecific binding to multiple molecules and the tendency for aggregation of QDs in the cytosol must be overcome before clinical application with their full potential.

3.4. Reporter gene labeling

Reporter gene imaging has been commonly applied to the non-invasive imaging of stem cell therapy by studying the survival, localization, and functional effects of exogenously administered stem cells. Imaging of gene expression in *living* subjects can be directed either at genes externally transferred into cells of organ systems (transgenes) or at endogenous genes, and the former one is used in most applications of reporter gene imaging at present. The principle of reporter gene imaging is relatively simple. In general, reporter genes are DNA sequences that encode for easily assayed proteins. In the case of imaging, reporter genes encode for a reporter protein that, when exposed to an imaging probe, produces an analytic signal which can be generates some form of signal that can be captured and quantified by an imaging modality such as MRI(21), PET(22), SPECT(16), or an optical charge-coupled device [6]. Reporter genes can be linked to a gene of interest (*i.e.*, creation of a promoter construct) such that the reporter protein provides a surrogate marker of that gene's activity.

In the fields of stem-cell-driven regeneration, some conventional reporter genes, such as green fluorescent protein (GFP) [7], firefly luciferase [23], renilla luciferase [24], and HSV1-tk [25] allow for localization in some small *living* animals. Stable transfection or transduction with reporter genes is useful in assessing kinetic survival status of the implanted cells because the reporter genes can be expressed as long as the cells are alive. However, the reporter gene approach in cell tracking requires genetic manipulations of the cells, which may lead to insertional mutagenesis. The advances in site-specific chromosomal integration mediated by phiC31 integrase may cast a new light in overcoming this obstacle [2]. Although small animals or animals transparent to light can be imaged with a cooled charged coupled device (CCD) camera, these imaging techniques are somewhat limited because of their lack of generalizability and detailed tomographic resolution.

4. Advances in molecular imaging for tracking stem cell therapy

Stem cell therapies offer enormous potential for the treatment of a wide range of diseases and injuries including neurodegenerative diseases, cardiovascular disease, diabetes, arthritis, spinal cord injury, stroke, and burns. More research teams are accelerating the use of other types of adult stem cells, in particular neural stem cells for diseases where beneficial outcome could result from either in-lineage cell replacement or extracellular factors. At the same time, the first three trials using cells derived from pluripotent cells have begun [12]. These early trials are showing roles for stem cells both in replacing damaged tissue as well as in providing extracellular factors that can promote endogenous cellular salvage and replenishment [26].

Clinical trials have demonstrated that stem cell therapy can improve cardiac recovery after the acute phase of myocardial ischemia and in patients with chronic ischemic heart disease [10]. Nevertheless, some trials have shown that conflicting results and uncertainties remain in the case of mechanisms of action and possible ways to improve clinical impact of stem cells in cardiac repair [27]. The public clinical trials database http://clinicaltrials.gov shows 238 clinical trials using MSCs for a very wide range of therapeutic applications. Although early clinical trials of stem cell therapy have showed positive effect, there remains much controversy about which cell type holds the most promise for clinical therapeutics and by what mechanism stem cells mediate a positive effect, and further research should be able to answer these questions.

4.1. Imaging of embryonic stem cells driven regeneration

Embryonic stem cells (ESCs) are pluripotent stem cells capable of self-renewal and differentiation into virtually all cell types [28]. Various lineages have been derived from human and mouse ESCs, including cardiomyocytes, neurons, hematopoietic cells, osteogenic cells, hepatocytes, insulin-producing cells, keratinocytes, and endothelial cells. Given their unlimited self-renewal and pluripotency capacity, ESCs have been regarded as a leading candidate source for novel regenerative medicine therapy. So far, ESCs transplantation has been widely investigated as a potential therapy for cell death-related heart disease, ischemic diseases, CNS disorders and diabetes. However, the bottleneck of application of ESC driven regeneration is high risk of teratoma formation *in vivo [3, 6].*

http://dx.doi.org/10.5772/53028

The concurrent development of accurate, sensitive, and noninvasive technologies capable of monitoring ESCs engraftment *in vivo* has greatly accelerated basic research prior to future clinical translation. Numerous imaging modalities have analyzed the behavior of embryonic stem cells that have been transplanted to regenerate tissues, which include MRI, bioluminescence imaging (BLI), fluorescence, PET, and multimodality approaches. Two main PET strategies for embryonic stem cell has been used——direct imaging [29] and indirect imaging [30]. Although the value of PET lies in its easy accessibility and high-sensitivity tracking of biomarkers, potential disadvantages of PET include repeated injection of radioactive substances into an organism with the potential to radiation accumulation [31] and adverse effect on ESCs viability and pluripotency capacity [32]. Additionally, the short half-lives of most current available radiotracers have limited their use for long-term tracing [33]. MRI has been used for tracking mouse ESCs [34] in the heart, hind limbs, brain, lung and kidney. Meanwhile, MRI is accessible for tracking ESCs engraftment, providing detailed morphological and functional information. Drawbacks of MRI include low sensitivity and being unable to quantify cell population. However, the use of CLIO-Tat peptides [35]is promising to overcome some of these limitations. Holding the significant advantage of high sensitivity (100-1000 cells, for more superficial anatomical sites), safety, low cost and the repeated tracking of small numbers of labeled cells in whole body distribution without background signal, BLI is widely used in this field. Zongjin Li, et al. have compared of BLI and MRI for tracking fate of hESCs and hESC derived endothelial cells (hESC-ECs) in animals, data of which prove that reporter gene of BLI is a better marker for monitoring ESCs and ESC-ECs viability and MRI is a better marker for high-resolution detection of cell location. Nevertheless, at present, bioluminescence imaging still lacks adequate tomographic resolution because of attenuation of photons within tissues [3]. An innovative approach to combine the strengths of optical fluorescence, bioluminescence, and PET is the creation and use of a fusion reporter [36] construct composed of RFP, Fluc, and HSV-tk. This fusion reporter construct has been adapted to research the spatio-temporal kinetics of hESC engraftment and proliferation in living subjects, without significant adverse effects on mouse ESC viability, proliferation, differentiation, or proteomic expression [37].

4.2. Imaging of mesenchymal stem cells driven regeneration

Mesenchymal stem cells (MSCs) are a heterogeneous subset of stromal stem cells that can differentiate into cells of the mesodermal lineage, such as bone, fat and cartilage cells, but they also have endodermic and neuroectodermic differentiation potential. The use of MSCs for clinical purposes takes advantage of their poor immunogenicity *in vitro*. Preclinical [38] and clinical [39, 40] studies have supported the possible use of MSCs obtained from allogeneic donors in the clinic. In preclinical researches, MSCs have been applied in tissue regeneration, including haematopoietic organs, heart, CNS, skin, kidney, liver, lung, joint, eye, pancreas and renal glomeruli. The current data indicate that bone-marrow-derived MSCs were first proposed for therapeutic purposes in regenerative medicine on the basis of their stem-cell-like qualities [41].

The versatility of the molecular imaging method could allow cellular tracking using single or multimodal imaging modalities. These single methods include direct labeling of cells for transplantation with iron oxide particles for MRI, with ^{18}F-hexafluorobenzene or ^{18}F-FDG for PET, or with ^{111}In-oxine or ^{111}In-tropolone for SPECT. Noninvasive MRI is fast becoming a clinical favorite, though there is scope for improvement in its accuracy and sensitivity. In that, use of superparamagnetic iron-oxide nanoparticles (SPION) as MRI contrast enhancers may be the best select for tracking MSC treatment delivery and monitor outcome [42, 43]. Indirect labeling relies on the expression of imaging reporter genes transduced into cells before transplantation. A classic example of using reporter gene tracing MSCs transplantation is the research by Zachary Love, et al. They have used a triple-fusion reporter system (fluc-mrfp-ttk) for multimodal imaging to monitor hMSCs transplanted into NOD-SCID mice. Signals from the cubes loaded with reporter-transduced hMSCs were visible by BLI over 3 mo, meanwhile, PET data provided confirmation of the quantitative estimation of the number of cells at one spot (cube) [44]. The reporter gene approach resulted in a reliable method of labeling stem cells for investigations in small-animal models by use of both BLI and small-animal PET imaging.

4.3. Imaging of neural stem cell therapy

Neural stem cells (NSCs)-driven regeneration has been proposed as a promising potential treatment option for CNS-related disease processes, including everything from cerebrovascular disease to traumatic brain injury to degenerative diseases of the CNS. Grafted NSCs differentiated into neurons, into oligodendrocytes undergoing remyelination and into astrocytes extending processes toward damaged vasculatures [45]. At present, Applications of NSCs therapy of neurological diseases, including Alzheimer's disease, Huntington disease, stroke, spinal cord injuries in preclinical researches have raised intense interest and the hope of radical new therapies in clinical.

In contrast to most tissues in adults, the central nervous system has a low regenerative activity, and neural stem cells reside in regions of the adult brain that are difficult to access by most imaging modalities [5] owning to tissue depth and the blood-brain barrier(BBB). The most promising techniques for monitor the fate of NSCs *in vivo* are MRI, PET and optical imaging. MRI has been used in clinical practice for the past 30 years to diagnose brain lesions and is therefore already a standard clinical adjunct for neuropathologies. Other than SPIO, which is the most studied and preferred contrast agent of MRI, magnetic resonance reporter genes [46] are another possible means of magnetic resonance labeling NSCs. However, this technique is still in its infancy, further study into the possibility of magnetic resonance reporter genes is needed before this technology can be used for NSCs. MRI has been used in tracing neural stem cells labeled with SPIO in patient with brain trauma [47]. The hypointense signal generated by the cells demonstrated cell trace from the implantation site to the periphery of the lesion the first week, and then disappeared by the seventh week, which the group attributed to NSC proliferation. PET has been used clinically for the past 20 years to assess for neurotransmitter changes in a wide variety of disease processes, including Parkinson's disease, Alzheimer's disease, Huntington's disease and psychiatric illnesses. *In vivo* PET imaging for NSCs requires the potential radiotracers in the brain owning the capacity of crossing BBB. A solution to the BBB problem could be the use of the xanthine phosphoribosyl transferase reporter enzyme PET system, which employs xanthine reporter probes that can cross the BBB [48]. With regard to *in vivo* NSCs imaging, bioluminescence is the most studied of the optical imaging techniques and has been employed in numerous small animal studies. Improvement of the existing imaging modalities, assessment of the effect of imaging modalities on cellular biology, and development of new techniques for *in vivo* NSC imaging, would open up the window of the use of NSCs for various neuropathologies.

4.4. Imaging of hematopoietic stem cell transplantation

Hematopoiesis is described to be the production of all types of fully differentiated daughter blood cells from ancestral great-grandmother hematopoietic stem cells (HSCs). HSCs studies and clinical applications have historically been ahead of other tissue stem cells and have generated most stem cell biology models. However, hematopoiesis is arguably among the most difficult of the mammalian stem-cell systems to image real-time *in vivo* [5]. In homeostatic conditions, the different short-lived cell types of blood are regenerated from a small population of HSCs [49], while a significant proportion of HSCs with long-term reconstitution potential is predominantly quiescent or divides infrequently. The HSC niche is most likely a complex, multi-component microenvironment of which the osteoblast is just one of the major constituents identified so far. Thus, non-invasive long-term imaging is more challenging in the bone marrow. Hematopoiesis is better understood than other stem-cell systems and has important clinical significance, but despite intensive research in the past decade, many basic questions are still unresolved [50]. MRI [51], bioluminescence imaging [52], and multiphoton fluorescence microscopy [53] had been applied in continuous observation of cellular behavior of HSCs. Mentionable, continuous observation of hematopoietic progenitor cells in the bone marrow was achieved at single-cell resolution by using multiphoton fluorescence microscopy after the transplantation, filling the gap of low single cell sensitivity and resolution of the first two modalities. The transplantation option of multiphoton fluorescence microscopy is clinically relevant because HSC transplantation is used to treat patients with hematological malignancies such as leukemia and multiple myeloma. Multiphoton fluorescence microscopy was also used to observe the homing of normal and malignant hematopoietic progenitor cells in the bone marrow and to characterize the specialized niches of these cells [54].

4.5. Imaging of endothelial progenitor cell therapy

Endothelial progenitor cells (EPCs) recruitment is often involved in the tissue injury triggered reparative processes, and contribute to healing ischemic tissues. Transplantation of

EPCs offers the potential for targeted treatment of ischemic diseases such as myocardial [55], hind-limb ischemia [56], and renal injury [57]. Considerable efforts have been made to monitor the fate of endothelial progenitor cells fate *in vivo* using the *in vivo* molecular imaging modalities, such as PET [58], computed tomography(CT) [59], MRI [56], BLI [60]. Micro-CT has been applied in studies of EPCs in rat, pig and human beings. In the research of homing and renal repair function of EPCs in renovascular disease [59], renal hemodynamics and function were assessed in pigs by multidetector computed tomography, showing that EPCs are renoprotective as they attenuated renal dysfunction and damage in chronic atherosclerotic renal artery stenosis, and consequently decreased the injury signals. Based on the previous research, maybe CT is promising in clinical application of endothelial progenitor-driven regeneration.

5. Ideal imaging modalities for stem cell therapy

Currently, none individual imaging modalities can fill the bill of flawless, without limitations in the spatial and/or temporal resolution or the time span and/or volume that can be observed in a single experiment. The use of direct labeling, with labeling agent such as SPIO or ^{18}F-FDG is hindered by signal decrease, as a result of radio-decay or cell division or cell dispersion. Additionally, the label may become dissociated from the exogenous stem cell. Thus, direct labeling may not be a reliable means of monitoring long-term cell viability. On the contrary, this approach is a valid method to observing the stem cell delivery and homing properties. Meanwhile, Reporter gene imaging offers unique capabilities for noninvasive and longitudinal measurement to determine cell biology and cell viability.

Fundamentally, the choice of modality depends on the questions being addressed (**Table 1**). If the objective of the research is to image the delivery and early cell localization and homing of stem cells in different organs, a direct labeling approach may be the answer, even though potential toxicity must be taken into account. MRI is among the least invasive of available imaging technologies, equipped with expensive new experimental machines, which provide almost the highest spatial and high temporal resolution for continuous single-cell delivery imaging. But the molecular sensitivity of MRI is lower than other modalities such as radionuclide imaging. Radionuclide imaging modalities (PET, SPECT) have been successfully and extensively used with high intrinsic sensitivity, although they may not provide sufficient spatial resolution. On the other hand, if observation of stem cell biology and interaction with microenvironment or long-term monitoring of cell viability is the goal, reporter gene imaging using optical imaging (bioluminescence, fluorescence), PET/ SPECT imaging, MR imaging appears to be a better option. For example, if a study is about ESCs derived myocyte, use of a reporter gene that is driven by a promoter that will only be activated when the cell has the features of an adult myocyte (*i.e.*, expresses the sarcomeric protein Troponin T) can provide the information of stem cell differentiation into goal histiocyte.

http://dx.doi.org/10.5772/53028

Goal	Strategy	Imaging modality	Spatial resolution	Depth	Sensitivity (mol/L)	Quantitative degree	*Clinical	Advantages	Disadvantages
Cell delivery	Direct visualization	Ultrasound	50–500μm	mm to cm	Not well characterized	+	Yes	Real-time, low cost	Limited spatial resolution
		MR fluoroscopy	1mm	No limit	10^{-3}–10^{-5}	++	Yes	3D datasets, soft-tissue contrast	Low spatial resolution
Early cell localization and homing	Direct cell labeling	QDs	100-400μm	<3cm	10^{-3}–10^{-9}	+	No	High sensitivity, multiplexing	Undefined effects on stem cell biology
		MRI (e.g.SPIO)	50–300μm	No limit	10^{-3}–10^{-5}	++	Yes	Combines morphological and functional imaging	Long scan and postprocessing time
		PET (e.g. , ^{64}Cu, ^{18}F-FDG)	1–2mm	No limit	10^{-11}–10^{-12}	+++	Yes	High sensitivity, quantitative translation	Low spatial resolution, radiation to subject
		SPECT (e.g. , ^{111}In-Oxine)	1–2mm	No limit	10^{-10}–10^{-11}	++	Yes	Can image multiple probes simultaneously	Low spatial resolution
Stem cell viability and biology	Reporter gene imaging	Bioluminescence (Flu, Rlu)	3–5mm	1–2 cm	10^{-15}–10^{-17}	+ ~ ++	No	Highest sensitivity, low-cost, high-throughput	2D imaging, limited translational research
		Fluorescence (RFP, GFP)	2–3mm	<1 cm	10^{-9}–10^{-12}	++	Yes	Detects fluorochrome in live and dead cells	Low spatial resolution, surface-weight
		MRI (e.g. , Transferrin)	50–300μm	No limit	10^{-3}–10^{-5}	++	Yes	Combines morphological and functional imaging	Long scan and postprocessing time
		PET (e.g. , HSV1-tk)	1–2mm	No limit	10^{-11}–10^{-12}	+++	Yes	High sensitivity, quantitative translational research	Low spatial resolution, radiation to subject
		SPECT (e.g. , NIS, ^{99}mTc)	1–2mm	No limit	10^{-10}–10^{-11}	++	Yes	Can image multiple probes simultaneously	Low spatial resolution

Table 1. The different imaging strategies of stem cell trafficking and guide to finding the appropriate molecular imaging modalities

6. Conclusions

Stem-cell-driven regeneration offers tremendous approach for the treatment of intractable diseases. Tracking the fate of implanted cells is vital to monitor the delivery and viability of the grafts over extended periods of time. Molecular imaging represents one such tool that can provide insight into cell survival and proliferation following transplantation into the tissue. The greatest potential for optimizing imaging approaches for regeneration research probably lies in applying new insights from stem-cell biology and the development of molecular imaging. As experimental techniques and molecular imaging technologies progress, the potential benefits of regenerative medicine should be a strong motivation to continuously improve imaging technology that will enable stem-cell-driven regeneration in mammals to be more understood. Efforts now should focus on the development of novel labeling agent and multimodality approaches to increase perception of regenerative medicine, and promote the clinical translation of these techniques.

Acknowledgment

This work was partially supported by grants from the National Basic Research Program of China (2011CB964903), National Natural Science Foundation of China (31071308), and Tianjin Natural Science Foundation (12JCZDJC24900).

The authors indicate no potential conflicts of interest.

Author details

Lingling Tong[1], Hui Zhao[2], Zuoxiang He[3] and Zongjin Li[1]

*Address all correspondence to: zongjinli@nankai.edu.cn

1 Department of Pathophysiology, Nankai University School of Medicine, Tianjin, China

2 Tianjin Key Laboratory of Food Biotechnology, School of Biotechnology and Food Science, Tianjin University of Commerce, Tianjin, China

3 Department of Nuclear Medicine, Cardiovascular Institute and Fuwai Hospital, Chinese Academy of Medical Sciences and Peking Union Medical College, Beijing, China

References

[1] Gu E, Chen WY, Gu J, Burridge P, Wu JC. Molecular imaging of stem cells: tracking survival, biodistribution, tumorigenicity, and immunogenicity. Theranostics. 2012;2(4):335-45.

[2] Li Z, Han Z, Wu JC. Transplantation of human embryonic stem cell-derived endothelial cells for vascular diseases. Journal of Cellular Biochemistry. 2009;106(2):194-9.

[3] Li Z, Suzuki Y, Huang M, Cao F, Xie X, Connolly AJ, et al. Comparison of Reporter Gene and Iron Particle Labeling for Tracking Fate of Human Embryonic Stem Cells and Differentiated Endothelial Cells in Living Subjects. Stem Cells. 2008;26(4):864-73.

[4] Huang NF, Okogbaa J, Babakhanyan A, Cooke JP. Bioluminescence imaging of stem cell-based therapeutics for vascular regeneration. Theranostics. 2012;2(4):346-54.

[5] Schroeder T. Imaging stem-cell-driven regeneration in mammals. Nature. 2008;453(7193):345-51.

[6] Su W, Zhou M, Zheng Y, Fan Y, Wang L, Han Z, et al. Bioluminescence reporter gene imaging characterize human embryonic stem cell-derived teratoma formation. Journal of Cellular Biochemistry. 2011(112):840–8.

[7] Li Z, Lee A, Huang M, Chun H, Chung J, Chu P, et al. Imaging survival and function of transplanted cardiac resident stem cells. Journal of the American College of Cardiology. 2009;53(14):1229-40.

[8] Weissleder R, Moore A, Mahmood U, Bhorade R, Benveniste H, Chiocca EA, et al. *In vivo* magnetic resonance imaging of transgene expression. Nat Med. 2000;6(3):351-5.

[9] Cai W, Chen X. Nanoplatforms for Targeted Molecular Imaging in Living Subjects. Small. 2007;3(11):1840-54.

[10] Hare JM, Traverse JH, Henry TD, Dib N, Strumpf RK, Schulman SP, et al. A randomized, double-blind, placebo-controlled, dose-escalation study of intravenous adult human mesenchymal stem cells (prochymal) after acute myocardial infarction. Journal of the American College of Cardiology. 2009;54(24):2277-86.

[11] Guenou H, Nissan X, Larcher F, Feteira J, Lemaitre G, Saidani M, et al. Human embryonic stem-cell derivatives for full reconstruction of the pluristratified epidermis: a preclinical study. Lancet. 2009;374(9703):1745-53.

[12] Li Z, Hu S, Ghosh Z, Han Z, Wu JC. Functional Comparison and Expression Profiling of Human Induced Pluripotent Stem Cell- and Embryonic Stem Cell-Derived Endothelial Cells. Stem Cells and Development. 2011;20:1701-10.

[13] Chang GY, Xie X, Wu JC. Overview of stem cells and imaging modalities for cardiovascular diseases. J Nucl Cardiol. 2006;13(4):554-69.

[14] Fu Y, Azene N, Xu Y, Kraitchman DL. Tracking stem cells for cardiovascular applications *in vivo*: focus on imaging techniques. Imaging in medicine. 2011;3(4):473-86.

[15] McClelland R, Wauthier E, Tallheden T, Reid LM, Hsu E. In situ labeling and magnetic resonance imaging of transplanted human hepatic stem cells. Mol Imaging Biol. 2011;13(5):911-22.

[16] Acton PD, Zhou R. Imaging reporter genes for cell tracking with PET and SPECT. Q J Nucl Med Mol Imaging. 2005;49(4):349-60.

[17] Li SC, Tachiki LM, Luo J, Dethlefs BA, Chen Z, Loudon WG. A biological global positioning system: considerations for tracking stem cell behaviors in the whole body. Stem Cell Rev. 2010;6(2):317-33.

[18] Rak-Raszewska A, Marcello M, Kenny S, Edgar D, See V, Murray P. Quantum dots do not affect the behaviour of mouse embryonic stem cells and kidney stem cells and are suitable for short-term tracking. PLoS One. 2012;7(3):e32650.

[19] Yukawa H, Watanabe M, Kaji N, Okamoto Y, Tokeshi M, Miyamoto Y, et al. Monitoring transplanted adipose tissue-derived stem cells combined with heparin in the liver by fluorescence imaging using quantum dots. Biomaterials. 2012;33(7):2177-86.

[20] Ranjbarvaziri S, Kiani S, Akhlaghi A, Vosough A, Baharvand H, Aghdami N. Quantum dot labeling using positive charged peptides in human hematopoetic and mesenchymal stem cells. Biomaterials. 2011;32(22):5195-205.

[21] Iordanova B, Ahrens ET. *In vivo* magnetic resonance imaging of ferritin-based reporter visualizes native neuroblast migration. Neuroimage. 2012;59(2):1004-12.

[22] Min JJ, Gambhir SS. Molecular imaging of PET reporter gene expression. Handb Exp Pharmacol. 2008(185 Pt 2):277-303.

[23] Li Z, Wu JC, Sheikh AY, Kraft D, Cao F, Xie X, et al. Differentiation, Survival, and Function of Embryonic Stem Cell Derived Endothelial Cells for Ischemic Heart Disease. Circulation. 2007;116(11_suppl):I-46-I-54.

[24] Xie X, Cao F, Sheikh AY, Li Z, Connolly AJ, Pei X, et al. Genetic modification of embryonic stem cells with VEGF enhances cell survival and improves cardiac function. Cloning and stem cells. 2007;9(4):549-63.

[25] Pomper MG, Hammond H, Yu X, Ye Z, Foss CA, Lin DD, et al. Serial imaging of human embryonic stem-cell engraftment and teratoma formation in live mouse models. Cell Res. 2009;19(3):370-9.

[26] Trounson A, Thakar RG, Lomax G, Gibbons D. Clinical trials for stem cell therapies. BMC medicine. 2011;9:52.

[27] Sanz-Ruiz R, Gutierrez Ibanes E, Arranz AV, Fernandez Santos ME, Fernandez PL, Fernandez-Aviles F. Phases I-III Clinical Trials Using Adult Stem Cells. Stem cells international. 2010;2010:579142.

[28] Li ZJ, Wang ZZ, Zheng YZ, Xu B, Yang RC, Scadden DT, et al. Kinetic expression of platelet endothelial cell adhesion molecule-1 (PECAM-1/CD31) during embryonic stem cell differentiation. J Cell Biochem. 2005;95(3):559-70.

[29] Tarantal AF, Lee CC, Batchelder CA, Christensen JE, Prater D, Cherry SR. Radiolabeling and *in vivo* imaging of transplanted renal lineages differentiated from human embryonic stem cells in fetal rhesus monkeys. Mol Imaging Biol. 2012;14(2):197-204.

[30] Sun N, Lee A, Wu JC. Long term non-invasive imaging of embryonic stem cells using reporter genes. Nat Protoc. 2009;4(8):1192-201.

[31] Frangioni JV, Hajjar RJ. *In vivo* tracking of stem cells for clinical trials in cardiovascular disease. Circulation. 2004;110(21):3378-83.

[32] Narsinh KH, Cao F, Wu JC. Molecular imaging of human embryonic stem cells. Methods Mol Biol. 2009;515:13-32.

[33] Jiang H, Cheng Z, Tian M, Zhang H. *In vivo* imaging of embryonic stem cell therapy. Eur J Nucl Med Mol I. 2011;38(4):774-84.

[34] Hong H, Yang Y, Zhang Y, Cai W. Non-invasive imaging of human embryonic stem cells. Curr Pharm Biotechnol. 2010;11(6):685-92.

[35] Lewin M, Carlesso N, Tung CH, Tang XW, Cory D, Scadden DT, et al. Tat peptide-derivatized magnetic nanoparticles allow *in vivo* tracking and recovery of progenitor cells. Nat Biotechnol. 2000;18(4):410-4.

[36] Wang L, Su W, Liu Z, Zhou M, Chen S, Chen Y, et al. CD44 antibody-targeted liposomal nanoparticles for molecular imaging nd therapy of hepatocellular carcinoma. Biomaterials. 2012;33:5107-14.

[37] Wu JC, Cao F, Dutta S, Xie X, Kim E, Chungfat N, et al. Proteomic analysis of reporter genes for molecular imaging of transplanted embryonic stem cells. Proteomics. 2006;6(23):6234-49.

[38] Zheng W, Honmou O, Miyata K, Harada K, Suzuki J, Liu H, et al. Therapeutic benefits of human mesenchymal stem cells derived from bone marrow after global cerebral ischemia. Brain Res. 2010;1310:8-16.

[39] Yamada Y, Nakamura S, Ito K, Sugito T, Yoshimi R, Nagasaka T, et al. A feasibility of useful cell-based therapy by bone regeneration with deciduous tooth stem cells, dental pulp stem cells, or bone-marrow-derived mesenchymal stem cells for clinical study using tissue engineering technology. Tissue Eng Part A. 2010;16(6):1891-900.

[40] Rush SM, Hamilton GA, Ackerson LM. Mesenchymal stem cell allograft in revision foot and ankle surgery: a clinical and radiographic analysis. J Foot Ankle Surg. 2009;48(2):163-9.

[41] Uccelli A, Moretta L, Pistoia V. Mesenchymal stem cells in health and disease. Nat Rev Immunol. 2008;8(9):726-36.

[42] Tang C, Russell PJ, Martiniello-Wilks R, Rasko JE, Khatri A. Concise review: Nanoparticles and cellular carriers-allies in cancer imaging and cellular gene therapy? Stem Cells. 2010;28(9):1686-702.

[43] Wang HH, Wang YX, Leung KC, Au DW, Xuan S, Chak CP, et al. Durable mesenchymal stem cell labelling by using polyhedral superparamagnetic iron oxide nanoparticles. Chemistry. 2009;15(45):12417-25.

[44] Love Z, Wang F, Dennis J, Awadallah A, Salem N, Lin Y, et al. Imaging of mesenchymal stem cell transplant by bioluminescence and PET. J Nucl Med. 2007;48(12): 2011-20.

[45] Daadi MM, Li Z, Arac A, Grueter BA, Sofilos M, Malenka RC, et al. Molecular and magnetic resonance imaging of human embryonic stem cell-derived neural stem cell grafts in ischemic rat brain. Mol Ther. 2009;17(7):1282-91.

[46] Zurkiya O, Chan AW, Hu X. MagA is sufficient for producing magnetic nanoparticles in mammalian cells, making it an MRI reporter. Magn Reson Med. 2008;59(6): 1225-31.

[47] Zhu J, Zhou L, XingWu F. Tracking neural stem cells in patients with brain trauma. N Engl J Med. 2006;355(22):2376-8.

[48] Doubrovin M, Ponomarev V, Serganova I, Soghomonian S, Myagawa T, Beresten T, et al. Development of a new reporter gene system--dsRed/xanthine phosphoribosyltransferase-xanthine for molecular imaging of processes behind the intact blood-brain barrier. Mol Imaging. 2003;2(2):93-112.

[49] Wilson A, Laurenti E, Oser G, van der Wath RC, Blanco-Bose W, Jaworski M, et al. Hematopoietic stem cells reversibly switch from dormancy to self-renewal during homeostasis and repair. Cell. 2008;135(6):1118-29.

[50] Schroeder T. Tracking hematopoiesis at the single cell level. Ann N Y Acad Sci. 2005;1044:201-9.

[51] Daldrup-Link HE, Rudelius M, Piontek G, Metz S, Brauer R, Debus G, et al. Migration of iron oxide-labeled human hematopoietic progenitor cells in a mouse model: *in vivo* monitoring with 1.5-T MR imaging equipment. Radiology. 2005;234(1):197-205.

[52] Lin Y, Cheung P, Roth JC, Wilson DL, Gerson SL. Imaging stem cell-derived persistent foci after *in vivo* selection of lentiviral MGMT-P140K transduced murine bone marrow cells. Mol Ther. 2011;19(7):1342-52.

[53] Junt T, Schulze H, Chen Z, Massberg S, Goerge T, Krueger A, et al. Dynamic visualization of thrombopoiesis within bone marrow. Science. 2007;317(5845):1767-70.

[54] Sipkins DA, Wei X, Wu JW, Runnels JM, Cote D, Means TK, et al. *In vivo* imaging of specialized bone marrow endothelial microdomains for tumour engraftment. Nature. 2005;435(7044):969-73.

[55] Yao Y, Li Y, Ma G, Liu N, Ju S, Jin J, et al. *In vivo* magnetic resonance imaging of injected endothelial progenitor cells after myocardial infarction in rats. Mol Imaging Biol. 2011;13(2):303-13.

[56] Agudelo CA, Tachibana Y, Noboru T, Iida H, Yamaoka T. Long-term *in vivo* magnetic resonance imaging tracking of endothelial progenitor cells transplanted in rat ischemic limbs and their angiogenic potential. Tissue Eng Part A. 2011;17(15-16): 2079-89.

[57] Patschan SA, Patschan D, Temme J, Korsten P, Wessels JT, Koziolek M, et al. Endothelial progenitor cells (EPC) in sepsis with acute renal dysfunction (ARD). Crit Care. 2011;15(2):R94.

[58] Higuchi T, Anton M, Saraste A, Dumler K, Pelisek J, Nekolla SG, et al. Reporter gene PET for monitoring survival of transplanted endothelial progenitor cells in the rat heart after pretreatment with VEGF and atorvastatin. J Nucl Med. 2009;50(11):1881-6.

[59] Chade AR, Zhu XY, Krier JD, Jordan KL, Textor SC, Grande JP, et al. Endothelial progenitor cells homing and renal repair in experimental renovascular disease. Stem Cells. 2010;28(6):1039-47.

[60] Fernandez-Ruiz V, Kawa M, Berasain C, Iniguez M, Schmitz V, Martinez-Anso E, et al. Treatment of murine fulminant hepatitis with genetically engineered endothelial progenitor cells. J Hepatol. 2011;55(4):828-37.

Section 2

Innovations in Medical Imaging Techniques

Chapter 5

Spin Average Supercompound Ultrasonography

Tsuicheng D. Chiu, Sonia Contreras and Martin Fox

Additional information is available at the end of the chapter

http://dx.doi.org/10.5772/53238

1. Introduction

Introduced to the medical field in the 1950s, ultrasound has applications across the spectrum of modern medicine including cardiology, urology, obstetrics, gynecology and abdominal imaging (kidneys, liver, spleen, gallbladder and pancreas excluding stomach and intestines which contain of air which blocks ultrasound). Vascular imaging is used especially for large vessels like the aorta. Ultrasound is also used as a guide in surgeries.

Although ultrasound is real-time, non-invasive, highly cost-effective [1], portable and uses non-ionizing radiation, its benefits are offset by penetration and resolution limitations. As a result, it has been coexists with computed tomography (CT) and magnetic resonance imaging (MRI) [2, 3]

The main goal of this research is to improve the quality and the usefulness of the ultrasound image. We present a supercompounding technique [4] which can be described as a two-dimensional spin average method. The supercompounding technique is one kind of spatial compounding. Unlike conventional compounding which typically uses a 30 degrees to 60 degrees compounding range, our spatial compounding technique which we have termed "supercompounding" uses a B-mode array that rotates around a target in a range of 120 degrees or greater. The experiments in the research use complete 360 degrees scanning to optimize results. We find that the quality of the ultrasound images is improved and whether the use of the ultrasound imaging can be extended to other applications. Our results suggest that, this technique will extend the limits of ultrasound imaging while preserving all its current benefits.

1.1. Ultrasound imaging system

The imaging system used in this research is the GE RT-3200 ultrasound imager, a relatively primitive early generation two-dimensional imager compared to modern equipment. The basic principles of commercial ultrasound are pitch and catch. The ultrasound waves are typically transmitted and received by transducers. In medical applications, reflection systems are virtually universal due to the ease of use of hand-held transducer. Such pulse-echo systems catch the reflected ultrasound waves and only one transducer is needed. Ultrasound waves are sent to an object and reflected with time delay between the transmission of the beams and the arrival of the reflected signals. All objects are taken with either a linear 7.5 MHz or a curvilinear 3.5MHz transducer. Although the GE RT-3200 is an early generation ultrasound imaging system, the results in the r should be evaluated with respect to the degree of image improvement. It is because the supercompounded image is integrated from hundreds of raw ultrasound images. If the quality of raw images is improved by modern equipments, with better compounding materials, it can result in an even better supercompounded images.

1.2. Types of ultrasound artifacts

Compared with CT and MRI, ultrasound images have lower signal-to-noise ratio because ultrasound waves are highly distorted when traveling through the tissues. The ultrasound image is constructed from the interactions between the transmitted ultrasound waves and the imaged tissues. Once the reflected ultrasound waves are distorted or compromised, the resultant image will incur artifacts that either omit or add erroneous information.

The following list states artifacts occurred in the experiments in this research and Figure 1 shows how they appear on the clinical ultrasound image.

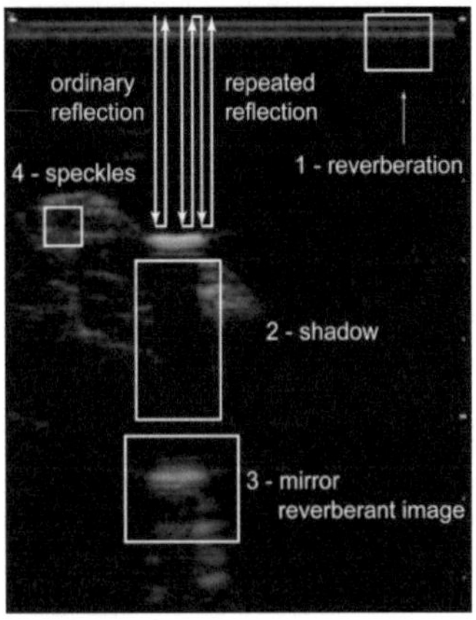

Figure 1. Artifacts: The object is a dissected rat thigh tightened with a supported wood stick placed in water bath and the image is taken using the 7.5 MHz linear transducer. Region 1 shows the reverberations, the reverberations are caused by the mismatched impedances between the wall of the water container (assembled by four 5 millimeters thick acrylic plates) and waters. Region 2 shows the shadow behind a side wall of the supported wood stick. Since the wood material is highly reflective, the stick blocks all ultrasound waves and it results the shadow. Region 3 shows a mirror reverberant image. It usually happens when a high reflective object is imaged. The reflected ultrasound waves are reflected again by the surface of the transducer and it makes the same ultrasound beams travel twice distance but with the same results. Therefore, the same or similar structures lies at the twice depth on the image. Region 4 shows speckles which come from the scattered ultrasound waves.

http://dx.doi.org/10.5772/53238

- Reverberation: Reverberations are multiple lines behind the physical objects normally found on the boundaries between two media, especially when the acoustic impedances of two materials are significantly mismatched as shown in Figure 2. The first and the second reflections represent the superficial and the deep boundaries of the second medium. The third to the nth reflections are the reverberations coming from the trapped ultrasound waves in the second medium. The fraction of the ultrasound waves that is reflected depends on the reflection coefficient between the two media.

- Shadows: Three scenarios cause shadows on ultrasound images. Shadows are caused either by a large impedance mismatch, a highly angled boundary or a highly absorptive material.

Unlike reverberations, where only parts of the ultrasound waves can penetrate through the boundaries and are trapped in the second medium, all the ultrasound waves can be totally blocked due to an even greater impedance mismatch. Since no waves penetrate the second medium, there is no information returning from the area behind the high reflective objects.

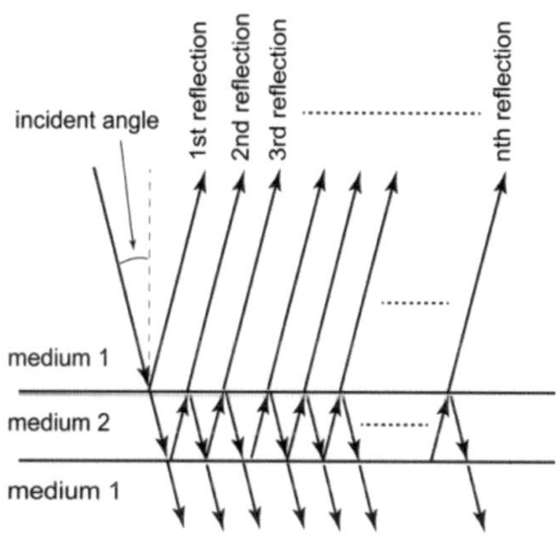

Figure 2. Illustration of reverberations. Reverberations show as multiple lines as the ultrasound waves bounce back and forth in the second medium, resulting from the mismatched impedances between the medium 1 and 2.

Acoustic absorptive materials can cause the shadowing effect for another reason. If ultrasound waves are totally absorbed by the target material, shadows will also result because no waves return to the transducer.

The third scenario is caused by the shape, not the material of the object. As illustrated in Figure 1, the incident ultrasound waves contact the boundaries and the reflected waves bounce back to the transducer. When the incident angle is large enough, the reflected ultrasound waves are not reflected back to the transducer. Large incident angle scan cause low intensities (parts of the reflected waves going back to the transducer) or even shadows (all waves redirecting away from the transducer) behind the boundaries on the image.

- Mirror reverberant images: A reverberant image occurs when the same structure appears twice. When the reflected ultrasound waves return to the transducer with enough energy to perform a second reflection on the surface of the transducer. It gives the same results with twice traveling distance for the same ultrasound waves; therefore, the ultrasound imaging systems are misled causing apparent imaging of nonexistent structures lying at the twice the depth of the original object.

- Speckles: Ideally when the ultrasound waves contact the object, the waves are either reflected or transmitted. However, small portions of the ultrasound waves can interfere coherently. The accumulation of random scatterings in the tissue volume results in intense fluctuations on the image that degrades its quality. The resultant speckle pattern can be modeled geometrically as a random walk of component phasor [6].

1.3. Point spread function

The response of an imaging device to a point object is described as a point spread function (PSF), a blurring process intrinsic to many imaging modalities. As a result, the acquired images can be convolved with a PSF. This phenomenon makes the general image function described by[7]:

$$i(x, y)= \iint h(x, y;\xi, \eta)i_r(\xi, \eta)d\xi d\eta \tag{1}$$

where i is the obtained image, h is a generalized PSF and $(x, y; \xi, \eta)$ are the output and input pair coordinates in input and output planes, with i_r being the spatial distribution or raw image before convolving with the PSF. The equation 1 shows a space variant PSF. The true spatial distribution is blurred by the PSF. PSFs are space variant in most ultrasound imaging systems, especially due to focusing, as illustrated in Figure 3. Since there is no closed form relationship between input and output signals, further image enhancement is difficult. In the most probable scenario, the algorithms that work at certain regions are not applicable to the whole image. Due to non-stationary PSFs, space variant algorithms have to be used. If the image has a regularized PSF, it can be expressed using the convolution operation:

$$i(x, y)= \iint h(x - \xi, y - \eta)i_r(\xi, \eta)d\xi d\eta \tag{2}$$

Space invariant algorithms can be used to improve its quality. Supercompounding provides an image with a more regularized PSF. "Regularized" implies that the lateral and axial resolutions are the same; indeed a circularly symmetric point spread function. This benefit can allow linear filtering to become more efficient and reliable and to simplify the image processing.

We propose an enhanced compounding technique which we term supercompounding. It generates integrated information collected around the object from wide acquisition angles into a single image. It has significant improvements in SNR, contrast and spatial resolution, artifact and speckle reduction and PSF regularization (more constant and symmetric PSF). It also has the ability to reconstruct complete edges of circular objects such as vessels and cysts which would appear as one or two semicircles on the conventional ultrasound images.

http://dx.doi.org/10.5772/53238

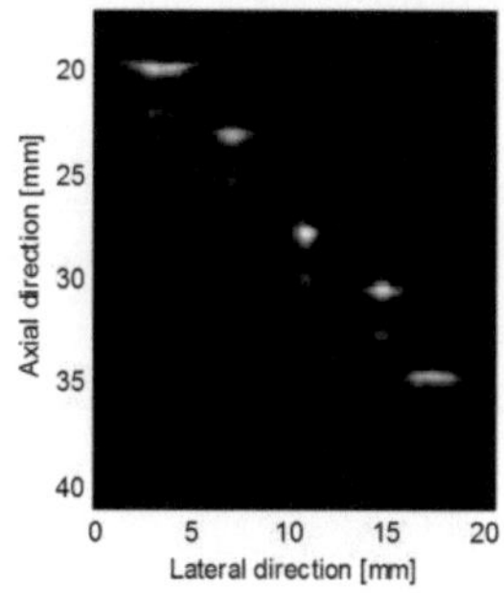

Figure 3. Variability of the PSF in the axial and lateral directions. The transducer is placed on the top of the image, and the focal distance is 27mm. The lateral resolution worsens with an increasing distance from the focal zone in either direction, superficial or deep.

2. Theory

2.1. Spatial compounding

Like in many other technological domains, researchers are still refining ultrasound imaging technology such as designing better transducers or faster systems trying to make ultrasonography more valuable. Most researches are aimed at improving on the basic paradigm of a focused scanned transducer array such as changing the geometry of element orders to make 2-D and 1.5-D arrays, increasing the numbers of the elements and reducing the sizes of the elements to improve resolution. Although the systems used today have much better resolution and cost effectiveness than prior systems, the technology is still limited by the physical behavior of sound waves. As a result, the medical application of ultrasonic imaging has seen evolutionary rather than revolutionary improvements. Combining ultrasonic imaging with spatial compounding could provide that revolutionary next-step. For instance, bones are highly reflective to sound waves. Current ultrasonic imaging techniques cannot penetrate bones, but in this research we explore large angle compounding methodologies that go around bones and other obstacles and have numerous additional benefits.

Several spatial compounding techniques, developed in the early 80's [8-10] combines multi-directional ultrasonic echoes into one image that represents the distribution of sound wave reflectivity within an area of interest. Several uncorrelated images [11] are combined in order to reduce speckle, avoid shadows, and increase contrast resolution. Combining N independent images reduces speckle contrast by an order of $\sqrt{N}$ [12, 13]. Diament et al. [14] used spatial compounding to identify stones in gall bladders and kidneys and Sehgal et al. [15] used spatial imaging to construct cross-sectional images of turkey and dog limbs. Improvements in computing, data acquisition and storage equipments, has increased the number of compounded images dramatically. The processing time is still long, however, and prevents the systems from operating in real-time in many cases. It could take two hours to do a 180-degree/110-image scan [16].

A simple example of compounding is illustrated in Figure 4. To acquire independent images without moving a transducer, the beams are electronically steered to create different incident angles. Changing the incident angle causes the obtained images to contain slightly different speckle patterns. In this case, the target of interest is a long disk-like ellipse. Placing the transducer on the top of the target Figure 4(b) results in missing information at the oblique angle. The image only contains top and bottom parts of the edges because the signal at oblique angles is reflecting away from the transducer. This phenomenon often happens when circular targets such as vessels are involved. To obtain a better contour of the target, compounding images from different incident angles such as Figure 4(a) and Figure 4(c) can help fill part of the missing edges. This type of compounding technique is usually embedded in the system without altering the ultrasound imaging techniques. Comparing the results in Figure 4(d) (with compounding) to 4(b) (without compounding), the boundaries is closer to be intact.

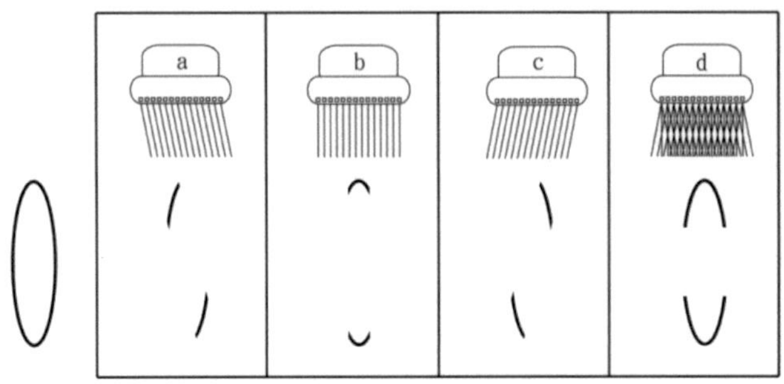

Figure 4. Illustration of conventional compounding: In panel b, the beams are generated at 90 ° to the surface. In panel a and c, the beams are steered to ± 12 °. The frames in panel a, b and c are compounded to construct a new image (frame d)

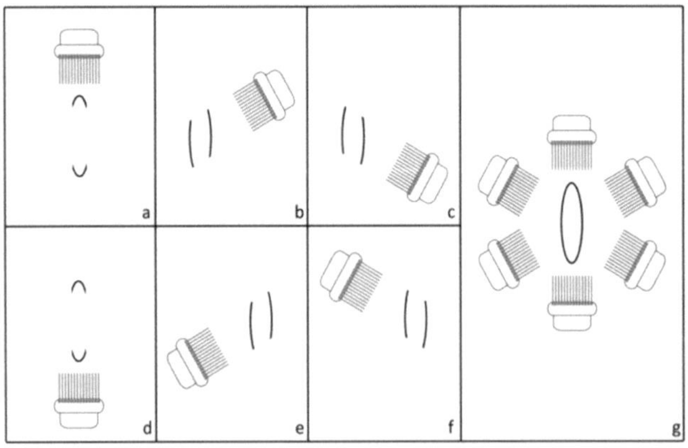

Figure 5. Illustration of supercompounding: the target is scanned from different angles on the same plane (panel a to panel f). The obtained images are compounded to construct a new image with better (complete) field of view of the target (frame g).

http://dx.doi.org/10.5772/53238

2.2. Supercompounding

The limitations of spatial ultrasound compounding technique stimulated research to produce an image with a complete edge (Figure 5). This concept was first used in the 80's became known as compounded ultrasound image in the 90's. In this work we investigate compounding capture angles greater than 120° and term this method as "supercompounding". In the present study, we develop a theoretical foundation for supercompounding based on our generalization of Bracewell's one-dimensional spin average concept [17, 18] to two-dimensions.

2.3. Spin average

The supercompounding technique used in this research is one kind of multi-angular spatial compounding but includes a much larger scanning range (up to 360°) than is typically employed. The target is scanned from different angles on the same plane in order to get uncorrelated data. The data contains information about the physical components as well as the artifacts. The reflected signal is variable and depends on both the incidence angle of the sound waves and the impedance mismatch within the subject. Unlike the artifacts, the primary subject of the imaging remains at the same position relative to the center of rotation while the transducer moves around the subject. Once the images are compounded together, the information of the physical components is permanent and the angular dependent artifacts are reduced.

2.3.1. One-dimensional spin average

The compounding method used in this research can be modeled using the spin average concept. One-dimensional spin average was illustrated by Bracewell [17, 18] and is given by

$$fs(r)=\frac{1}{2\pi}\int_0^{2\pi} f(r\cos\theta)d\theta \tag{3}$$

where $fs(r)$ is the resultant function once $f(x)$ is spin averaged, r is the radius from the center of rotation and α is the angle from axial-x. Assuming $f(x, y)$ is a two-dimensional function which is a *rect* function in x-direction but independent in the y-direction. Figure 2.3 illustrates the one-dimensional spin average of a designed function stated by

$$f(x,\ y)=f(x)=rect(x/2a) \tag{4}$$

where $|x|$ is less than a, $f(x)$ is set up to one; otherwise, $f(x)$ is zero. The value of the function indicates the height of a surface above the (x, y)-plane, and the cylindrical ridge in the y-direction shows the independence of y.

Instead of spinning the function, Figure 6 shows the source travelling around the center of the spinning function along the radius r at uniform speed to return to the starting point. The travel path is a cycle of radius r on (x, y)-plane. The spin averaged function $fs(r)$ is the integral of the values passing during the course of one rotation, which gives the average heights of function *f(x)*. For this particular case, the close form solution can be derived into

$$fs(r)=1-(2/\pi)\cos^{-1}(a/r)H(r-a) \tag{5}$$

$$H(r-a)=\begin{cases}0 & if r<a\\ 1 & if r>a\end{cases} \tag{6}$$

where fs*(r)* is the spin averaged function and *H* is a step function. The profile of the spin-averaged *rect* function is illustrated in Figure 7. When the translation distance is less than *a*, the travel path is on the plate form at all times. The spin-averaged values equal to one. If the translation distance is beyond *a,* the decrease of the spin-averaged value follows $fs(r)=1-(2/\pi)\cos^{-1}(a/r)$.

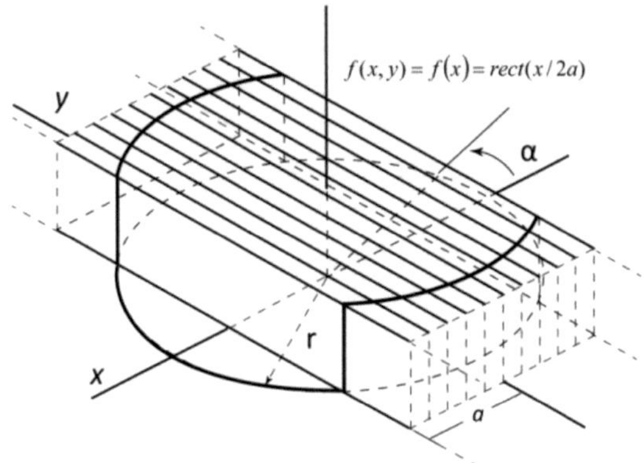

Figure 6. The illustration of equation (4): the bold curve is the travel path and its projection is a cycle of radius r on the (x, y) plane.

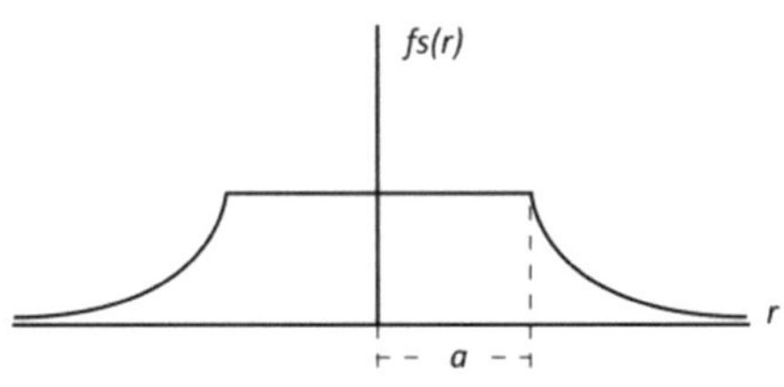

Figure 7. Profile of spin-averaged rect function: the spin averaged value starts to drop when r reaches distance a.

Alternately, we can treat the spin average as a long exposure of sound waves recorded on one image but not displayed in real time. Since sound waves are longitudinal, the beams coming from the transducer can be considered linear sources of sound, each one corre-

http://dx.doi.org/10.5772/53238

sponding to an axial line in the acquired image. When the function is being spun, the resultants are overlapped on the previous image. After one rotation, the superimposed image is the final spin average function.

2.3.2. *Two-dimensional spin average*

Since the y-direction is not independent in ultrasound imaging systems, we generalize Bracewell's one-dimensional spin average to two-dimension [19]. The expanded spin average function is re-written

$$f_2s(r)=\frac{1}{2\pi}\int_0^{2\pi} f(r\cos\theta,\ r\sin\theta)d\theta \tag{7}$$

The two-dimensional spin average function is no longer independent in the y-direction; therefore, the term of $r\bullet sin\alpha$ *is included in equation* 7. As comparison to one-dimensional spin average function, we have a one-dimensional rect function times a two-dimensional circ function illustrated as Figure 8 and the profile shows in Figure 9.

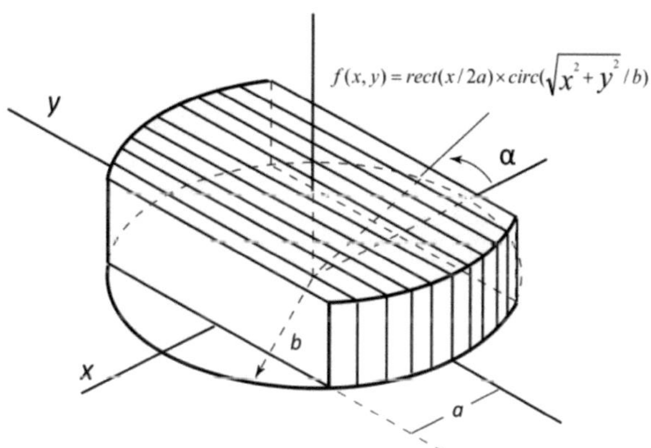

Figure 8. The illustration of equation (7): f(x,y)is a rect function in x direction and a two-dimensional circ function with radius b.

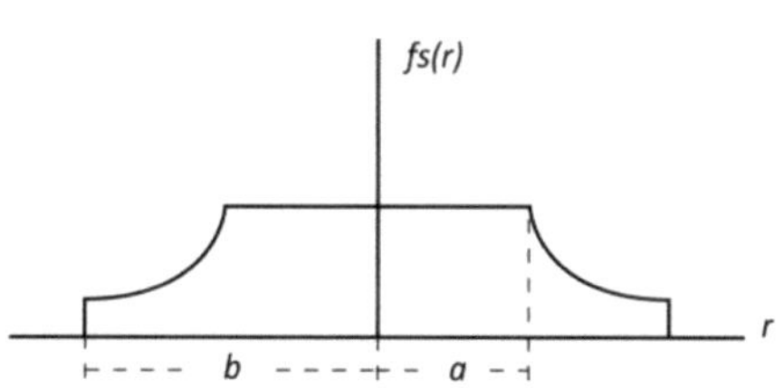

Figure 9. The profile of the two-dimensional spin averaged function

If we travel at the radial distance (r) where less than a, we are always on the top of the two-dimensional function. The value stays high. When travel at the radial distance where greater than a but less than b, the spin average value decreases and drop to zero when r equals to b.

To illustrate the concept on ultrasound image, we use numerical spin averaging on a stretched two-dimensional Gaussian function (G) which is written

$$G(x, y) = a exp\left[\frac{-(x - 4b)^2 - (y - b)^2}{2\sigma^2}\right] \quad (8)$$

where G represents two-dimensional Gaussian function and a is the amplitude of the function which is set to 255. σ and b are set to 4.5 and 0.2. The distribution along the x-axial is four times broader than the distribution along y-direction to simulate the PSF of a typical ultrasound system. Resolution is usually better in the axial direction than in the lateral. The stepping angle of spinning is 27.69° and it gives us thirteen images for spin-averaging. The results are shown in Figure 2.7.

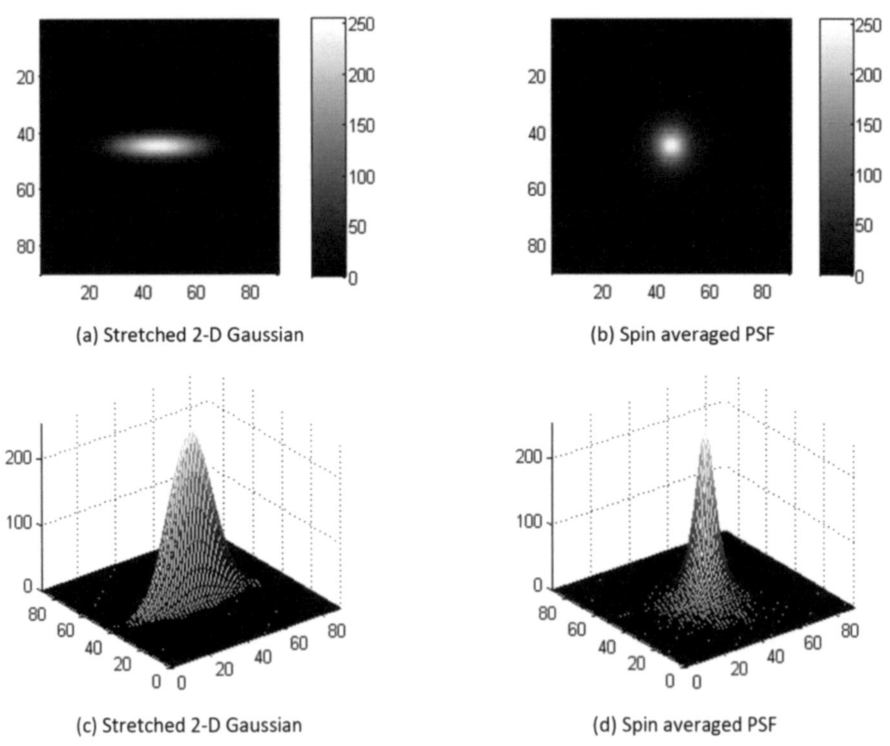

Figure 10. Spin averaging a stretched two-dimensional Gaussian function.

Figure 10(a) and 10(b) are two-dimensional images and 10(c) and 10(d) are three-dimensional images before and after spin-averaging respectively. Comparing 10(a) and 10(b) the image has different widths in x and y directions. After spin averaging, the resultant is more concentrate, symmetric and point-like. The profiles of the axial and lateral resolutions of 10(a) and spin averaged function of 10(b) are shown in Figure 11.

The profile of the spin average PSF (solid line) is located between the outer and inner dashed line, which represent the lateral and axial resolutions respectively. After spin-averaging, the new image becomes more isotropic. Lateral resolution is improved but axial resolution is reduced. However, the axial resolution is reduced but as return a regularized and space invariant PSF is gained. As a result, the system becomes less space-variant and the images can be further enhanced by efficient linear image techniques.

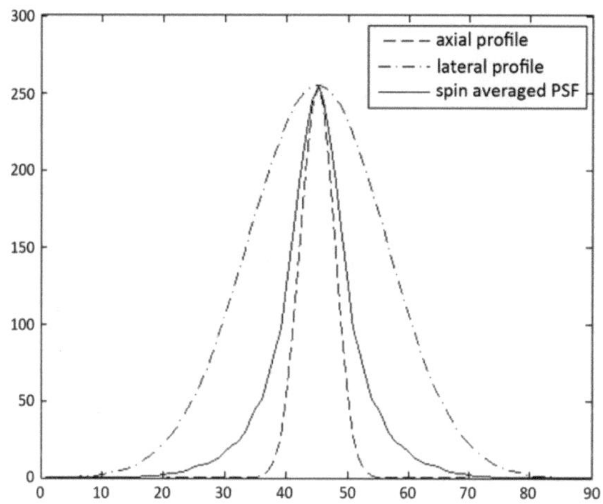

Figure 11. Profile: a. outer dashed line - lateral resolution of the stretched 2-D Gaussian function (x-direction), b. inner dashed line - axial resolution of the stretched 2-D Gaussian function (y-direction) and c. solid line - the spin averaged resolution.

In an ultrasound image, the function values (heights) while spin-averaging show the intensity of the reflected signal. In practice, these signals not only contain the information we want, but artifacts as well. Therefore, facing heights that change rapidly during the spinning will result in a high the standard deviation, which could indicate an angular dependent artifact. On the other hand, if the heights are maintained while spinning, the standard deviation is low. Thus the possibility of having a physical component located at that point is high. Therefore, spin average keeps a fairly high amount of intensity values of the physical components, and reduces the intensity of artifacts. Hence, the contrast resolution is enhanced.

2.4. Regularized point spread function

Spin average reduces artifacts, reveals the true shapes of physical components and regularizes the point spread functions which means having a more symmetric, more uniform and tighter PSF which is less space invariant. For practical purposes, the quality of results is inversely related to the size of the travel step α. The regularization of the PSF function is shown in Figure 12. In this illustration, a metal pin head is used to simulate a point target.

In Figure 12(a) the PSF resultant picture shows an upside down triangle with long wings. Since the physical shape of the target is a point, the level of artifacts will be high. The axial reverberation is angular dependent artifacts, and the size of lateral resolution is limited by both the transducer and different focal zones. By reducing the stepping angle of spinning α from 0° (360°) to 60°, and then to 30°, the compounded PSF shrinks to a point (Figure 12(b), (c)). This suggests that the spin average can remove the angular dependent artifacts and distortion caused by focusing.

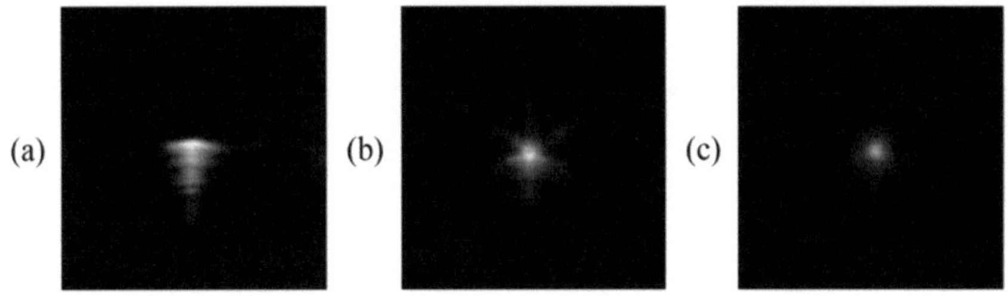

Figure 12. The PSF of a metal pin head (a) the original PSF without spin average - $\alpha = 0°$ (b) the PSF with 6 images compounded - $\alpha = 60°$ (c) the PSF with 12 images compounded - $\alpha = 30°$

3. Materials and methods

3.1. Introduction

The experiment setup focuses on utilizing a conventional ultrasound imaging system (GE RT-3200) to test the spin average theory and the supercompounding concept. The experimental apparatus – the three-dimensional moving platform – is designed in two parts, image acquisition and image processing.

Since a complete spin average is an integral between 0 and 2π, the images or data has to be acquired around the targets of interest. In order to do so, either a transducer has to be rotated around the targets or the targets themselves have to be rotated around the center point. The latter option – objects rotating around a center point – is used in this experiment to achieve better results in demonstrating the concept of the spin average theory and supercompounding technique. One reason to favor this option is that the rotation of the targets of interest allows us to accomplish the goal without moving or vibrating the transducer. Another reason is that the transducer will always have solid contact with the surface of the target container. As a result, our objects are mounted on a rod connected to a DC gear motor controlled by a micro-controller.

The same micro-controller also controls image acquisition. Once the target is rotated to the designed angle, the micro-controller triggers the frame grabber to capture the image and to store the results in a specific order. Such order is the index for quantifying the rotational degree of the images.

Since the conventional ultrasound images are usually shown in the vertical axial direction, the transducer is positioned at the top of the image shown as Figure 13. In order to have all images aligned in the same coordinate system, a coordinate transformation (derotation) has to be applied on each image at a specific angle based on the rotation index around the center of the rotation. After derotation, all images are ready for the recombination, which completes the supercompounding process.

3.2. Work flow

The work flow of the experiment is as illustrated in Figure 14(a). The target is submerged in a water tank illustrated as Figure 14(b), muffled with foam material on the rear, lateral, and bottom sides to reduce the surplus reflection of sound waves. The sound wave form is generated and detected by the ultrasound transducer and the results are sent to the ultrasound console (GE RT-3200) for detection and processing to form real time ultrasound images. These images are simultaneously shown on the screen of the RT-3200 and the display of the frame grabber. Once the micro-controller drives the subject to the designed angle, it triggers the frame grabber to capture and store a still image, which then moves on to the next designed angle; the process repeats until the micro-controller completes a 360 degree scanning. These still images are stored in sequence as the rotation index. The whole set of images is used to construct one final supercompounded ultrasonography.

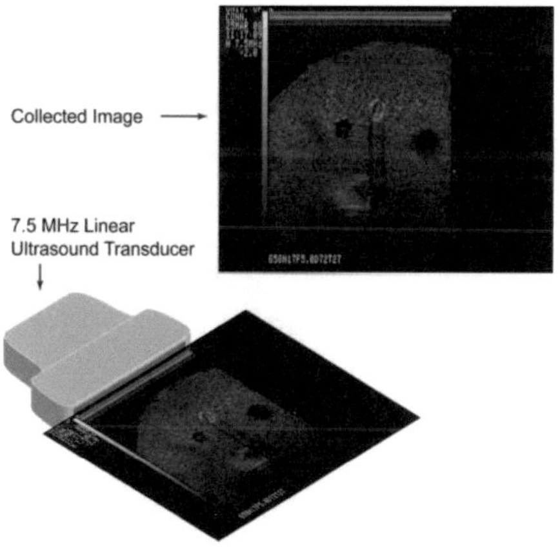

Figure 13. Illustration of the relative positions between the collected image and the ultrasound transducer. The image shows the vertical axial direction with the image plane perpendicular to the surface of the ultrasound array. The specific 7.5 MHz linear ultrasound array shown above has 128 elements. With two times of zoom-in setting, it covers two-thirds field of view.

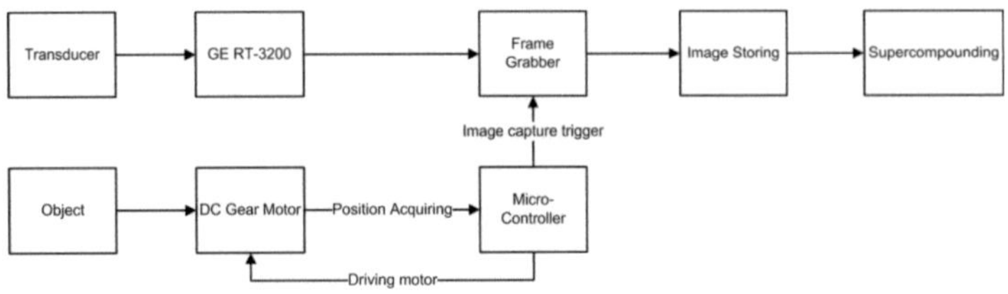

(a) Work flow

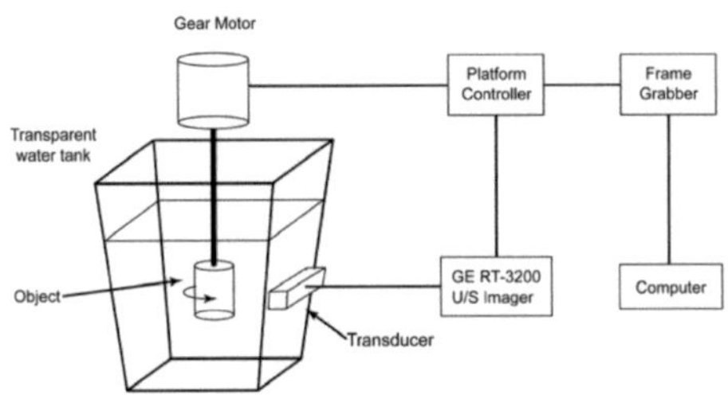

(b) Illustration of the experiment setup

Figure 14. The work flow and the illustration of the experiments setup. The target of interest is mounted on the output shaft of the DC gear motor. Micro-controller controls the rotation of the motor. Once it is rotated to the designed angle, the micro-controller sends capturing signal to the frame grabber to store the image that is concurrently being received from the GE RT-3200 ultrasound console.

3.3. Processing of ultrasound images

3.3.1. Software

The software used to process the raw image data for supercompounding is MATLAB (matrix laboratory). MATLAB is a numerical computing environment that allows matrix manipulations, plotting functions and data and implementation of algorithms to solve the mathematic issues. Behind the mathematic operations, it is also a tool to create a user interface, correlating with programs written in other languages, such as C++.

The reasons why MATLAB is used to process the resultant images are (1) the image itself is a matrix and (2) manipulating matrices is one of the major strengths of MATLAB. With many built-in tool boxes, most of the ordinary image operation can be accomplished easily.

3.3.2. Images

The image is pixelized data. Each pixel (point) in the image corresponds to an intensity value ranging from 0 to 255, the dynamic range of the display. In an ultrasound imaging system, the image is black and white, or in the so-called "gray scale". "Zero" represents black and "255" represents white. Between black and white there are different shades of gray illustrated as Figure 15.

http://dx.doi.org/10.5772/53238

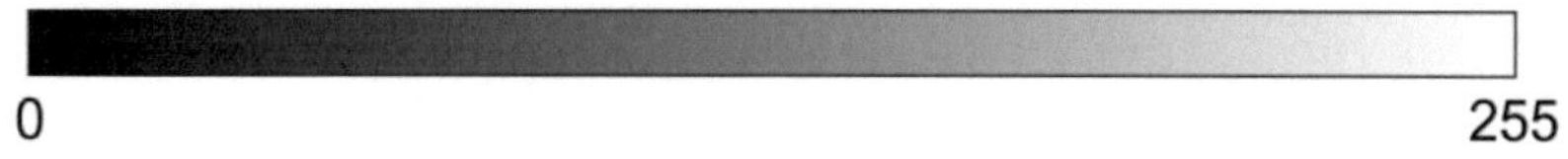

Figure 15. Illustration of the dynamic range of a gray scale image. Values between absolute black and white are divided into 255 levels. These levels are called "gray levels".

The resulting images are stored as bitmap image files (bmp) in a 24-bit bitmaps format including three color layers (green, blue and red). Bitmap data (pixel array) describes the image pixel by pixel. 24-bit represents 24 bits per pixel. For instance, the recorded ultrasound image in the experiment is 640 pixels by 480 pixels. That leads to 307,200 pixels in total. Each pixel is 24 bits, which gives us 7,372,800 bits per image, 921,600 bytes (1 byte = 8 bits) or 900 k (1 k = 1024 bytes) in other words.

Since the ultrasound images used in the experiment are black and white (gray scale) images, the data recorded in the three color layers are the same. To reduce image processing time, only one layer of data is used. The layers are segregated and only the green layer is kept. It leads to a smaller image size – 300k (one-third of 900k).

3.3.3. Image rotation

As is stated in the discussion in section 3.1, to process the spin average concept, involved images must be in the same coordinate system. Each individual image has to be derotated around the center of rotation (corresponding to the relative position between the ultrasound transducer and the output shaft of the gear motor shown as Figure 16).

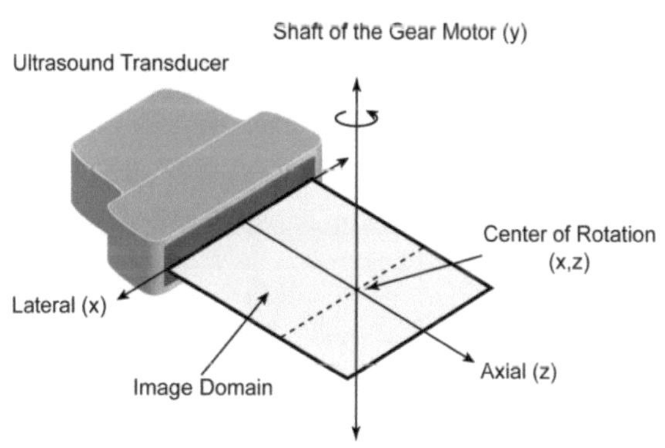

Figure 16. Illustration of the relative position between the shaft of the gear motor and the ultrasound transducer. In the experiment, the object is mounted on the output shaft of the gear motor and is rotated at the center of rotation.

Figure 17 (a) and (b) illustrate how a triangular object is imaged. (a) is taken when the object is at the starting position. In order to perform spin average concept, the object has to be imaged from other angles. (b) is collected when the object is rotated 30 degrees counter clockwise around the center of the rotation. (c) and (d) are the results of (a) and (b) respectively. As the results shown in (c) and (d), the objects are shown in two different coordinate systems. Therefore, a coordinate transformation has to be performed on the images to keep the objects in the same coordinate system. A 30-degree-clockwise rotation is performed on Figure 17 (d) to transform the image to the same coordinate system as (e) which is 0 degree rotation from (c). Since the coordinate transformation is the second time of rotation and is in the opposite direction to neutralize the first time of rotation, we call it derotation.

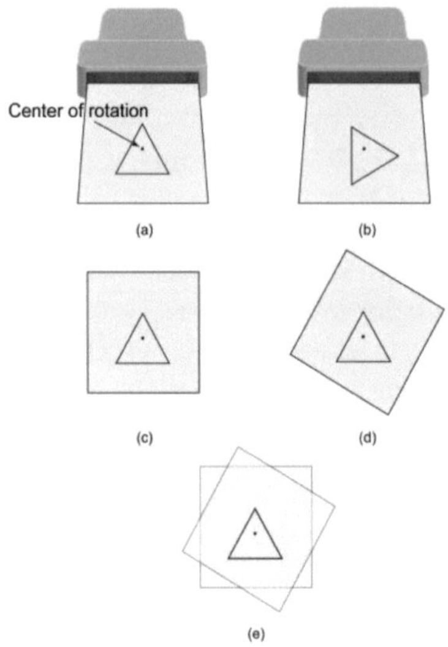

Figure 17. Illustration of derotation. (a) and (b) illustrate how a triangular object is rotated and then imaged. (c) and (d) are the images after derotation. (e) is the compounded image of (e) and (f).

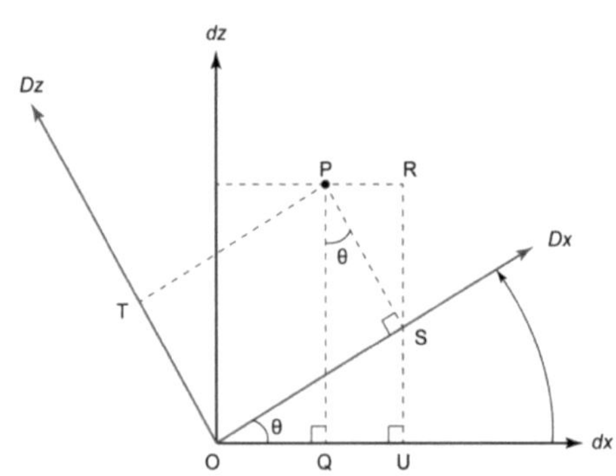

Figure 18. dx and dz are the initial axes and Dx and Dz are the rotated axes by θ. P is the demonstration point and O is the origin.

All images are electronically derotated around the center of rotation in MATLAB. Coordinates mapping the derotated images to the initial position can be obtained using the standard formula for axes rotation [20]:

http://dx.doi.org/10.5772/53238

$$\begin{cases} Dx = dx\cos\theta + dz\sin\theta \\ Dz = dz\cos\theta - dx\sin\theta \end{cases} \tag{9}$$

where dx and dz are distances of the pixel from the center of rotation, Dx and Dz the new coordinates after transposition. The relationship between initial and rotated axes (shown as Figure 18) can be derived geometrically.

The coordinates of P on dx-dz plane is $(\overline{OQ},\ )\ \overline{QP}$ and is $(\overline{OS},\ \overline{PS})$ on Dx-Dz plane.

$$\begin{cases} \overline{OQ} = \overline{OU} - \overline{QU} = \overline{OS}\cos\theta - \overline{PS}\sin\theta \\ \overline{PQ} = \overline{RS} + \overline{SU} = \overline{PS}\cos\theta + \overline{OS}\sin\theta \end{cases} \tag{10}$$

The relation in general form is denoted as following equations.

$$\begin{cases} dx = Dx\cos\theta - Dz\sin\theta \\ dz = Dz\cos\theta + Dx\sin\theta \end{cases} \tag{11}$$

Equation 11 can be solved and rewritten as equation 9.

3.3.4. *Supercompounding*

As discussed in section 2.3 and 2.4, the supercompounding technique is based on the two-dimensional spin average concept. To satisfy equation 7 in practice, the discrete method is used in the present study. By rotating the object and summing a multiplicity of images, we can approximate a continuous spin average. In theory, the rotational stepping degree θ is infinitely small. In practice, the angular stepping degree of the motor represents the travel step in the theory and equation 7 can be rewritten discretely as the following equation,

$$f_2s(r) = \int_0^{2\pi} f_d(r\cos\theta,\ r\sin\theta)d\theta \tag{12}$$

$$f_2s\left(r\right) = \frac{1}{N}\sum_{M=1}^{N} f_d(r\cos M\theta,\ r\sin M\theta) \tag{13}$$

where $f_2s(r)$ is the two-dimensional spin average function, f_d represents the image domains after the derotation process, θ is the stepping degree, M is 1,2,3,…,N and N is the total number of the derotated images (N=2π/θ). Either equation 7 or 12 is described in the polar coordinate system. To process the concept on the images which is described as a pixel grid, Cartesian coordinate system can be used to further simplify the process illustrated in the following equation,

$$f_{2S}\left(Dx,\ Dz\right)=\frac{1}{N}\sum_{M=1}^{N} f_{d,M}(Dx,\ Dz) \tag{14}$$

where Dx and Dz are coordinates in Cartesian system after the derotation transformation and $f_{d,M}$ represents the numbers of derotated images. Once the raw images are derotated properly, they can be substituted into equation 13 easily. The process can be broken down into three phases, (1) derotate raw images, (2) superimpose derotated images and (3) average the result. The illustration and the example of the supercompounding process are shown as Figures 19 and 20.

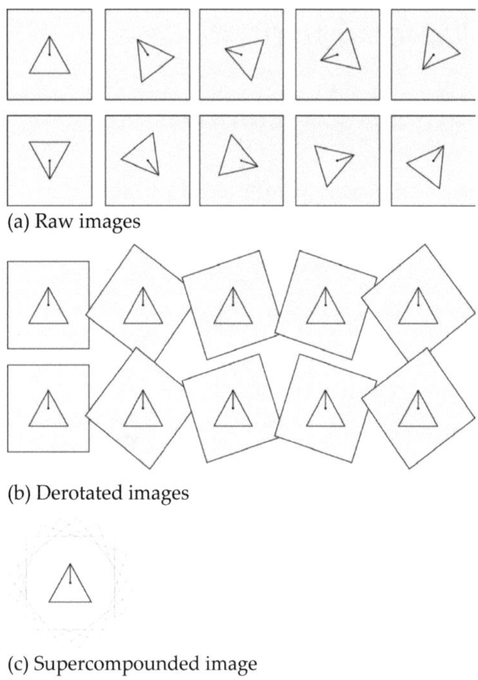

Figure 19. Illustration of the supercompounding process. The triangular object is rotated every 36 degrees counterclockwise and it makes the clockwise derotation. The supercompounded image is the superimposed image of all derotated images.

4. Results

In this research, two objects are studied: the metal pin heads and the dissected porcine aortic root. Each object is chosen for different purposes and together allows us to observe the performances of the spin average concept and the supercompounding technique under different circumstances. These selected objects also represent some issues that conventional ultrasound imagers face, which include the following:

- Non-circular point spread function (PSF): As stated in section 2.4, the PSF is not a circular point in the conventional ultrasound imagers. This is because the lateral resolution is several times worse than the axial resolution. Therefore, after the image convolves with the PSF, the output image from the ultrasound system could be several times more blurred in the lateral direction than in axial. To evaluate the supercompounded PSF, the metal pin head is selected.

- Circular object: Circular objects generally do not appear circular on ultrasound images. The edges of the two-side walls are usually missing because the incident ultrasound waves are reflected away-from instead of back-to the transducer. The ultrasound system cannot receive any signals coming from those regions and causes the image to dropout at oblique angles. The dissected porcine aortic root is used to test the imaging performance of circular objects like blood vessels or cysts. The tests of the aortic roots are collaborated experiments with Dr. Wei Sun [21] (Biomedical Engineering, University of Connecticut).

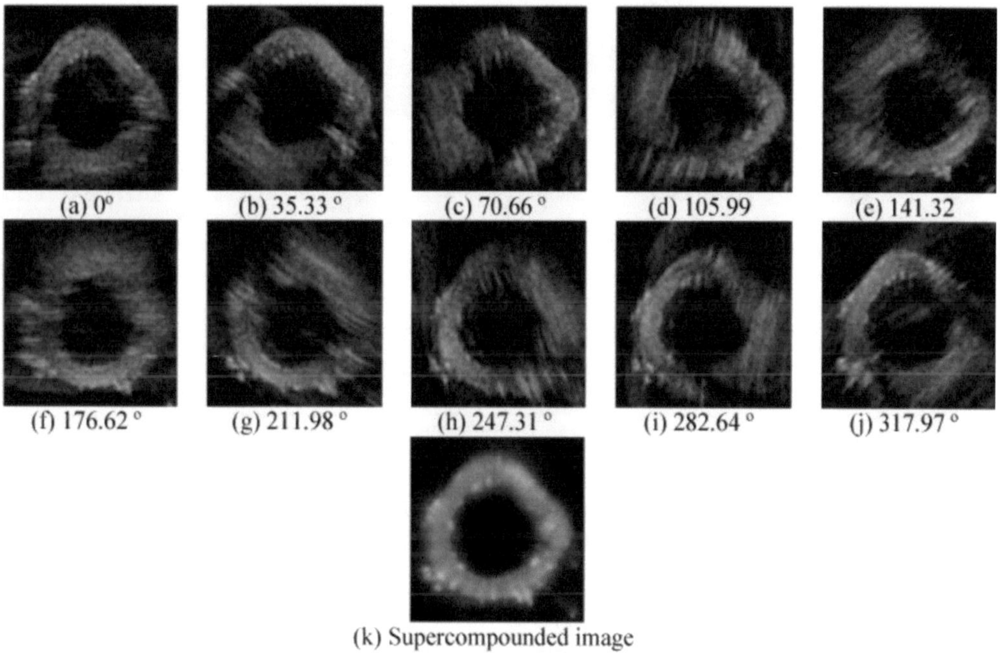

Figure 20. Example of supercompounding process with a porcine aorta. The results of (a) to (j) are the part of the derotated images taken from the every 1.68 degrees. (k) is the supercompounded image superimposed from 214 derotated images. Note multiple nodes of enhanced echogenicity become clear after supercompounding.

4.1. Imaging of metal pin heads

The metal pin heads used in the study are 0.5 millimeter diameter pin heads. They were selected for their small size and for their material, which is highly reflective when placed in water due to the acoustic impedance mismatch. Sound waves that hits this material cause massive reverberation, i.e. multiple reflections, in which create parallel lines under the object on the ultrasound images. Therefore, in addition to observing the offset of improving the point spread function, this test can be used to observe how supercompounding handles reflective material layers. Figure 21 is one of the raw images of the metal pin heads. The metal pin heads are arranged as a capital letter 'L'. All images are taken with the 7.5MHz linear transducer.

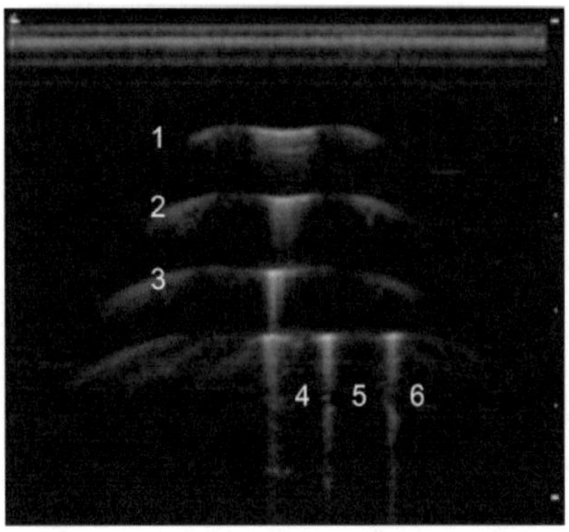

Figure 21. Metal pin heads are arranged as a letter L. The six objects are shown as "T" like shape instead of point like. The axial artifacts are caused by the reverberations inside the metal pin heads. The reverberations mislead the ultrasound imager that there are the same objects in consecutive depths. It makes multiple lines behind the objects. The pin number 1 to 3 and group 4, 5 and 6 are aligned at different depths. The focal zone is 27 millimeter in depth. It is at the middle of the pin number 3 and group 4, 5 and 6; therefore, the pin number 1, 2 and 3 are superficial to the focal point and the group 4, 5 and 6 are deep to the focal point.

Figure 21 shows artifacts on the image of six objects caused by reverberation. The objects are the metal pin heads and they should appear point like instead of a T-shaped with long tails (reverberations) and wings (side lobes). As stated in section 2.4, the point spread function is space variant in most conventional ultrasound imagers and causes size differences for the same objects depending on how far the object is away from the focal zone. In Figure 21, each pin represents the point spread function at one spatial position. The measurements of dimensions are described in Table 1.

Pin number	Lateral size	Axial Size	Depth
1	46 px	3 px	11.30 mm
2	31 px	4 px	17.99 mm
3	11 px	3 px	25.32 mm
4	13 px	4 px	31.80 mm
5	13 px	3 px	31.80 mm
6	13 px	3 px	31.65 mm

Table 1.

Pins 1-6 are all either three or four pixels in axial size regardless on reverberation artifacts. This translates to an average size of 0.56 ± 0.086 mm.

The lateral sizes, however, vary depending upon the depths and the distance from the focal zone. The pin closer to the focal zone (27 mm) has better lateral resolution. The average size in the lateral direction is 3.59 ± 2.38 mm, which is seven times larger than the actual size. The best result is the pin number 3. It is 1.7 mm away from the focal zone (27mm – 25.32mm = 1.7mm), and with a lateral size is 1.83 mm, it is still three times larger than the actual size of the metal pin head. Figure 22 compares the raw image with the supercompounded image constructed from 214 derotated raw images.

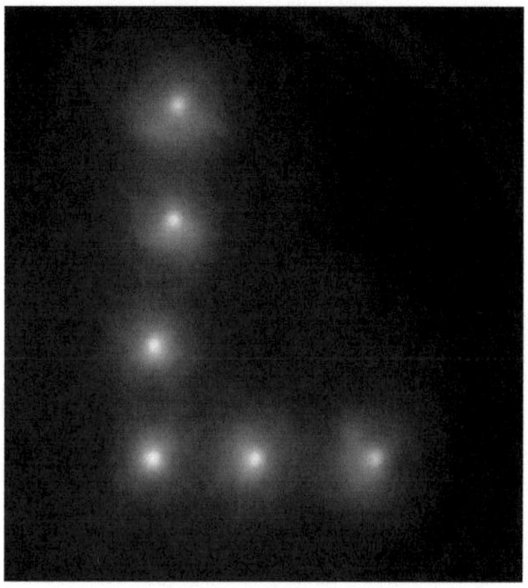

Figure 22. Supercompounded image. Comparing to Figure 4.1, the artifacts are significantly reduced and the result shows each point has similar circular shape and is tighter and more symmetric.

In Figure 22, six points appear instead of the T-shape. The artifacts from reverberation are significantly reduced as well. The measurements are included in Table 2.

Pin number	Lateral size	Axial Size	Depth
1	5 px	6 px	N/A
2	5 px	5 px	N/A
3	5 px	5 px	N/A
4	4 px	6 px	N/A
5	4 px	4 px	N/A
6	4 px	4 px	N/A

Table 2.

The average size in lateral direction is 0.86 ± 0.09 mm and 0.835 ± 0.15 mm in the axial. They are one and half times larger than the actual size of the pin head in all directions. As discussed in section 2.5, the supercompounded PSF should be closer to the axial resolution.

4.2. Imaging of dissected porcine aortic root

The study objects in this section are dissected porcine aortic roots. Each target is scanned under different pressures and levels (Figure 23), and the images are taken during the inflation test of the aortic root. The inflation test simulates the mechanical response of the aorta under different blood pressure ex-vivo. Different stress levels are simulated when the hydrostatic pressure supply inflates the target.

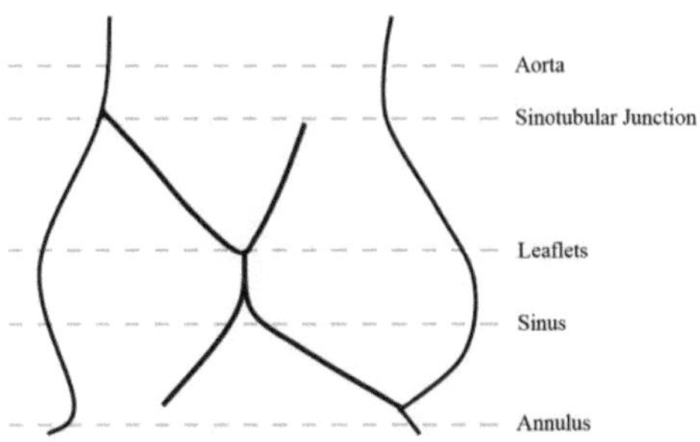

Figure 23. Illustration of aortic root. The root is scanned at five different levels named aorta, sinotubular junction, leaflets, sinus and annulus.

The study is focused on the geometry of the aortic valve, which can be used as a standard model to calculate volume changes during the inflation test. The raw images are collect with the 7.5MHz linear transducer. In this research, after derotating and spin averaging the 214 pictures, the resulting supercompounded picture at aorta level is shown in Figure 24 and Figure 25.

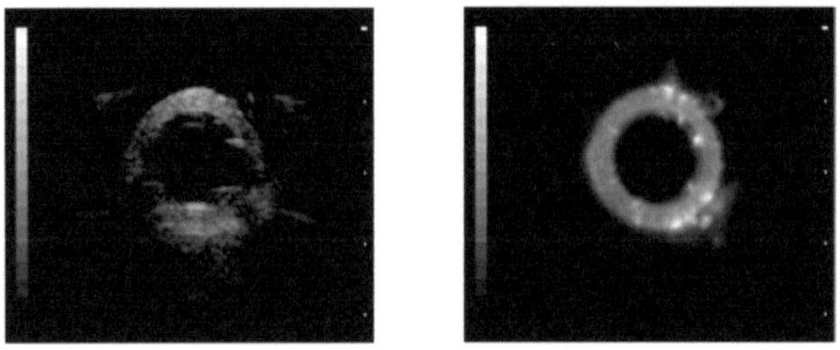

(a) raw image (b) Supercompounded image

Figure 24. The dissected porcine aortic root at aorta level.

The raw B-scan image Figure 24(a) shows sound waves that are dropped-out (region 2 and 3 in Figure 25) at the oblique angles to the normal line of the tissue structure interface. This phenomenon happens when circular shape objects (such as vessels) or spherical objects (such as cysts) are imaged. The supercompounded image (Figure 24(b)), constructed by multi-angular images with an independent viewpoint, exposes each segment of boundary to normal incidence, thus reducing dropout. The entire vessel is symmetrical and intact and spots like echogenicities (arrows in Figure 25) become visible in the supercompounded image. The supercompounding technique enables the observation and study of these echogenicities and their properties.

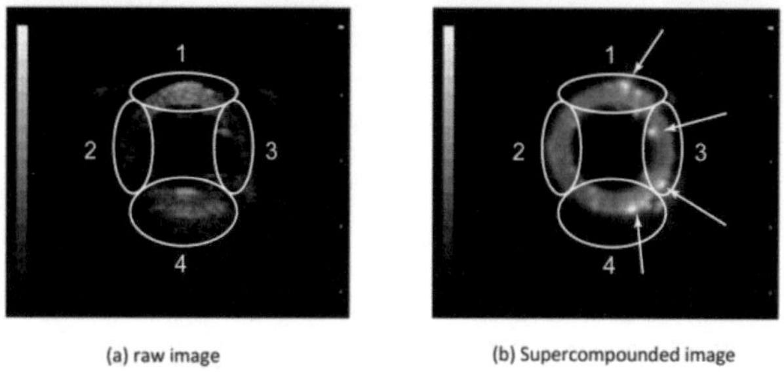

Figure 25. Comparison results of the dissected porcine aortic root at aorta level. Region 1 is the superficial area. It is close to the focal zone. It makes the best part of result on the raw image. Region 2 and 3 are the dropout areas. Because of the shape of structures in the regions are at the oblique angles to the incident ultrasound waves, the ultrasound waves are not reflected back to the transducer. It makes missing edges on the image. Region 4 is the out of focal zone area. Due to the worse PSF and the attenuation of the ultrasound waves, the structures in the area are not described accurately comparing to the same region on the supercompounded image. In the region 4 of the supercompounded image, the structures are clear and sharp, but they are blurry and several times larger on the raw image. The arrows point out the echogenicities which are not appeared on the raw image.

Not only can supercompounding fill the portions of tissues missed by conventional ultrasound imagers, but also can markedly reduce speckle noise in the image. The results shown in Figure 26 and Figure 27 are the aortic roots at leaflets level. Professionally trained eyes might be able to distinguish between an aortic root and the leaflet. Untrained eyes will find it hard to determine the boundaries and the size of the root.

In the raw image Figure 26 (a), the boundary is not clear especially away from the focal zone (region 5 in Figure 27) where is deep to the focal zone of the image. The supercompounded image Figure 26 (b) shows clear edges and details. We can now easily determine the location of the leaflets (region 2, 3 and 4 in Figure 27). The supercompounded image offers a better field of view as well, making the image more valuable and easier to read.

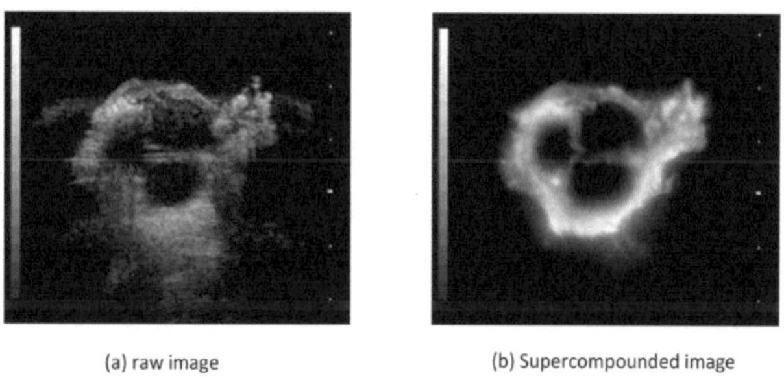

Figure 26. The dissected porcine aortic root at leaflets level.

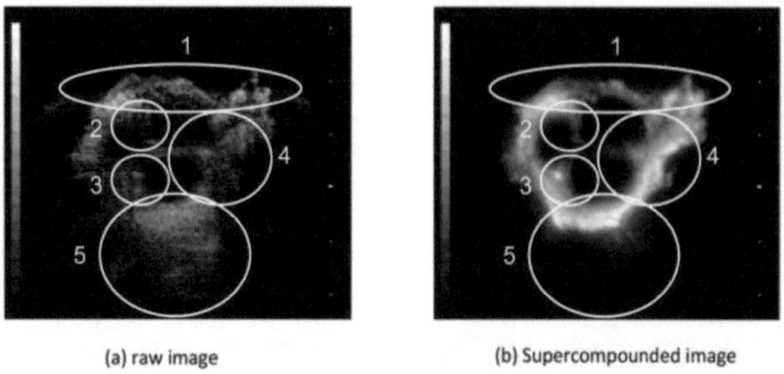

Figure 27. Comparison results of the dissected porcine aortic root at leaflets level. Region 1 is the area having the best result which is close to the focal zone. Region 2, 3 and 4 are the areas show three leaflets. As the result on the supercompounded image, three leaflets appear clearly. However, on the raw image, only the region 4 indicates or suggests a leaflet. The other two in the region 2 and 3 are barely recognized as leaflets. Region 5 is the deep area. It is out of the focal zone. Affected by the worse PSF and the attenuation of the ultrasound waves, the structures are not even close to the real object in the region.

5. Discussions and conclusions

Supercompounding is an innovative and still developing space compounding technique. It can be applied to traditional ultrasound imaging systems. As shown as this research, the supercompounding technique can provide dramatic improvement to the quality of ultrasonography of typical biologic tissues. The speckle, artifacts and reverberation are reduced, and we are able to visualize complete edges especially at oblique angles to the front of beam direction. However, these are not the only benefits of supercompounding. By utilizing the two-dimensional spin average theory it was shown that supercompounding can improve spatial resolution by regularizing the point spread function. It is a critical improvement to have an ultrasound image with a regular or space invariant point spread function that can potentially enhance performance by application of linear systems of signal processing algorithms.

Validation of supercompounding includes two main activities: ultrasound image acquisition and supercompounding processing. Ultrasound image acquisition includes the design and the construction of a three-dimensional moving platform. The platform allows the imaged object to rotate 360 degrees for testing the spin average concept and also to move in three directions for constructing a three-dimensional voxel set of information of the object, a set that could be used to produce a three-dimensional image.

The supercompounding processing has evolved in two sub branches: preprocessing and post-processing algorithms.

- Preprocessing technique produces a supercompounded image from derotating and combining the acquired raw image set. It is considered a preprocessing because the proposed supercompound imaging overcomes some of the physical limitations of ultrasound signals. It reduces speckles, shadows and reverberations and gives a regularized point

http://dx.doi.org/10.5772/53238

spread function across the ultrasound images. For example, a shadowed region in conventional ultrasound cannot be restored since the data is simply not present, or the point spread function may obscure fine details beyond the ability of post-processing to retrieve it. Another aspect to consider is that post-processing may be based on preconceived notions of what certain image regions should look like, thus providing inaccurate information of the imaged anatomy. Consequently, we consider the use of preprocessing techniques to be preferable as they provide "true" improvements in SNR and resolution [22].

- A regularized point spread function makes post-processing algorithms [22] (image enhancements) more beneficial to the supercompounded image, especially for linear systems algorithms like image deconvolution. By utilizing the two-dimensional spin average theory, supercompounding is shown to improve spatial resolution by having a regularized and tighter point spread function. Due to space variant resolutions in both axial and lateral directions, the point spread function of ultrasound image changes. Therefore, it is essential to have an ultrasound image with a regularized point spread function for further application of many signal processing algorithms. There is less need to make an assumption of the space invariant point spread function or to discretize the processed image into small pieces working windows when we process the ultrasound images.

- For example, a regularized point spread function can simplify the frequency filtering or deconvolution process which is one of the most straight forward and effective image sharpening methods. As discussed in section 2.1, the obtained image can be modeled as the result of a raw image convolving with a point spread function. This convolution is a blurring process. In order to get back to the original sharp image, the reverse process, namely "deconvolution", is required to restore the image before it convolves with the point spread function. However, it is not directly applicable on ultrasound images because of the space variant point spread function. Therefore, the deconvolution is applied regionally or not at all. Since the supercompounded image has a symmetric and regularized point spread function, the deconvolution process can be applied to the whole image without segmenting it [4, 23, 24]. Thus supercompounding provides a higher quality preprocessed image and also makes post-processing applications more viable and effective.

5.1. Supercompounding applications

The results in this study suggest that the spin average concept and the supercompounding technique can dramatically improve the quality of the ultrasound images. The following list points out three ways to utilize the supercompounding technique in clinically:

- Extremities: The supercompounding applicant could be utilized on extremities. It is easy to gain 360 degrees access around the extremities and usually the ultrasound waves can at least penetrate half of the thickness of the extremities (from superficial skins to the bones in the middle) even with higher frequency ultrasound transducers. It could potentially be a great way to diagnose and evaluate abnormalities of the muscles and the tendons, especially for sport medicine.

- Neck: The supercompounding technique could also be used on the neck for diagnosis of carotid atherosclerosis. If plaque builds up in the body's arteries, the condition is called atherosclerosis. Once the built up plaques narrow the common carotid arteries, the patient is under a high risk of cerebral flow reduction or stroke because of the reduced blood flow. The diagnosis is often evaluated by CT or multidetector-row CT angiography (CTA) [25] which utilizing ionizing radiation. Supercompounding ultrasound could offer a safer way to make the same diagnosis. The plaque is often calcified which particularly late stage can make it highly reflective. It can show high intensity on the ultrasound image. Plaques can be identified relatively easily. With the help of the supercompounding technique, the disease could be diagnosed more cost-effective and without exposing patients to the ionizing radiations once a proper mechanical supporting apparatus is designed for 360 degrees scan around the neck.

- Abdomen: Ultrasound imaging is widely used to image certain organs in the abdomen such as the liver, kidneys and pancreas. However, the evaluation is highly related to experiences and training of the radiologist. For instance, a patient who has liver cancer could have different kind of reports depending on the image reading whether by radiologists or other professionals. Imaging can provide information on extend of metastasis often diagnosis of cancer is made. Abdominal ultrasound imaging usually is performed with low frequency transducer and has low resolution results. It is radiologists' responsibilities to discover the abnormalities. With the help of supercompounding, it could reduce the odds for such error. It would be easier for radiologists to identify abnormalities. Abdominal imaging is made challenging due to the thickness of the belly and the bowels (small and large intestines) which are filled with gas which blocks ultrasound propagations. Therefore, ultrasound in the abdomen is limited to a few "windows" where the probe can bypass the intestines and gain access. Even with the 3.5 MHz transducer (which is close to the lowest frequency presently used for ultrasound imaging), it is hard for the ultrasound waves to penetrate through the whole abdomen. There are two possible solutions to the task: one is to perform partial supercompounding and the other is to further lower the ultrasound frequency. The partial supercompounding might not help construct an image with complete edges of the object, but it could still be much better than one single raw image according to the spin average concept.

The second solution is to image the abdomen with lower ultrasound frequency such as 1-2MHz. The ultrasound waves might be able to penetrate through; however, the resolution might be worse than using 3.5MHz transducer since for such low frequency, the corresponding wavelength of sound (at 1MHz) is 154mm, assuming the speed of sound is 1540 m/s in soft tissue. It means the two objects have to be at least 154mm away from each other to be identified as different objects on the ultrasound image when 1MHz transducer is used. Comparing two supercompounded images constructed from raw images scanned by the 7.5MHz and the 3.5 MHz transducers, there is no significant resolution reduction between the two supercompounded images, which is highly noticeable when we compare the two

http://dx.doi.org/10.5772/53238

raw images from the two transducers. This suggests that the resolution of the supercompounded images is not affected as much as the traditional raw images when we lower the frequencies of the ultrasound transducers. It is potentially a good way of obtaining a satisfactory resolution of the supercompounded image with lower frequency transducer without sacrifice of ultrasound penetration.

5.2. Conclusions

Advances in the technology of transducers, semiconductor devices, and computers have supported the implementation of enhancement techniques and the development of the industry of ultrasound in general. The present ultrasound imagers can provide higher signal-to-noise ratio and utilize transducer arrays with increasing numbers of elements. Consequently, the quality of the images has improved significantly especially compared to the earlier generation ultrasound imager used in the study (GE RT-3200). However, there has been no major breakthrough from physics point of view. The limitations of ultrasound imaging still remain such as the trade-off between penetration and frequency (resolution), space variant point spread function and sound wave self interference (speckle). These limitations sometime have become part of the ultrasound imaging, and by well training, radiologists or sonographers can work around them to some degree.

If it is possible to obtain higher quality tomographic images of the human body with ultrasound, the use of this technology can be extended to other applications where currently CT and MRI are used and make diagnosis more accurate, safer and more cost-effective for radiologists or sonographers. The proposed supercompounding imaging of ultrasound is a good approach to make ultrasound imagers perform beyond their present limitations. It works in harmony with the technology of modern ultrasound imagers. Supercompounding will benefit from better ultrasound transducers. The advantages would be to avoid the exposure of the patients to ionizing radiation and the availability of high quality soft tissue medical imaging at reduced cost. The unique sensitivity of ultrasound to soft tissues also makes it qualitatively superior to X-rays for many applications and it is a much faster modality than magnetic resonance. Overall we feel this technology could provide the impetus for an entire new generation of ultrasound imaging.

Author details

Tsuicheng D. Chiu[1], Sonia Contreras[2] and Martin Fox[3]

1 Biomedical Engineering, University of Connecticut, Storrs, CT, USA

2 Electrical and Electronic Engineering Program, Universidad Tecnologica de Bolivar, Bolivar, Colombia

3 Electrical & Computer Engineering, University of Connecticut, Storrs, CT, USA

References

[1] R. H. Gottliev, "Imaging for Whom: Patient of Physician?," American Jorunal of Roentgenology, vol. 185, pp. 1399-1403, 2005.

[2] J. J. Cronan, "Ultrasound: Is There a Future in Diagnostic Imaging?," Journal of the American College of Radiology, vol. 3, pp. 645-646, 2006.

[3] J. F. Moreau, "Re: "Ultrasound: Is There a Furture in Diagnostic Imaging?"," Journal of the American College of Radiology, vol. 4, pp. 345-357, 2007.

[4] T. Chiu, et al., "Supercompound imaging with Weiner deconvolution," in Proc. SPIE 7265, Orlando, FL, 2009.

[5] I. P. Herman, Physics of the Human Body. New York: Springer, 2006.

[6] R. F. Wagner, Smith,S.W.,Sandrik,J.M. and Lopez,H., "Statistics of Speckles in Ultrasound B-Scans," IEEE Trans. on Sonics and Ultrasonics, vol. 30, pp. 156-163, 1983.

[7] A. K. Jain, Fundamentals of Digital Image Processing. Englewood Cliffs, NJ: Prentice Hall, 1989.

[8] G. Wade, "Ultrasonic Imaging by Reconstructive Tomography," Acoustical imag., vol. 9, pp. 379-431, 1980.

[9] J. Greenleaf and R. Bahn, "Clinical Imaging with Transmissive Ultrasounic Computerized Tomography," IEEE Trans. Biomed Eng, vol. 28, pp. 177-185, 1981.

[10] D. E. Robinson and P. C. Knight, "Computer reconstruction techniques in compound scan pulse-echo imaging," Ultrasonic Imaging, vol. 3, pp. 217-234, 1981.

[11] C. B. Burckhardt, "Speckle in Ultrasound B Scans," IEEE Trans. Sonics Ultrason., vol. SU-25, pp. 1-6, 1976.

[12] P. M. Shankar, "Speckle Reduction in Ultrasound B-Scans Using Weighted Averaging in Spatial Compounding," Ultrasonics, Ferroelectrics and Frequency Control, IEEE Transactions on, vol. 33, pp. 754-758, 1986.

[13] Trahey, et al., "Speckle pattern correlation with lateral aperture translation: experimental results and implications for spatial compounding," IEEE Trans. UFFC, vol. 33, pp. 257-264, 1986.

[14] M. Diament and M. Malekzadeh, "Ultrasound and Diagnosis of Renal and Ureteral Calculi," J Pediatr, vol. 109, pp. 980-983, 1986.

[15] C. Sehgal, et al., "Ultrasound Transmission and Reflection Computerized Tomography for Imaging Bones and Adjoining Soft Tissues," in IEEE Ultrason Symp, Chicago, IL, 1988, pp. 849-852.

[16] J. R. Jago and T. A. Whittingham, "Experimental Studies in Transmission Ultrasound Computed Tomography," Physics in Medicine and Biology, vol. 36, pp. 1515-1527, 1991.

[17] R. N. Bracewell, Two-Dimensional Imaging. Englewood Cliffs, NJ: Prentice Hall, 1995.

[18] R. N. Bracewell, Fourier Analysis and Imaging. New York: Kluwer Academic/ Plenum Publishers, 2003.

[19] M. Fox, et al., "SHARP: Sonographic Histology by Axial Rotation of Projections," in 11th New England Doppler Conference, 2004.

[20] R. Lewis, Practical Digital Image Processing. London: Ellis Horwood, 1990.

[21] E. Sirois, Chiu, D., Fox, M., Sun, W., "Aortic Root Inflation Testing Utilizing the Supercompounding Algorithm for Ultrasonic Images," in Proc. of Biomedical Engineering Society, St. Louis, 2008.

[22] S. Contreras, "Compounding and Hexagonal Filtering for Ultrasound Enhancement," Ph.D., Biomdeical Engineering, University of Connecticut, Storrs, 2011.

[23] J. Nebeker and T. R. Nelson, "Enhancement of compounded ultrasound images with spatial filtering," in Proc. SPIE 7265-34, Orlando, FL, 2009.

[24] T. Chiu, et al., "Sharpening Ultrasonography by Compounding and Deconvolution," in Proc. of 34th NEBEC, Brown University, 2008.

[25] M. Wintermark, et al., "High-Resolution CT Imaging of Carotid Artery Atherosclerotic Plaques," American Journal of Neuroradiology, vol. 29, pp. 875-882, 2008.

Chapter 6

Ocular Movement and Cardiac Rhythm Control using EEG Techniques

María Viqueira, Begoña García Zapirain and
Amaia Mendez Zorrilla

Additional information is available at the end of the chapter

http://dx.doi.org/10.5772/55375

1. Introduction

There exist different methods to analyze and study biomedical signals. Some of these methods are based on medical imaging, involving Magnetic Resonance Imaging (MRI), Computed Tomography (CT), Nuclear Scintigraphy, etc. This techniques show the image of a specific part of the human body. But there exits other methods which study the different signals based in 1-dimensional analysis, such as Electroencephalography (EEG), Electrocardiography (ECG), etc. These do not show an image, but they also show relevant information.

These techniques are not only used to detect any anomaly, but in the case of the EEG, it is also possible to develop communication systems by Brain Computer Interface (BCI) [1]. The BCI technology has numerous applications which can improve the quality of life of those people who need external help at the time of communication or controlling their movements.

EEG records the electrical activity along the scalp produced by the neurons. This activity happens since the brain cells communicate each other giving place to tiny electrical impulses.

The impulse begins with a chemical discharge which origins a current in the membrane of the emitting cell. Once the impulse gets the extreme of the connection between cells, the neuron secretes a protein that inhibits or excites another neuron.

After receiving the signal, the neuron releases ions to the outside of the cell. When lots of ions are expelled at the same time they can stimulate other neurons. At the time this wave of ions gets to the electrodes, the ions can attract or push the metal of the electrodes. This difference of pressure can be measured by a voltmeter and the record of this activity along time is the EEG signal.

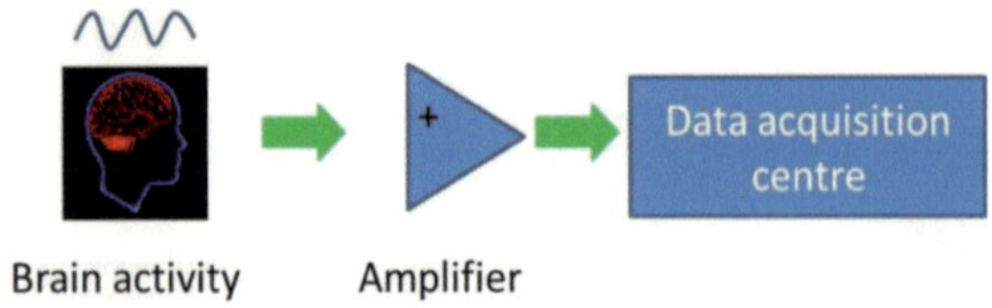

Figure 1. EEG operation

Different studies show that, with the correct training, it is possible to control different external devices with the BCI technology. In [2], Galán et al. present a study where two users have to control a wheelchair using a system based in BCI. They have concluded that the success has been higher after learning the interaction with the system.

With respect to the communication, the most used technique is the detection of the P300 wave as result of a photostimulus [3]. In these cases, the user has to watch one keyboard where the columns and rows are illuminated randomly. If the letter the person is watching is illuminated, the brain sends a signal as a response to that photostimulus. This answer is called P300.

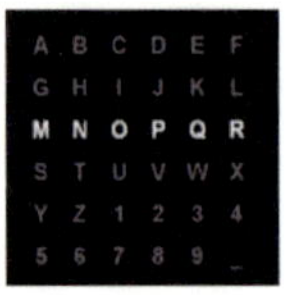

Figure 2. Keyboard used for the detection of P300. Source: http://www.bbci.de/competition/ii/albany_desc/albany_desc_ii.html

In [4] the authors use a system based on evoked potential to control one robotic arm. The system illuminates different actions which can be made by the arm. To know which action the user is focused, they detect the P300 and the N2pc.

There are also different applications of BCI technology in different games, such as Mindball [5], which consist on moving a ball depending on the brain activity: the more relaxed and focused the user is, the more the ball will move.

But electrodes are not only used to measure brain signals, but they also register the electrical activity from other parts, such as the heart (ECG) or the skeletal muscles (EMG). It is also possible to pick up the muscular activity, as it could be the measurement of the eye movements (EOG).

We have decided to use an EEG as electrocardiograph (ECG) and as electrooculography (EOG). The used device is the same for both applications: a portable EEG with 4 different channels.

This device was initially acquired to work in one application in which it was necessary to carry a portable EEG. Due to its portability, it can collect data during long periods of time and outdoors.

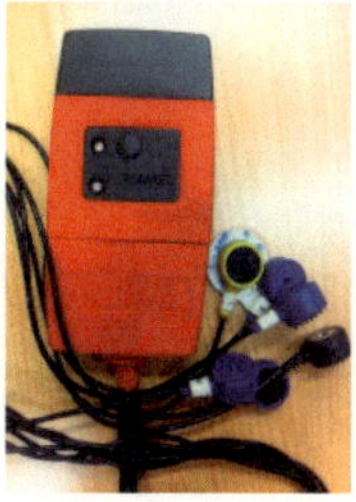

Figure 3. PET 4.0: EEG of 4 channels

The electrooculography (EOG) is based on the electrical activity of the eyes movement and it has been used for the user's communication. There are other applications based on the eye movements to control devices. They detect the user's iris, so it can know the position the user is looking through the coordinates of the iris. In [6] the study presents a method to control a wheelchair with one camera establishing three points as reference: the eyes and the nose. This three points form a triangle.

The ECG is a register of the electrical activity of the heart in order to know if there is any anomaly depending on the heart behavior.

We have used two different placements of the electrodes:

- Bipolar placement: each channel represents the difference between two adjacent electrodes. This montage has been used for the EOG.
- Referential or monopolar placement: each channel represents the difference between one electrode and another one established as reference. The ECG has been acquired with this montage.

The chosen electrodes are adhesive because of their facility to be placed both in the face as well as in the breast. The diameter of each electrode is 24 millimeters.

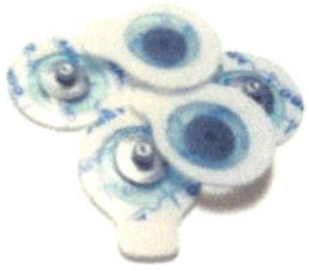

Figure 4. Kendall Arbo electrodes. Source: http://www.brainquiry.com/KendallArbo.html

The electrodes are responsible for registering the voltage inside a single cell. An electric impulse, known as the action potential, is an electric discharge which travels along the cellular membrane. The action potential is used to transport the information between the tissues. Although they can be generated for different kind of corporal cells, the most active are the cells of the nervous system [7].

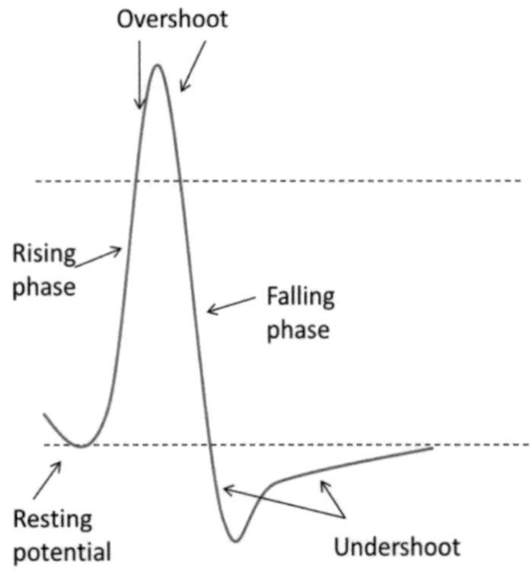

Figure 5. Action potential

For the monitoring and the posterior analysis we have developed two user's interface in Matlab: one for the ECG and another one for the EOG.

2. Relation between EEG and EOG

During the register of an EEG, there can appear different signals called artifacts. These signals can be originated by multiple causes: muscular movements, skin impedance, technical problems, etc. One of the causes of these artifacts can be the ocular movement, such as eye blinking. This electrical activity is registered in the frontal region of the brain, being FP1, FP2 the channels where can best be appreciable.

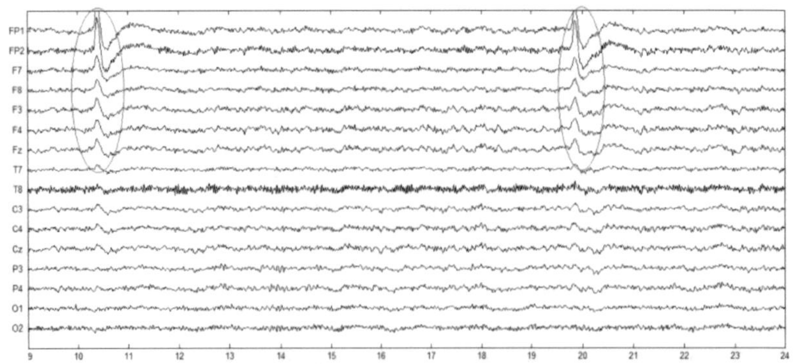

Figure 6. EEG with two eye blinking

But to register the eye activity it is not necessary to place the electrodes on the head, it can be registered placing the electrodes in the face, which is called EOG.

An EOG is a method to register the eyes movement by placing little electrodes near the eyes muscles. Under normal conditions there exists a potential difference (10μV to 5 mV approximately) between the cornea and the Bruch´s membrane, located on the back of the eye. This is known as cornea-retinal potential. The cornea corresponds to the positive extreme and the retina corresponds to the negative of the dipole.

Figure 7 represents the differential of potential between the cornea and the retina:

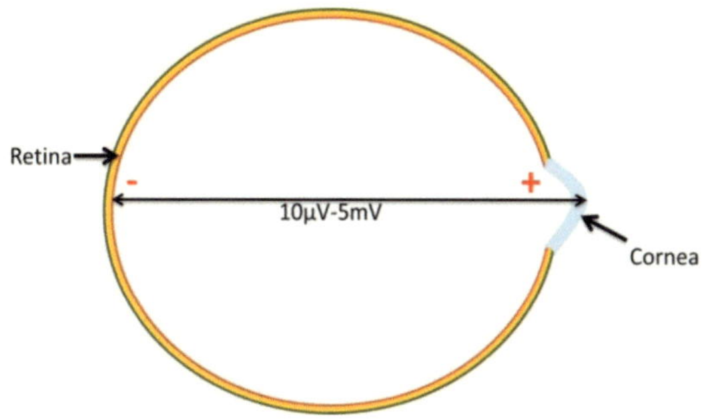

Figure 7. Cornea - retinal potential

Figure 8 show the behavior of the eye as a dipole:

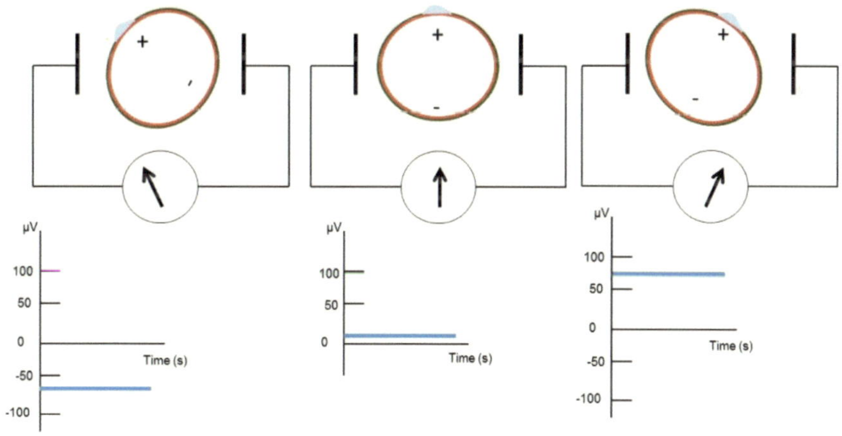

Figure 8. Eyes movement potential

In [8] it is well explained the different kinds of eye tracking systems and the evolution of them. For studying the eyes movement the criteria for divide the different techniques is different. There are three different kinds of eye tracking:

- Invasive technique: this technique uses a special contact lens with an incorporated mirror or a magnetic field senor. The data acquired are more detailed because it is in contact with the eyeball, but is more uncomfortable because the user has to wear the contact lens.
- Electrical potential: it uses electrodes placed around the eyes to detect the movement [9]. It is a robust method to measure the ocular movements when there are eyes blinking or change of the gaze. The main disadvantage is that it may become uncomfortable and the register can be affected by the electrodes movement. One of the main advantages is that it registers the eye movement with closed eyes so they can be used in the analysis of sleeping problems [10] and [11]. The EOG is within this kind of eye tracking.
- Non - invasive technique: there is no contact with the eyes. The eyes movement is located through a camera or an optical sensor. The infrared light generates different reflections of the cornea of the user's eyes known as Purkinje images [12] and [13].

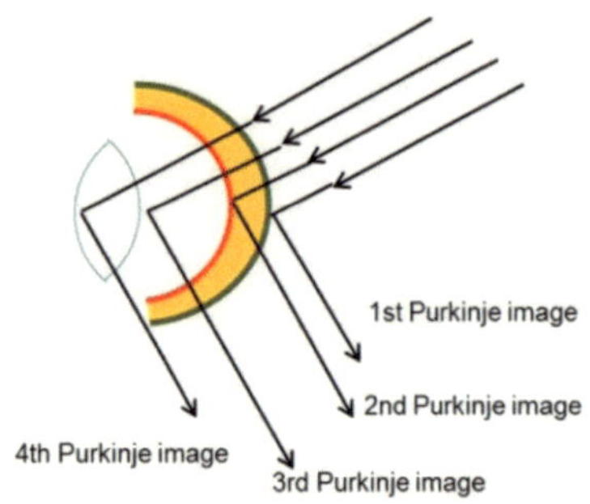

Figure 9. Purkinge images

The montage of the electrodes is bipolar: we register the difference between two electrodes. As the device is a 4 channel EEG, we have used them to perform 2 different positions: one for register if the user is looking on the left or on the right; and a second one to check if the user is looking up or down. The reference electrodes are placed in the ears.

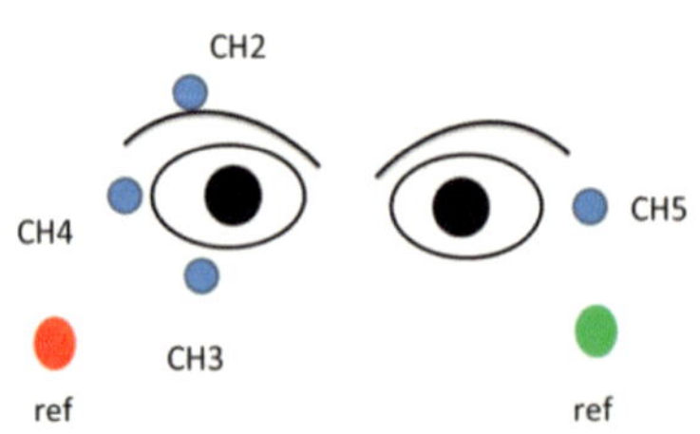

Figure 10. Electrodes position of EOG

The difference between channels 2 and 3 shows whether the user is looking up (positive) or down (negative). The difference between channels 4 and 5 determines if the user has looked to the left (positive) or to the right (negative).

http://dx.doi.org/10.5772/55375

The final application will have one user interface divided into two tasks:

- Communicate between the device and the main application via Bluetooth.
- Interpret what the user wants to express.

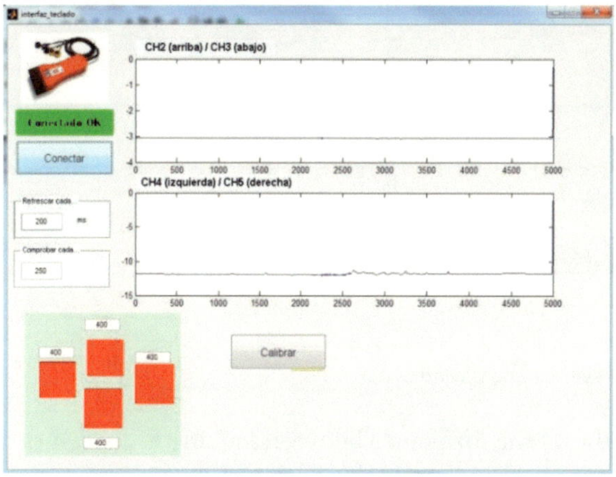

Figure 11. User's interface of EOG

For the first task, we have used the API provided by the fabricant. To allow the user's communication, the application will show the same keyboard as Figure 12:

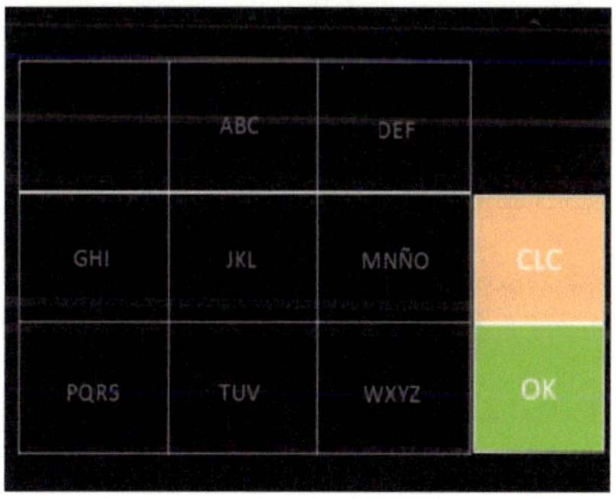

Figure 12. Keyboard

The user moves one circle through the keyboard by moving his eyes to the left, to the right, up or down. Once the user selects "OK", the application will use the T9 dictionary to interpret the correct word. The dictionary has been programmed taking in count the words which meaning is related with expressing feelings and emotional states.

Figure 13 show the difference between looking up and looking down. The subtraction of CH2 and CH3 accentuates the difference between the eye movements.

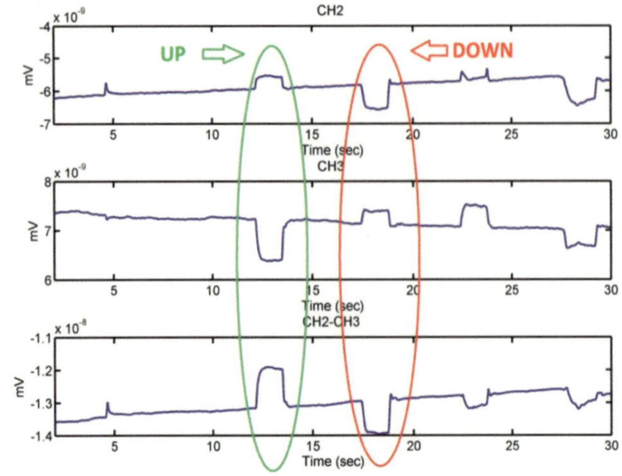

Figure 13. Difference between looking up and down

In Figure 14, which shows the difference between looking to the left or to the right, it can be seen that the situation is similar than looking up and down: looking to the left produces an increment of the signal value, while looking to the right decrements it.

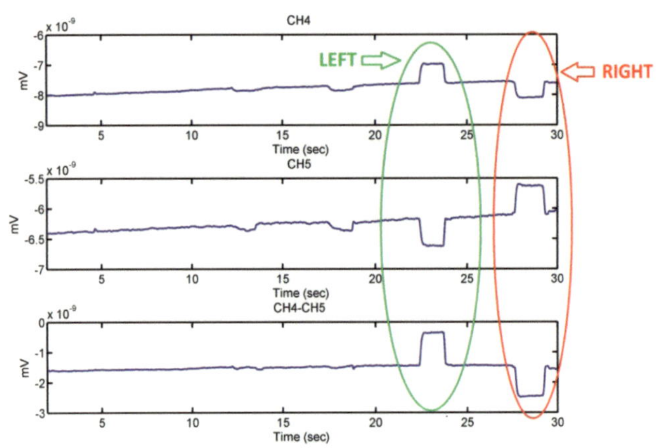

Figure 14. Difference between looking to the left and to the right

3. Relation between EEG and ECG

An ECG is the graphical representation of the electrical activity precedent from the heart. It is a non - invasive method to study and to analyse the condition of the heart with the aim of detecting possible anomalies or diseases.

In order to synchronize the cyclical contraction of the heart, the fibers of the cardiac muscle transmit electrical impulses.

The electrical activity is the potential difference generated by the cardiac cells (each cell acts as a voltage generator) which are appreciable on the skin surface, where the electrodes pick up this activity in order to get a graphical representation.

This representation shows 4 significant parts:

"P Wave": the cardiac cycle begins with the depolarization, which leads on the contraction of the atriums in order to deposit the blood in the ventricles. The sinus node (SA node) indicates the atrium muscles that they have to contract to begin the sequence. The potential action is propagated through the specialized cells of the cardiac muscle to the AV nodule.

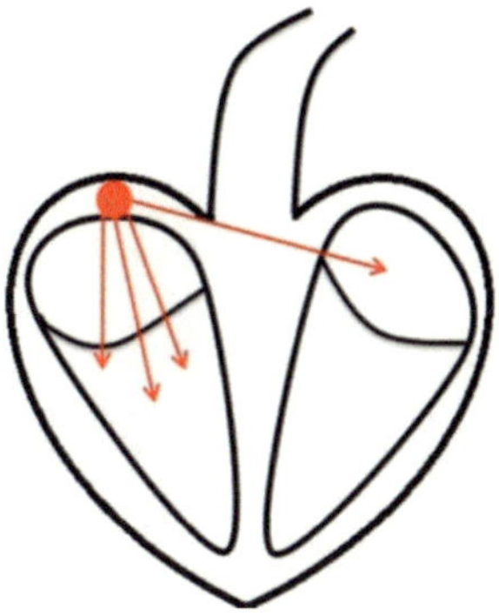

Figure 15. Atrial systole

"QRS complex": the wave of depolarization arrives to the ventricles through the Bundle of His and the Purkinje fibers, producing the contraction of the ventricles.

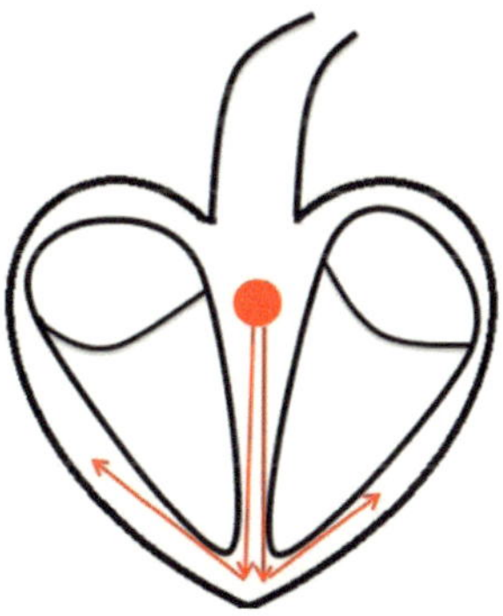

Figure 16. QRS complex

"ST segment": indicates the time between the end of the contraction of the ventricles and the beginning of the resting period.

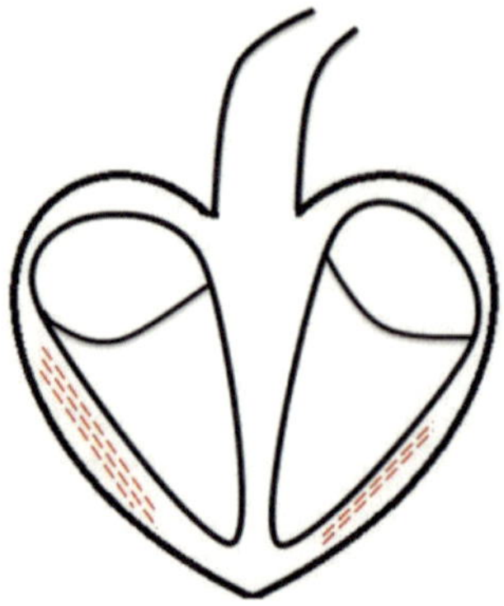

Figure 17. ST segment

"T wave": indicates the repolarization of the ventricles.

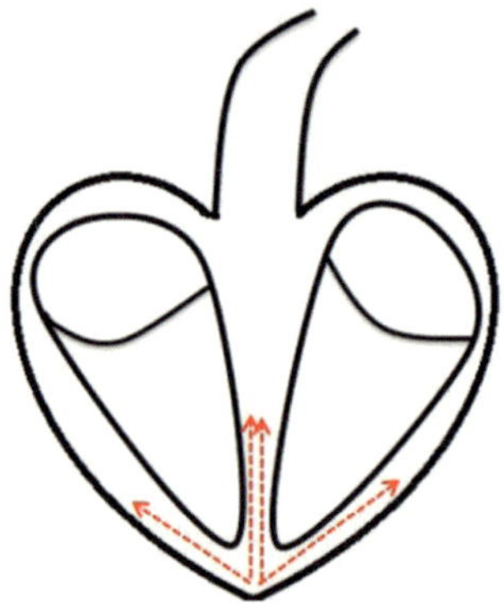

Figure 18. T wave

Figure 19 is the representation of a normal ECG. There can be appreciated the different waves explained before.

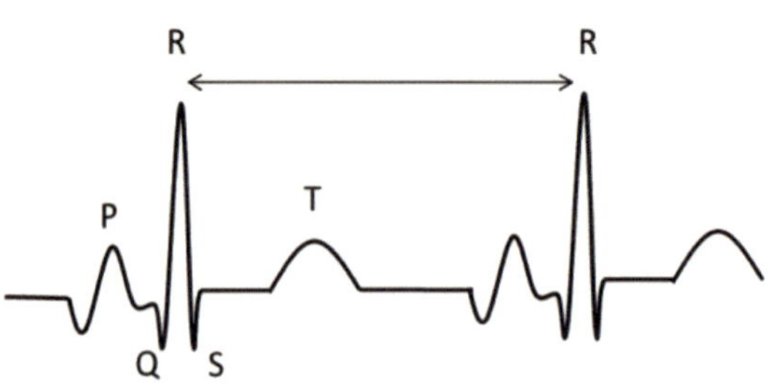

Figure 19. Heart signals

When the electrical impulse arrives to a cardiac cell it provokes the interchange of ions inside the cell, giving place to a change of polarity. The action potential is the base for the depolarization and polarization of the myocardium: it is what generates the electrical impulse.

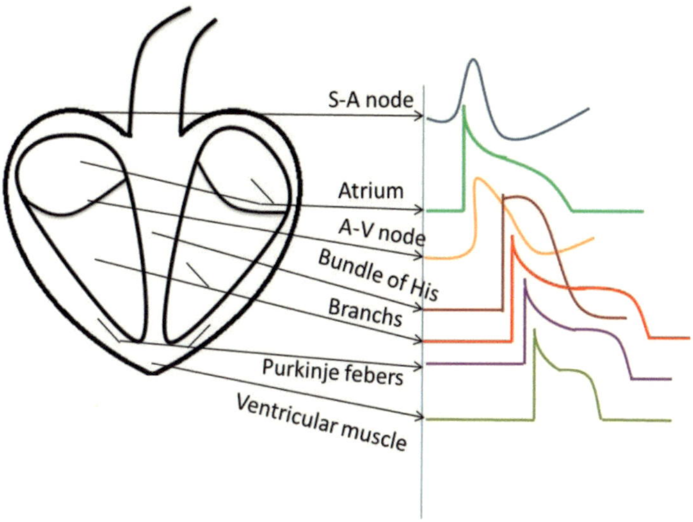

Figure 20. Cardiac action potential

The electrodes are places along the trunk of the users, taking the shoulders as reference. Figure 21 shows the position of the electrodes for the correct register of the ECG.

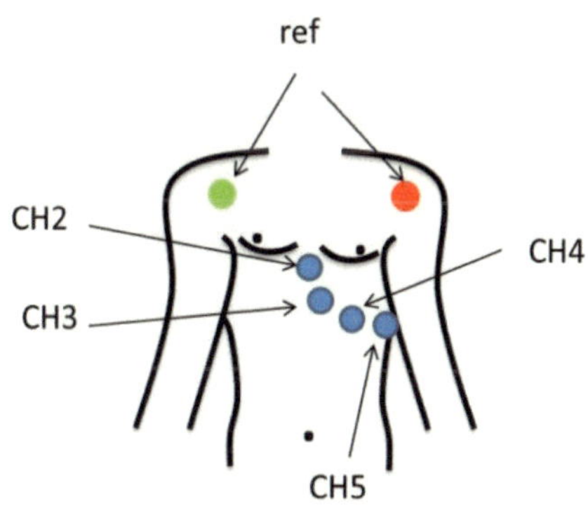

Figure 21. Electrodes placement

The user's interface has the aspect of Figure 22. The user can select the channels in both graphs.

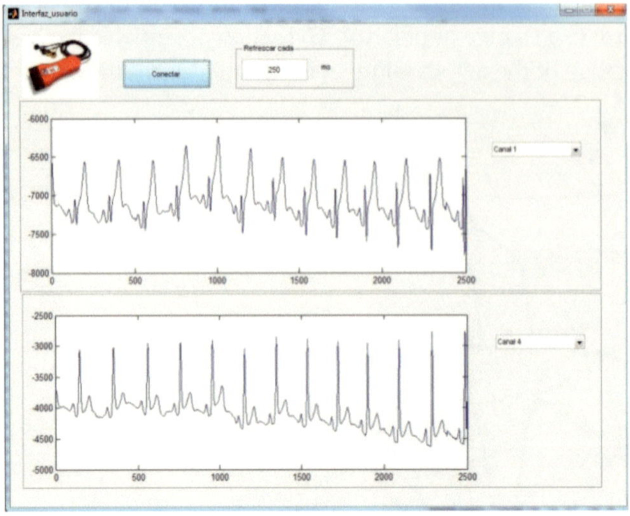

Figure 22. User's interface for ECG

4. Practice examples

4.1. EOG

In this section, it will be described how the EOG has been used to move a mark along a keyboard on the screen in order to help the people who are not able to communicate with the rest due a disease.

First of all, the application calibrates the position of the electrodes and establishes the correspondent thresholds to know the position of the eyes. After that, it will show the keyboard the user will use for the communication.

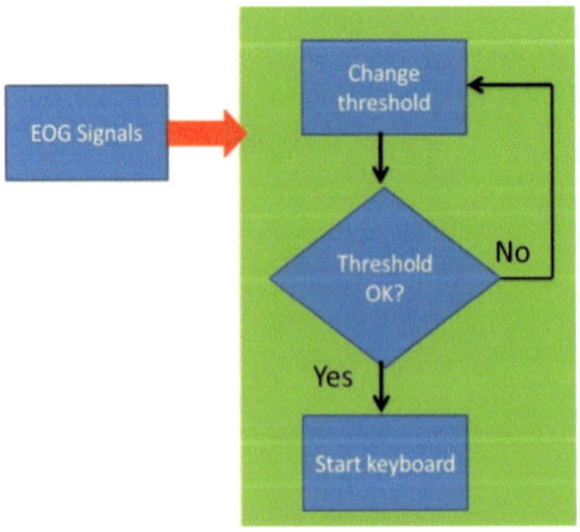

Figure 23. General diagram

http://dx.doi.org/10.5772/55375

Once the application shows the keyboard, it will do the operations described in Figure 24 and Figure 25 to know if the user has made any action with the eyes.

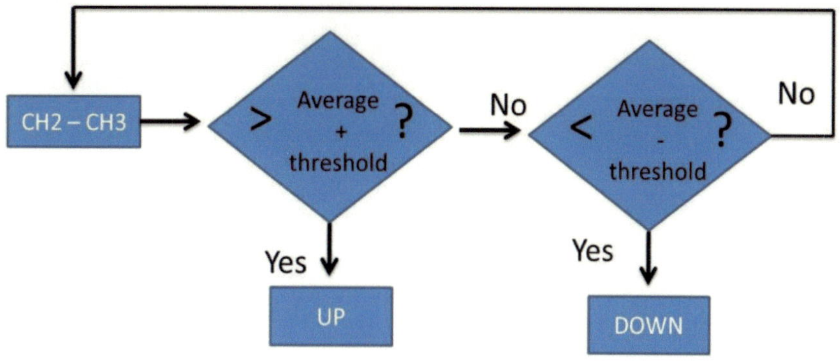

Figure 24. Up and down criterion

The signal is obtained during 200ms and then the application calculates the average during this time interval. After that, it compares if there has been an enough increment or decrement to detect if the user has moved the eyes intentionally.

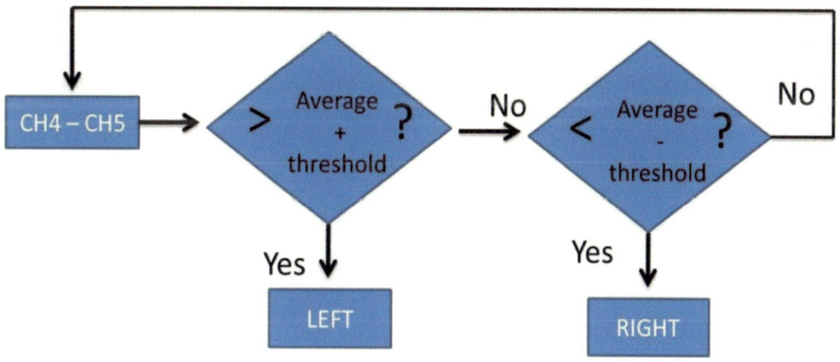

Figure 25. Left and right criterion

Figure 26 and Figure 27 show the calibration state of the EOG before showing the keyboard. The first two images correspond to looing up (yellow rectangle) and down (green rectangle).

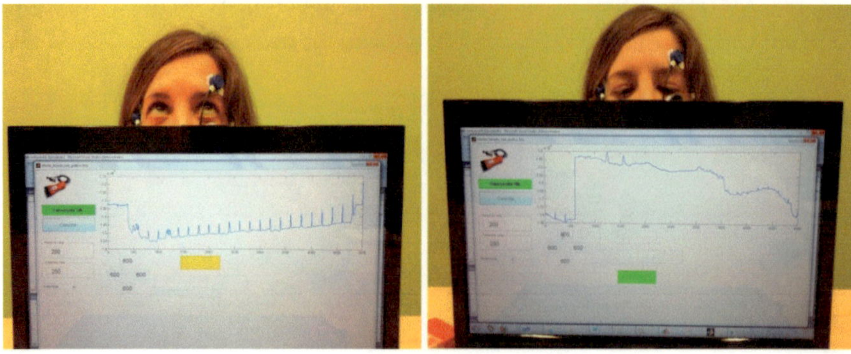

Figure 26. Looking up and down

Below, the pictures show the user looking to the left (dark blue) or to the right (cyan).

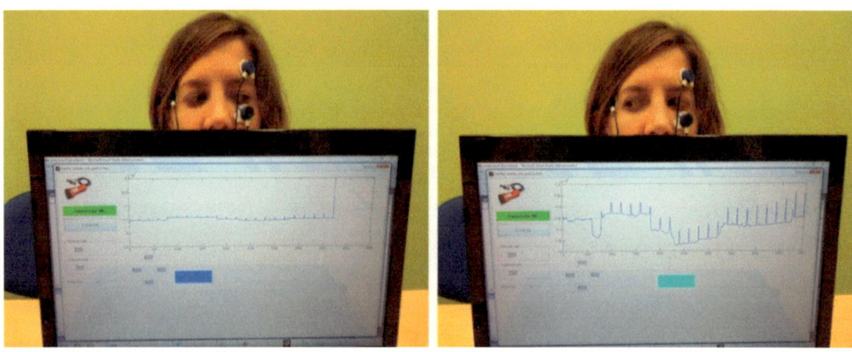

Figure 27. Looking to the left and to the right

The EOG has been tested with 5 different users (3 female, 2 male) with ages between 23 and 30. They have been asked to spell 5 different words: WATER, FISH, SUN, DOG and MIND.

4.2. ECG

This section describes the ECG used to monitor the heart activity and to detect possible anomalies. In this case, the montage is monopolar, so we can obtain information from 4 different points (4 channels), establishing as a reference the user's shoulders. The signals the ECG records are smoothed before being monitored.

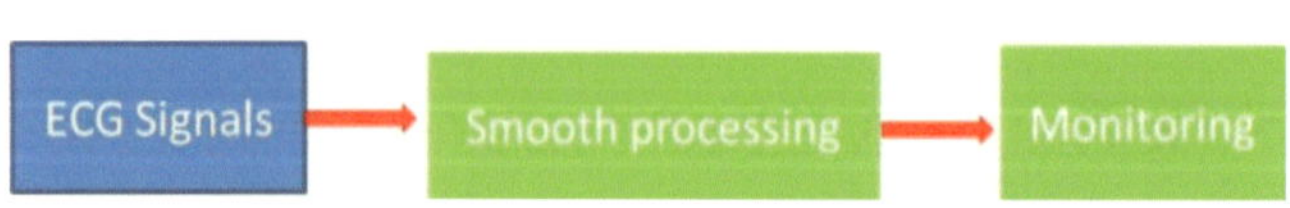

Figure 28. General diagram of ECG monitoring

http://dx.doi.org/10.5772/55375

After acquiring the signal (Figure 29), it is filtered with a Butterworth bandpass filter between 15Hz and 50Hz to detect the QRS complex (Figure 30).

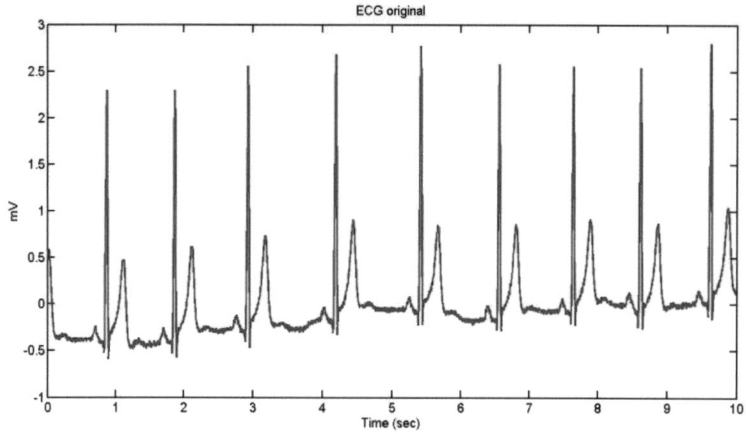

Figure 29. Original ECG

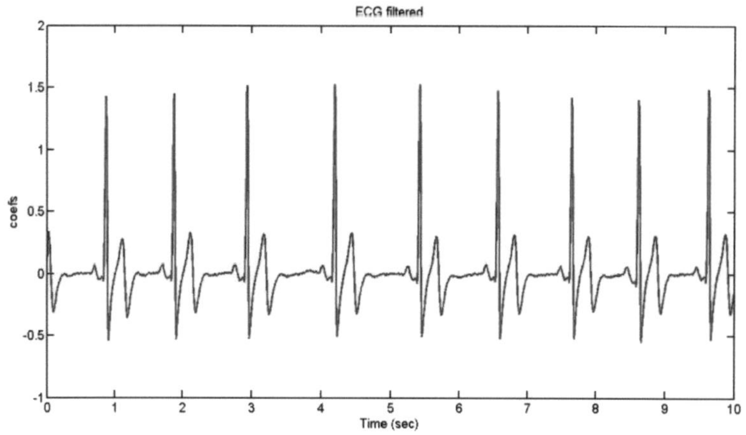

Figure 30. Butterworth filter

Once the signal has been filtered, we have established a threshold to facilitate the detection of the R wave (Figure 31):

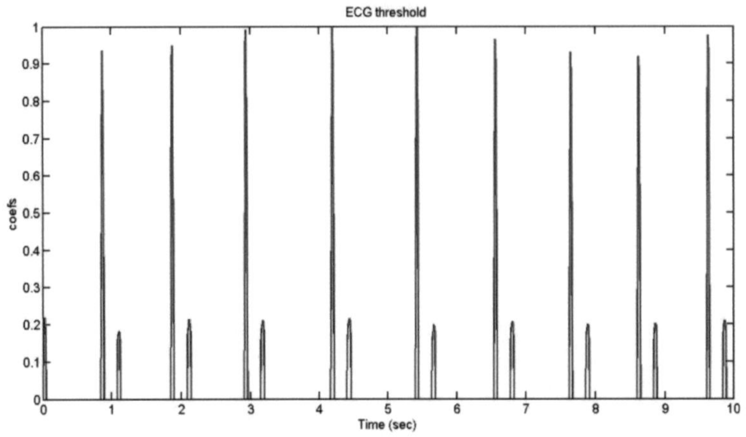

Figure 31. Signal after establishing the threshold

$$\textit{if data}\ (i) < 2^{*}\textit{average} - \textit{data}\ (i) = 0$$

5. Results

5.1. EOG

We have asked the users to move a circle along a keyboard to spell five different words. We have divided the results into areas: the spelling of the whole word and the spelling of the single letters.

It has been established that if the user expends more than three attempts to move the mark, the objective letter is considered as an error.

Table 1 shows the obtained results for the different users:

	User 1	User 2	User 3	User 4	User 5
WATER	o	o	o	o	o
FISH	x	o	x	x	o
SUN	o	o	o	o	o
DOG	o	o	o	o	o
MIND	o	o	x	o	o
Average letter	78.95%	100%	84.21%	89.47	100%
Average word	80%	100%	60%	80%	100%

Table 1. Spelled words by users

http://dx.doi.org/10.5772/55375

Table 2 contains the average of each word by letter and by users. The number inside the parenthesis indicates the total number of letters of each word involving the five sessions (five different users).

	Average by letters	Average by users
WATER (25)	100%	100%
FISH (20)	65%	40%
SUN (15)	100%	100%
DOG (15)	100%	100%
MIND (15)	90%	80%

Table 2. Average of each word

After establishing different thresholds, it is possible to select the wished letter controlling the movement with the eyes with an average of the 90.53%.

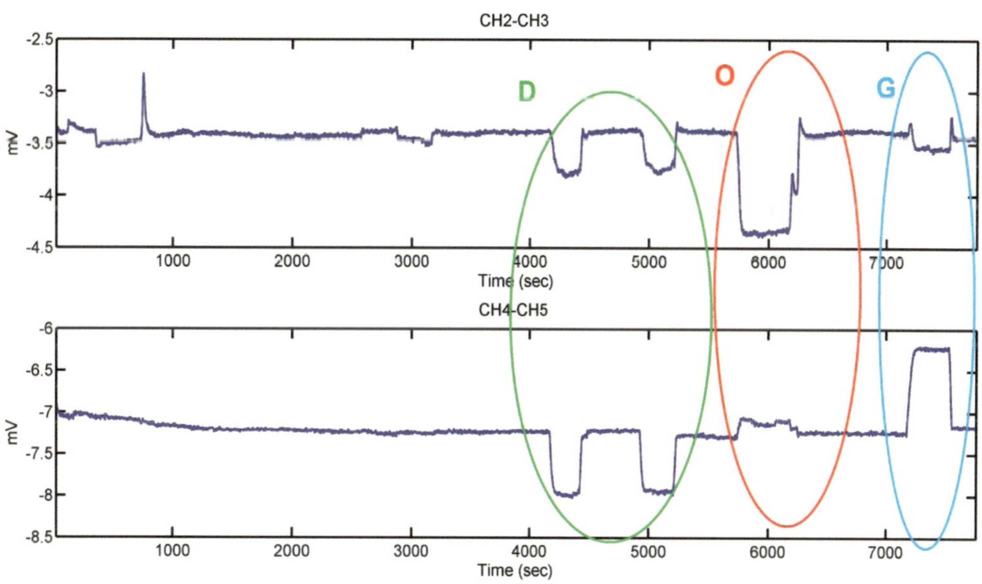

Figure 32. Eye movements for the word DOG

Figure 32 and Figure 33 present the different movements for the spelling of the words DOG and WATER respectively.

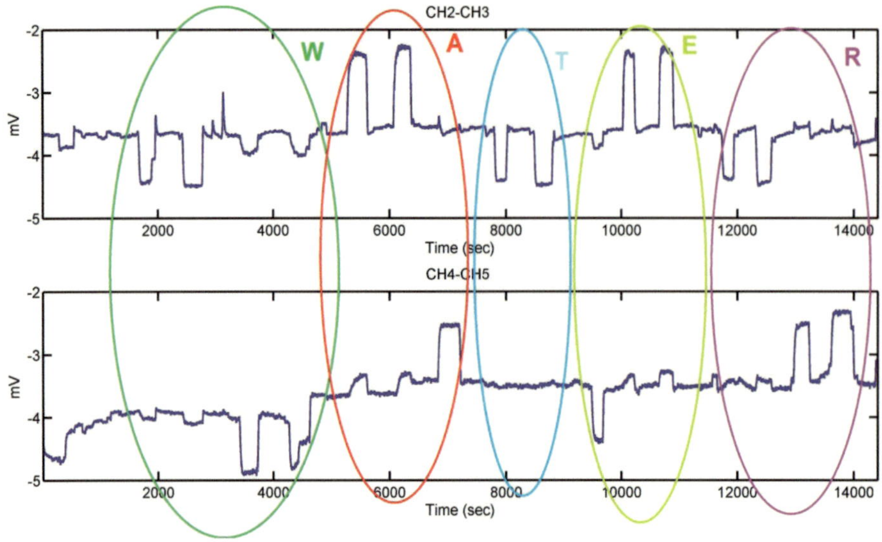

Figure 33. Eye movements for the word WATER

The following two graphs are presented where the word FISH is correctly spelled (Figure 34) and wrongly spelled (Figure 35).

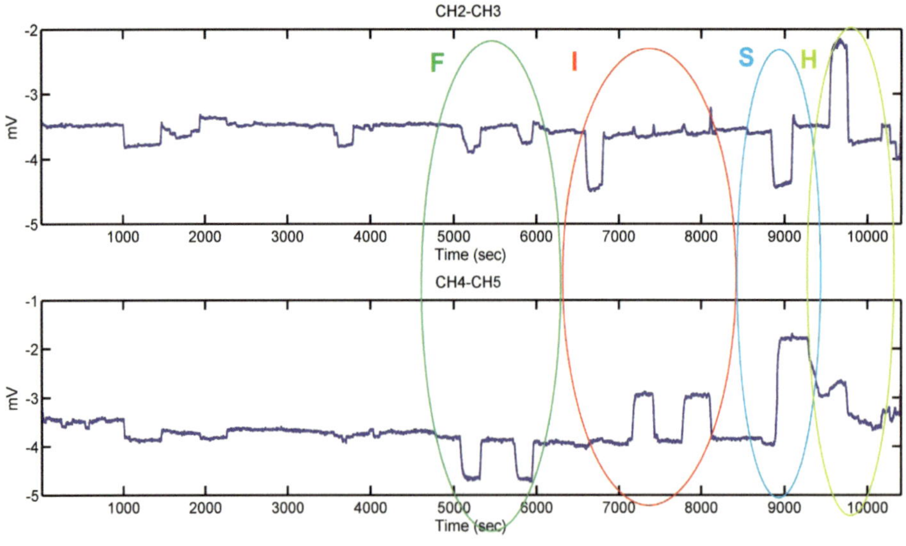

Figure 34. Word FISH well spelled

It can be seen that an exception has happened with the EOG at the time the user was spelling fish.

http://dx.doi.org/10.5772/55375

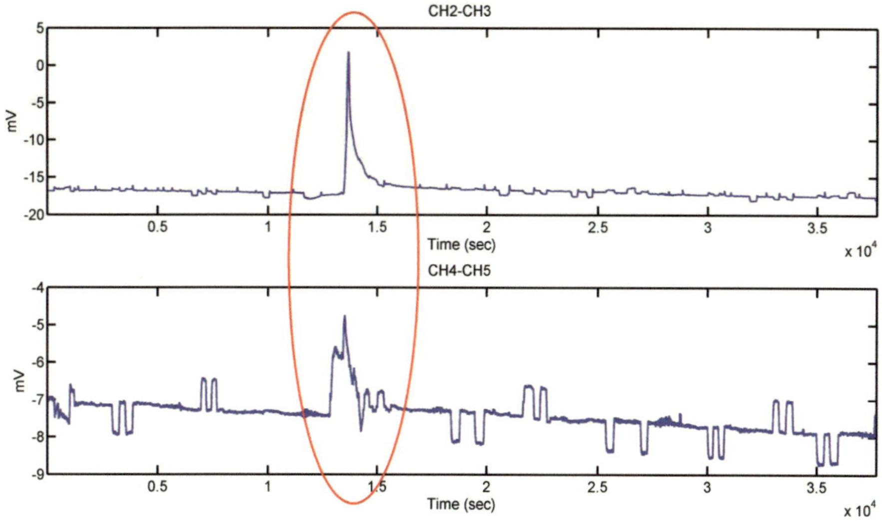

Figure 35. Word FISH bad spelled

5.2. ECG

The ECG allows the detection of the principal waves for the posterior analysis of anomalies.

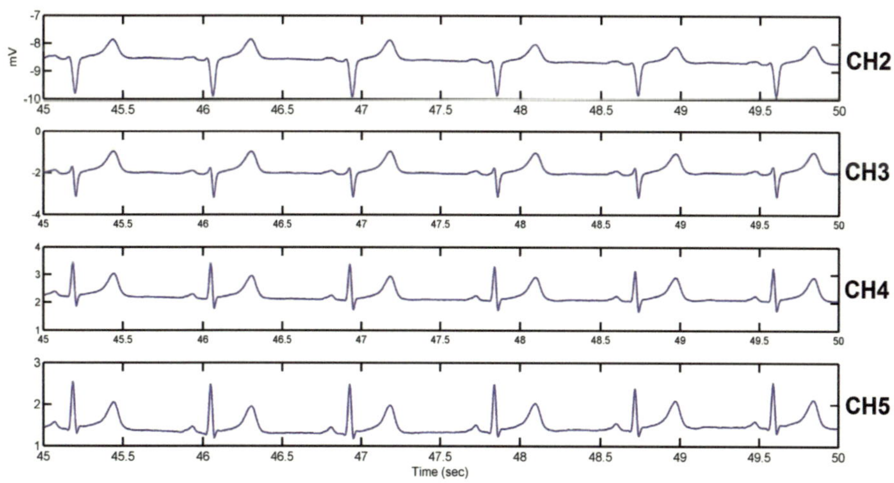

Figure 36. Normal ECG

The ECG shown in Figure 37 presents a premature ventricular contraction after the T wave.

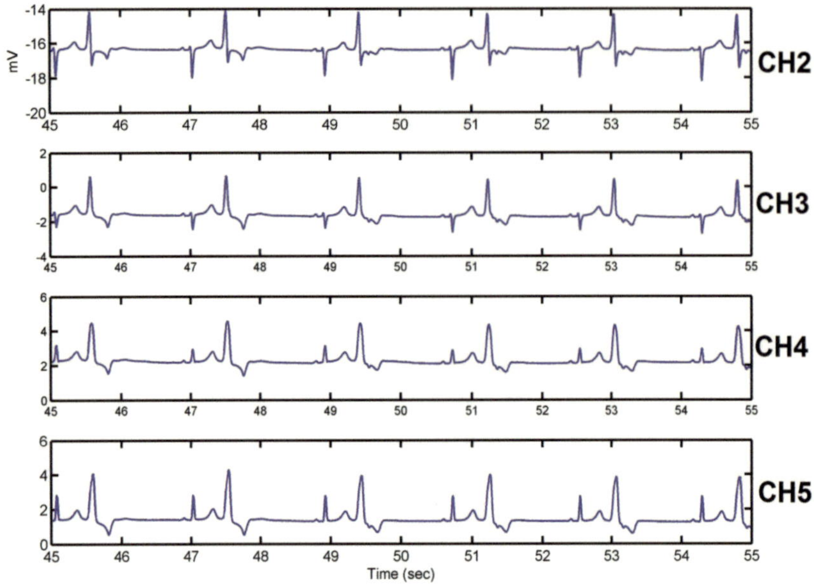

Figure 37. ECG for different channels with anomaly

Figure 38 contains an ECG with arrhythmias: the cardiac frequency presents an alteration in the second 83 and the second 86.

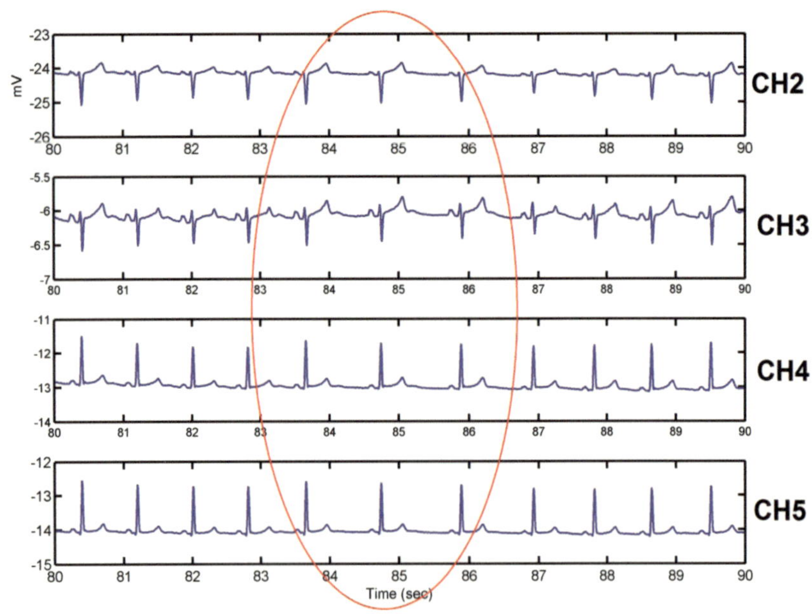

Figure 38. ECG for different channels with arrhythmias

http://dx.doi.org/10.5772/55375

The three graphs explained above correspond to three different users, showing the channels acquired for the 4 electrodes. The first one presents a normal ECG while the other two present two kinds of anomalies: premature ventricular contraction and arrhythmia.

Comparing the normal ECG with the rest, it can be seen that there are differences between the form of the wave and the RR intervals. In the second graph, there is a beat which is advanced in respect of a normal frequency. Because of that, the second graph presents few numbers of RR intervals (6 beats in 10 seconds).

Regarding to the third graph, the form of the waves is similar than the normal ECG, but the heart frequency is not constant: it can be appreciated that the heart frequency is not constant due to a little pause between the seconds 83 and 86.

6. Conclusions

As it has been demonstrated, the sensors used in BCI have an extra potential for applications which need high sensitivity.

The signals recorded by an EEG, an EOG and an ECG are bioelectrical signals; that is why the techniques to obtain the electrical activity of the brain, the eye movements and the heart activity are very similar. In the three cases, it is necessary to place electrodes in order to measure the biologic potentials.

The electrical activity of the eyes and the heart movement can be better appreciated than the activity from the brain. Because of that, it has been possible to use one EEG device as ECG and EOG as the resolution to distinguish the different signals is less than in an EEG. On the contrary, it could be not possible to use as EEG a device which has not been designed for that.

The election of the type of electrodes that are needed to be used is very important depending on the signal to measure and the needed resolution. The chosen electrodes are good for the recording of an EOG and an ECG, but their resolution may not be sufficient in some EEG applications.

Regarding to the EOG, the users have communicated the different letters with an average of 90.53%. With the appropriate training, the times of spelling could be reduced and it would be possible to increase the hit rate.

As future work there could be three different lines:

- Use the EEG for analyzing more bioelectrical signals, for example EMG.
- Analyze the signals in real time in order to detect any possible anomaly.
- Improve the results of the EOG adding new functions to the interface and check the most adequate trainings to increase the percentage of success.

Acknowledgements

Finally, we would like to thank to those people who has helped to develop the application, especially to Eneko Lopetegui, because his advices and knowledge.

Author details

María Viqueira, Begoña García Zapirain and Amaia Mendez Zorrilla

Deustotech-LIFE, Universidad de Deusto, Bilbao, Spain

References

[1] Graiman, B, Allison, B. Z, & Pfurtscheller, G. Brain-Computer Interfaces: Revolutionizing Human-Computer Interaction. Springer-V. New York: (2011).

[2] Galán, F, Nuttin, M, Lew, E, Ferrez, P. W, Vanacker, G, Philips, J, et al. A brain-actuated wheelchair: asynchronous and non-invasive Brain-computer interfaces for continuous control of robots. Clinical neurophysiology®: official journal of the International Federation of Clinical Neurophysiology. (2008). Sep; , 119(9), 2159-69.

[3] Guger, C, & Edlinger, G. How many people can control a brain-computer interface. Journal of Neuroscience letters. (2010). , 462, 94-8.

[4] Sirvent, J. L, Azorín, J. M, Iáñez, E, Úbeda, A, & Fernández, E. Interfaz Cerebral no Invasiva Basada en Potenciales Evocados para el Control de un Brazo Robot. Revista iberoamericana de automática e informática industrial. (2011). Apr; , 8(2), 103-11.

[5] Lin, T. A, & John, L. R. Quantifying Mental Relaxation with EEG for use in Computer Games. In: International Conference on Internet Computing. Las Vegas, NV, United States, June 26- 29: (2006).

[6] Purwanto, D, Mardiyanto, R, & Arai, K. Electric wheelchair control with gaze direction and eye blinking. Artificial Life and Robotics. (2009). Dec 15; , 14(3), 397-400.

[7] Bear, M. F, Connors, B. W, & Paradiso, M. A. Neuroscience: Exploring the Brain. Third. Philadelphia: Lippincott Williams & Wikins; (2007).

[8] Duchowski, A. T. Eye Tracking Methodology: Theory and Practice. Second edi. New York: Springer; (2007).

[9] Muthmainnah, N, Noor, M, & Ahmad, S. Simulation Analysis of Different Strength Levels of EOG Signals. In: International Conference on Computer and Communication Engineering. Kuala Lumpur, Malaysia, July 3- 5, (2012). , 3-5.

[10] Liang, S-F, Chen, Y-H, Kuo, C-E, Chen, J-Y, & Hsu, S-C. A fuzzy inference system for sleep staging. In: 2011 IEEE International Conference on Fuzzy Systems. Taipei, Taiwan, June 27- 30: (2011)., 2104-2107.

[11] Tagluk, M. E, Sezgin, N, & Akin, M. Estimation of sleep stages by an artificial neural network employing EEG, EMG and EOG. Journal of medical systems. (2010). Aug; , 34(4), 717-25.

[12] Talukder, A, Morookian, J, Monacos, S, Lam, R, Lebaw, C, & Bond, A. Real-time Non-Invasive Eyetracking and Gaze-point Determination for Human-Computer Interaction and Biomedicine. In: SPIE Defense and Security Symposioum, Optical Pattern Recognition. Orlando, FL, United States, April 12-16, (2004).

[13] Weigle, C, & Banks, D. C. Analysis of eye-tracking experiments performed on a Tobii T60. In: Woods AJ, McDowall IE, Corner BD, Rogowitz BE, Börner K, Eschbach R, et al., editors. Proceedings of the SPIE. Visualization and Data Analysis. San José, CA, United States, January 28- 29, (2008).

Chapter 7

Novel Imaging Techniques in Gastrointestinal Endoscopy in the Upper Gastrointestinal Tract

Rehan Haidry and Laurence Lovat

Additional information is available at the end of the chapter

http://dx.doi.org/10.5772/53807

1. Introduction

The advent of high definition endoscopy has transformed the management of pre-malignant and early malignant diseases of the esophagus and upper gastrointestinal tract. The ability to view the mucosa in detail whereby the cellular architecture can be viewed has enabled the endoscopist to make in-vivo histopathological diagnoses, which in turn will direct the management of the pathology instantly. In this chapter, we describe the various techniques available from high definition white light endoscopy, through chromoendoscopy and confocal endomicroscopy. We describe the characteristics and staging of lesions of the esophagus including Barrett's esophagus (BE) and associated esophageal adenocarcinoma. Furthermore, we describe how endoscopy can be used to define Barrett's and squamous dysplasia. Finally, we describe the classification and staging of early cancers of the esophagus and explore the role of endoscopic ultrasound. We also examine the role of emerging radiological techniques such as virtual colonography that act as adjuncts to current practice and will no doubt help to focus the expertise of skilled endoscopists towards interventional endoscopy rather than routine diagnostic procedures.

Accurate diagnosis and staging of benign and malignant lesions of the esophagus requires an in-depth understanding of current endoscopic techniques and the latest technology. The endoscopic optical technology has evolved rapidly in the last decade such that the resolution of the 'CCD" chip is up to 1.4 million pixels. The images are further enhanced by optical filters and post image processing technology allowing detailed views of the mucosal architecture. This in turn allows improved accuracy of diagnosis. We explore the roles of high definition white light endoscopy, chromoendoscopy, confocal endomicroscopy and EUS in the diagnosis and staging of esophageal neoplasia.

2. White Light Endoscopy (WLE)

This process has several limitations. White light endoscopy is not sensitive enough to detect neoplasia in pre-cancerous conditions in the upper GI tract. For example in Barrett's esophagus, the standard approach is to take one biopsy in every quadrant of the Barrett's segment every 1-2 cm and send for histopathological review [1]. If biopsies are taken every 2 cm, the average number per procedure is 12 and if taken every 1cm, this number will double. Even with an efficient endoscopy setup, it takes around 30 seconds per biopsy so the procedure takes up to 30 minutes to perform. It is also very time consuming for the pathologist, needing up to 30 minutes to evaluate a set of biopsies from a single endoscopy. Dysplasia and early BE neoplasia result in subtle changes that may not often be visible with WLE examination. In addition, random biopsies have significant sampling error since intestinal metaplasia and dysplasia have a patchy distribution and only a small fraction of the BE segment is sampled in this way. Even the most rigorous biopsy protocols including those using jumbo biopsy forceps survey less than 1% of the esophageal mucosa and still miss up to one third of cases with high-grade dysplasia (HGD) or early cancer [2-5].

3. Chromoendoscopy

The use of chromoendoscopy in the GI tract was first described in 1977 [6], and involves the topical application of stains or pigments to improve visualization of the mucosa during endoscopy. The basics of performing chromoendoscopy require only a small number of items: staining agents, spray catheters, water rinses, and mucolytic agents. There are three main types of stains that are used:

i. Absorptive stains (methylene blue, Lugol's solution)

ii. Contrast stains (indigo carmine, acetic acid)

iii. Reactive stains such as congo red or phenol

There are two essential principles in chromoendoscopy: mucus removal and dye application. The former is achieved by using water, or occasionally some centers have advocated the use of a mucolytic agent; N-Acetylcysteine [7-9]. This can be achieved by flushing the agent through the working channel, using a spray catheter or even administering it as an oral solution before the endoscopic procedure. Once the mucus is cleared, the dye can then be applied.

3.1. Methylene Blue (MB) chromoendoscopy

MB, an absorptive dye, is probably the most investigated stain for evaluation of BE. MB is applied topically at a concentration of 0.5-1.0% and is absorbed by goblet cells present in metaplastic Barrett's epithelium. Much of the early work on MB has been performed by Canto's group [10]. The first series published in 1996 assessed 14 patients with Barrett's

http://dx.doi.org/10.5772/53807

esophagus and 12 control patients. Methylene blue stained specialized columnar epithelium in 18 of the 26 patients, including those with intramucosal carcinoma (1), high-grade dysplasia (1), and indefinite/low-grade dysplasia (6). The overall sensitivity of methylene blue staining for the biopsy finding of specialized intestinal metaplasia was 95%. The same group then went on to a prospective, sequence randomized, trial of MDMB versus standard surveillance endoscopy with 2cm quadrantic biopsy [11]. 41 patients were studied with each procedure performed by separate endoscopists within an interval of 3 to 4 weeks. The average number of biopsies was significantly lower with MBDB than 2cm quadrantic biopsy but the MB staining added a mean of 7 minutes (range 2 to 12 minutes) to the endoscopy procedure. Dysplasia or cancer was diagnosed in significantly more biopsy specimens (12% [12,13] vs. 6%, p = 0.004) and patients (44% vs. 28%, p = 0.03) by MBDB than by random biopsy technique.

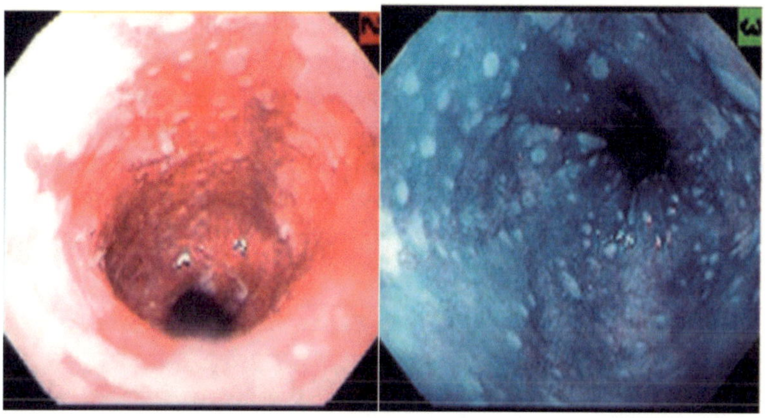

Figure 1. Example of diffuse staining. Esophagus seen before and after staining with diffuse, uniform methylene blue staining [14].

The problems with MB in BE is that dysplastic areas do not stain. Furthermore even areas which do not harbor IM do not absorb the dye. This makes it difficult for the endoscopist to decide on which areas to target the biopsies during the procedure. There are also some issues with the uniformity of the dye. It has been examined in both long and short segment BE [12,13,15]. Two patterns of staining have been documented - diffuse and focal. Canto *et al.* [15] found that most patients with long segment BE exhibited diffuse staining, whereas Wo *et al.* [16] observed focal staining in their cohort of patients with long segment BE. Similar results have been found when examining short segment BE by Sharma *et al.* [17] who found that the majority of their patients with short segment BE stained diffusely. In contrast, in 30 patients with short segment BE assessed by Kiesslich's group [18], only 80% demonstrated staining in a focal pattern.

A recent meta-analysis assessing the diagnostic yield of MB in detecting intestinal and dysplasia in BE looked at 9 published studies that included 450 patients. Despite controlling for differences in technique and quality of published data, the meta-analysis showed no significant benefit of MB chromoendoscopy compared with random biopsies in detecting SIM, dysplasia or early esophageal cancer [19].

Unfortunately MB is inconvenient to use. It must be left in contact with the mucosa for 3 minutes followed by vigorous washing to clear away excess dye. As a result the endoscopic appearances are unpredictable, subjective and not reproducible

3.2. Acetic acid chromoendosocpy

Acetic acid 2.5% (AA) when sprayed onto Barrett's mucosa causes a reversible acetylation of nuclear proteins to occur. This leads to an acetowhitening reaction, with increased opacity of the mucosal surface. It also causes vascular congestion and improves surface pattern evaluation. There is a growing body of evidence that magnification chromoendoscopy with acetic acid improves the diagnosis of specialized intestinal metaplasia. The technique is advantageous as it is both safe and inexpensive. When topically applied to multilayered squamous epithelium the acetic acid is progressively neutralized by mucus covering the epithelium and the underlying stroma and the vascular network are protected [20]. In single layered columnar lined esophagus the acetic acid reversibly alters the barrier function of the epithelium and reaches the stroma and vascular network. This leads to swelling of the mucosal surface and enhancement of the surface architecture. There is also enhancement of vascular pattern due to congestion of the capillaries. Transient changes to the structure of cellular proteins may also occur.

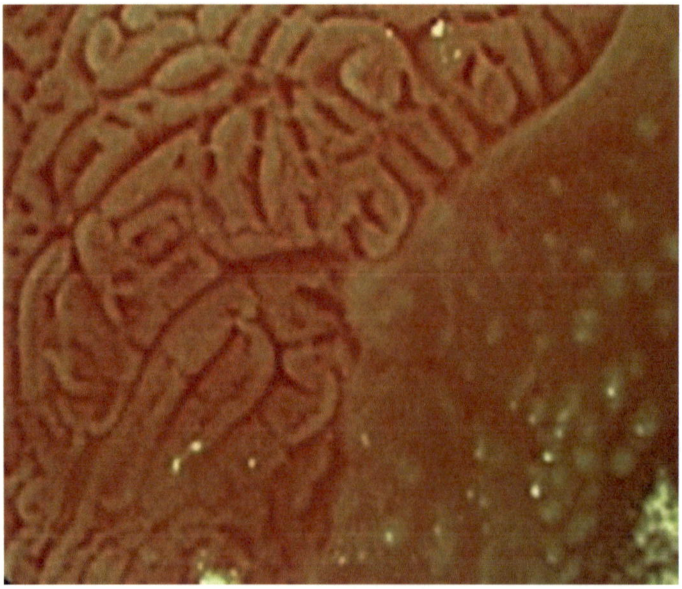

Figure 2. Acetic acid used to visualise Barrett's oesophagus, ridge pattern signifying Intestinal metaplasia

All of the studies using acetic acid have combined magnification endoscopy to study the pit pattern of the mucosa. Classification is based on Guelrud's description of four typical pit patterns; gastric patterns (pattern I = pits with a regular and orderly arranged circular dots; pattern II = reticular pits that are circular or oval and are regular in shape and arrangement); SIM patterns (pattern III = fine villiform appearance with regular shape and arrangement; pattern IV = thick villous convoluted shape with a cerebriform appearance with regular shape and arrangement).

In the first prospective cohort study of 49 patients, sensitivity for specialized intestinal metaplasia = 96.5%, specificity = 88.7% and overall accuracy was 92.2% [21]. Using modified criteria, a second study of 67 patients demonstrated sensitivity 88.5%, specificity 90.2% and diagnostic accuracy of 90% [22]. Reaud *et al.* studied 28 patients with a type III or IV pattern with sensitivity for SIM of 95.5%, specificity 42.9 % and diagnostic accuracy of 75% [23].

A further randomised crossover study using acetic acid for the detection of Barrett's metaplasia in 32 patients was performed by Hoffman *et al.* [24]. Patients were randomized to either standard video endoscopy with quadrantic biopsies or to magnifying endoscopy with acetic acid. All patients were re-examined after 14 days post initial endoscopy with the corresponding procedure. The investigators found that magnifying endoscopy enabled the prediction of Barrett's epithelium with a sensitivity of 100% and specificity of 66% and accuracy of 83.8%. The biopsies obtained following exposure to acetic acid yielded a significantly higher percentage of tissues containing Barrett's metaplasia (78%) compared to random biopsies (57%). Again this study had no dysplasia cases and the authors recognized this as a limitation of the study.

In a very recent landmark study by Longcroft-Wheaton *et al.* [25] from Portsmouth in the United Kingdom, the efficacy of acetic acid has been investigated in detecting Barrett's dysplasia. Data were collected from 190 patients with Barrett's esophagus examined over a 3 year period at a tertiary referral center from procedures performed by a single experienced endoscopist. Patients were first examined with white light gastroscopy and visible abnormalities were identified. Acetic acid (2.5%) dye spray was used to identify potentially neoplastic areas and biopsy samples were collected from these, followed by quadrantic biopsies at 2 cm intervals of the remaining Barrett's mucosa. The chromoendoscopic diagnosis was compared with the ultimate histological diagnosis to evaluate the sensitivity of acetic acid chromoendoscopy. Acetic acid chromoendoscopy had a sensitivity of 95.5% and specificity of 80% for the detection of neoplasia. There was a correlation between lesions predicted to be neoplasias by acetic acid and those diagnosed by histological analysis ($r = 0.98$). There was a significant improvement in the detection of neoplasia using acetic acid compared with white light endoscopy ($P = 0.001$).

3.3. Indigo carmine chromoendoscopy

Whilst Indigo carmine has been used in many studies looking at colonic neoplasia, it has not been studied to such a degree in the esophagus. As in the colon, it is not absorbed by esophageal and Barrett's mucosa, but accumulates in the pits and valleys between cells, highlighting the architecture. It is a contrast agent which can highlight mucosal irregularities and has been very helpful in the colon. However, results have been less encouraging in the esophagus.

Sharma *et al.* showed that using indigo carmine and high resolution endoscopy 3 distinct patterns can be recognized at endoscopy: ridged and/or villous, circular, and irregular and/or distorted [26]. Barrett's epithelium was most commonly identified in the ridged-villous pattern, whereas high-grade dysplasia was found entirely in the irregular/distorted pattern. An irregular/distorted pattern either throughout the entire segment of Barrett's esophagus or in combination with a ridge/villous or circular pattern had a sensitivity or 83%, a specificity of 88%, a positive predictive value of 45%, and a negative predictive value of 98% for high-grade dysplasia.

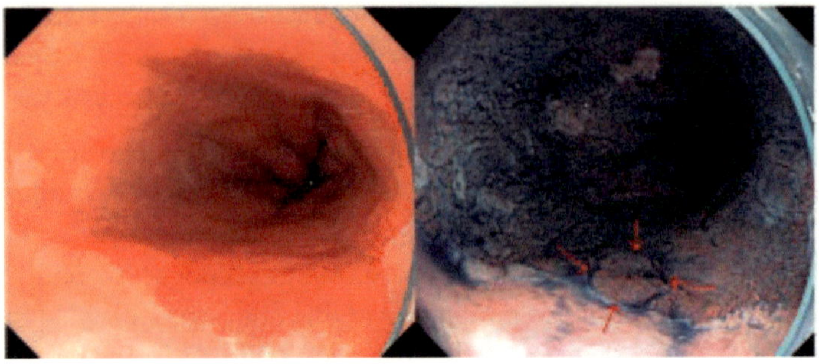

Figure 3. High–resolution white–light imaging (left) and indigo carmine chromoendoscopy (right) of a small mucosal lesion (type IIb) at the 6–o'clock position (arrows), detected in a patient with Barrett's esophagus. This area was regarded as suspicious after spraying of indigo carmine. High grade dysplasia was found in the corresponding biopsy specimens [27].

4. HD WLE & optical enhancements

Video endoscopy relies on a charge coupled device (CCD) chip to enhance image resolution and magnification. Standard definition (SD) WLE is rapidly being replaced by the introduction of high definition endoscopes. Video endoscopes use white light from a xenon or halogen source for illumination. The reflected light is captured by a CCD chip at the tip of the instrument in order to reconstruct the images. Conventional SD endoscopes are equipped with CCD chips that produce an image signal of 100,000 to 400,000 pixels which is displayed in SD format. The chips currently in use in HD endoscopes produce resolutions that range from 850,000 to 1.3 million pixels. In order to generate a true HD image, each component of the system (e.g. the endoscope CCD chip, the processor, the monitor, and transmission cables) must be HD compatible.

4.1. Enhanced imaging systems – Olympus Narrow Band imaging (NBI)

Conventional WLE uses the entire spectrum of visible light (400-700mm) to examine tissue. *Narrow band imaging (NBI)* developed by Olympus Medical Systems (Olympus, Japan) is a new advance in endoscopy that uses optic filters to isolate two specific bands of light: 415 nm blue and 540 nm green. By isolating these two bands of light and taking into account their absorptive and reflective properties on the mucosal surface, an image that enhances visualization of superficial mucosal and vascular structures is created. The quality of the surface pit pattern morphology is also clearly enhanced by this technology. It enables the endoscopist to switch between conventional white light and NBI views easily and quickly during the procedure, thus making the procedure itself less messy and cumbersome compared to chromoendoscopy. By depressing a lever on the endoscope, the focal distance of the lens at the tip of the endoscope can be adjusted electronically thus enabling the endoscopist to achieve a maximal magnification of 115X in real time.

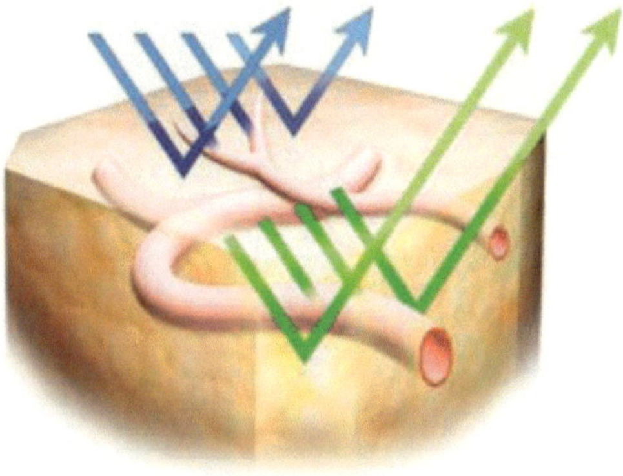

Figure 4. NBI uses two discrete bands of light: One blue at 415nm and one green at 540nm. Narrow band blue light displays superficial capillary networks, while green light which penetrates more deeply into tissue displays subepithelial vessels and when combined offer an extremely high contrast image of the tissue surface.

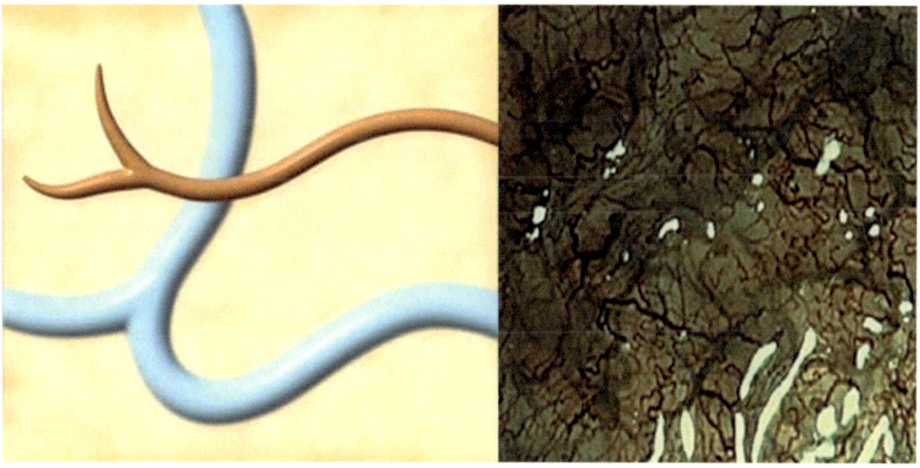

Figure 5. NBI image on the monitor: Capilaries on the surface are displayed in brown and veins in the sub surface are displayed in cyan.

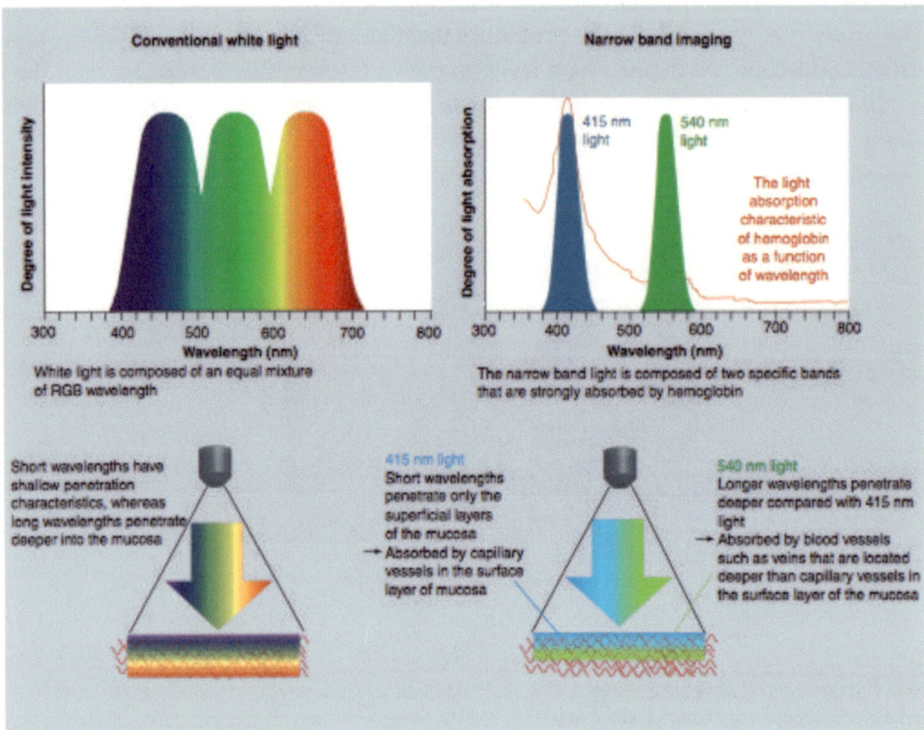

Figure 6. Light filtering in the narrow-band imaging system. The white light is split into two narrow bands: a blue narrow band of 415 nm and a green narrow band of 540 nm.

Although many studies have shown the benefit of NBI over conventional WLE in detecting HGD and early esophageal cancer, others have questioned whether NBI achieves any incremental improvement beyond that of HRE-WLE. Wolfsen *et al.* investigated whether NBI targeted biopsies could detect advanced dysplasia using fewer biopsy samples compared with conventional endoscopy using the four-quadrant biopsy method with a prospective, blinded, controlled tandem study [28]. The study revealed that NBI detected dysplasia in 57% of patients compared with 43% in the conventional endoscopy with four-quadrant biopsy group, with higher grades of dysplasia detected in the NBI group ($P < 0.001$). In addition, more biopsies were taken in the four-quadrant biopsy group compared with narrow-band targeted biopsies (mean 8.5 versus 4.7; $P < 0.001$). A study by Kara *et al.* investigated chromoendoscopy versus NBI, both in combination with high resolution endoscopy, in a prospective, randomized crossover study with 14 patients [29]. The sensitivity of chromoendoscopy and NBI was 93% and 86%, respectively, compared with 79% for four-quadrant biopsies with conventional endoscopy in the diagnosis of high-grade dysplasia or early cancer (EC) in patients with BE. Although chromoendoscopy and NBI identified additional lesions (chromoendoscopy two additional lesions in two patients; NBI four additional lesions in three patients), they did not increase per patient sensitivity for identifying HGD/EC.

Interestingly, in an inter-observer agreement study by Curvers *et al.* there was moderate inter-observer agreement for classification of mucosal morphology by NBI (0.40–0.56) [30]. Although there was improvement in image quality with NBI compared to HRE, NBI provided no significant improvement in inter-observer variability and yield for detecting neoplasia. The yield of HRE-WLE for neoplasia was 81%, 72% for NBI, and 83% for the HRE-WLE with NBI. The addition of enhancement techniques did not improve the yield of neoplasia in this series.

More recently Curvers *et al.* have performed a review of studies that analyzed NBI images for accuracy in differentiating HGD/cancer from low-grade dysplasia (LGD) or non-neoplastic Barrett's esophagus [31]. In a meta-analysis that included 149 areas with HGD/cancer and 607 areas with LGD or non-dysplastic Barrett's esophagus, NBI had a sensitivity for HGD/cancer of 97% (95% CI 89– 99%) and a specificity of 94% (60–99%), and an accuracy of 96% (72–99%). Consequently, the use of 'targeted' biopsy techniques using image enhancement techniques has potential time and cost savings. They recognize however that these findings may not be generalizable as these studies were performed in high-risk populations.

4.2. Comparing high definition WLE to enhanced imaging systems (NBI)

The majority of studies looking at NBI compare its efficacy in relation to other endoscopic modalities such as chromoendoscopy or autofluorescence as well as HD-WLE. There are limited data directly comparing the efficacy of NBI versus HD-WLE in the diagnosis of dysplasia/early cancer in patients with Barrett's esophagus. A very recent randomized control trial from 2012 by Sharma *et al* [32] compared the use of HD WLE and NBI for detection of IM or dysplasia in patents with BE. Patients referred for BE screening or surveillance at three tertiary referral centers were prospectively enrolled and randomized to HD-WLE or NBI followed by other procedures in 3-8 weeks. During HD-WLE, four quadrant biopsies every 2 cm, together with targeted biopsies of visible lesions (Seattle protocol), were obtained. During NBI examination, mucosal and vascular patterns were noted and targeted biopsies were obtained. 123 patients with BE (mean age 61; 93% male; 97% Caucasian) with mean circumferential and maximal extents of 1.8 and 3.6 cm, respectively, were enrolled. Both HD-WLE and NBI detected 104/113 (92%) patients with IM, but NBI required fewer biopsies per patient (3.6 vs 7.6, $P < 0.0001$). NBI detected a higher proportion of areas with dysplasia (30% vs 21%, $P = 0.01$). During examination with NBI, all areas of HGD and cancer had an irregular mucosal or vascular pattern. This important study demonstrates that NBI targeted biopsies can have the same IM detection rate as an HD-WLE examination with the Seattle protocol while requiring fewer biopsies. In addition, NBI targeted biopsies can detect more areas with dysplasia. Regular appearing NBI surface patterns did not harbor high-grade dysplasia/cancer, suggesting that biopsies could be avoided in these areas.

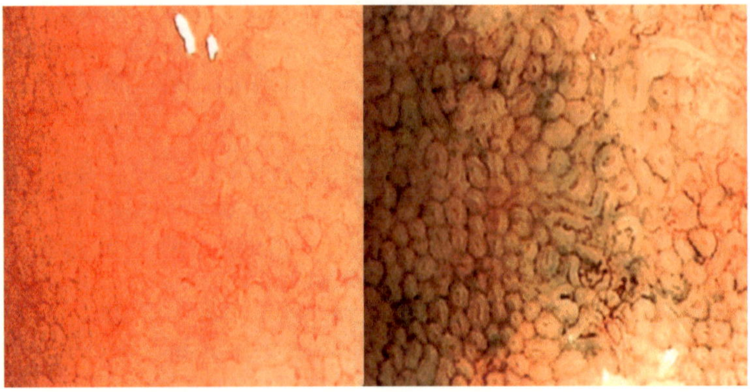

Figure 7. High magnification white light endoscopy-round pits in keeping with columnar mucosa without intestinal metaplasia with corresponding area on right image seen with narrow band imaging (NBI) and magnification

4.3. Enhanced imaging systems – Pentax medical i-scan

A new endoscopic image enhancement technology, *i-scan,* has been developed by PENTAX (HOYA Corporation), Japan. i-Scan uses the EPKi processor technology which enables resolution above HDTV standard, with distinct digital filters for special post processing online imaging, which can provide detailed analysis. i–Scan is a novel endoscopic post processing light filter technology using sophisticated software algorithms with real time image mapping technology embedded in the EPKi processor. The computer controlled digital processing provides resolution of about 1.25 mega pixels per image. Different elements of the mucosa are enhanced by pressing a button on the hand piece of the high definition endoscope. i–Scan can be used for surface analysis to recognize lesions using three modes of image enhancement. These are:

i. *Surface enhancement (SE)/ i-scan 1* – enhancement of the structure through recognition of the edges

ii. *Contrast enhancement (CE)/ i-scan 2* – enhancement of depressed areas and differences in structure through colors presentation of low density areas

iii. *Surface and Tone enhancement (TE)/ i-scan 3*– enhancement tailored to individual organs through modification of the combination of RGB components for each pixel

i-scan images are as bright as conventional WLE images and therefore i-scan can observe larger areas in a distant view than NBI. i-scan does not need magnifying endoscopy to observe the demarcation between normal and abnormal tissue. i–scan can be switched on and effected quite simply and instantaneously by pushing a button, therefore it is an easy method for screening or detailed inspection, and may reduce both time and costs. The sensitivity and specificity of i-scan in detecting dysplasia in Barrett's patients is yet to be investigated.

http://dx.doi.org/10.5772/53807

There is as of yet no formal i-scan classification system for BE mucosal patterns. However using those devised for other modalities such as NBI, endoscopists are able to direct and target therapy to subtle anomalies based on these validated classification systems. There is however a growing body of work showing the increased accuracy of i-scan in the colon in detecting adenomatous polyp [33].

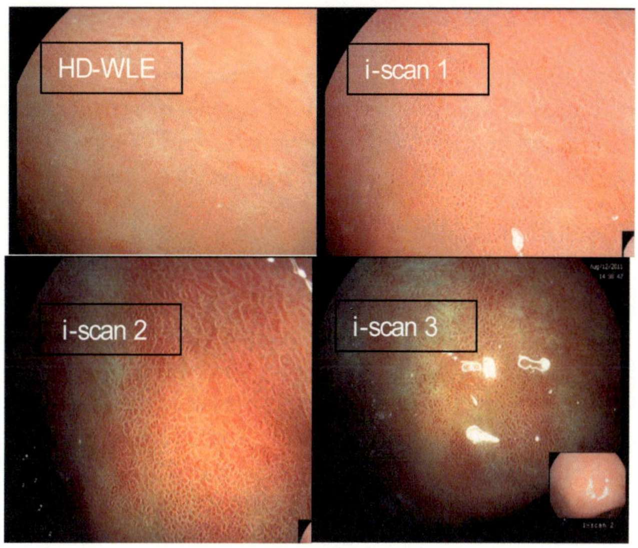

Figure 8. Pentax Images of an area of BE mucosa with IM using the various enhancement settings

4.4. Flexible spectral imaging color enhancement (FICE)

Unlike NBI, which utilizes a physical filter, FICE (Fujinon, Japan) is a post processor technology which captures spectral reflectance by a color CCD video endoscope. This is sent to a spectral estimation matrix processing circuit contained in the video processor. The reflectance spectra of corresponding pixels that make up the conventional image are mathematically estimated. From these spectra, it is feasible to reconstruct a virtual image of a single wavelength. Three such single-wavelength images can be selected and assigned to the red, green, and blue monitor inputs, respectively, to display a composite color-enhanced multi band image in real time. In practice this can be used like narrow band imaging to remove data from the red part of the waveband and narrow the green and blue spectra

A prospective cohort study of 72 patients demonstrated that the identification of Pallisade vessels using FICE provided a clear demarcation between Barrett's mucosa and the gastric mucosa which was superior to standard white light endoscopy [34]. This study did not attempt to diagnose dysplasia and used transnasal Fujinon endoscopes. These are very small with a more limited field of view and no optical magnification.

In a small prospective cohort study of 57 patients which compared FICE with random biopsy in patients with suspected HGD or early cancer arising in BE, a sensitivity of 92% and specificity of 97% for FICE was achieved [35]. There was HGD or early cancer in 24/57 patients. However the investigators used acetic acid in addition to FICE.

5. Mucosal classification systems for dysplasia in BE

There are now several recognized mucosal classification systems that have been described in the literature. They have formed the basis for further extensive work attempting to validate numerous optical enhancement modalities for neoplasia in BE. 2 of the very first systems were defined by Guelred *et al.* and Endo *et al.* in 2001 and 2002.

Guelrud *et al* [36] in 2001 described a technique they named enhanced-magnification endoscopy, which combines magnification endoscopy with instillation of acetic acid. They classified Barrett's mucosa into 4 patterns: I, round pits; II, reticular (circular or oval pits); III, villous (fine villiform appearance without visible pits); and IV, ridged (thick villi with convoluted cerebriform appearance without visible pits). This initial study by Guelrud *et al.* included 49 patients undergoing endoscopic surveillance for short-segment Barrett's esophagus. At the time the study was conducted, a magnification endoscope with standard resolution and a magnification power of 35x was used. A spray catheter was used to apply approximately 10 to 15 mL of 1.5% acetic acid onto the distal oesophagus. This technique added an estimated 5 to 8 minutes to the length of a standard endoscopic examination. The 4 different mucosal surface patterns were observed, and one biopsy specimen was taken from each representative pattern. All patients with Barrett's esophagus had a villiform mucosal pattern that correlated with the finding of intestinal metaplasia on histopathologic evaluation of the biopsy specimens. The yield of biopsy specimens in the detection of intestinal metaplasia was correlated with the endoscopic pattern. Biopsy specimens from Pattern I mucosa revealed fundic epithelium, and this pattern served as a control for the analysis. Biopsy specimens from Pattern II mucosa revealed cardia mucosa in 90% of cases; intestinal metaplasia was found in two of 18 samples. Analysis showed that Pattern III and Pattern IV mucosa contained intestinal metaplasia in 87% and 100% respectively of biopsy specimens. The overall accuracy of enhanced magnification endoscopy for the detection of intestinal metaplasia was 92%; the positive predictive value of Patterns III and IV was 87.5%.

In 2002 Endo *et al.* [37] examined 67 regions in Barrett's mucosa and described 5 patterns. These patterns were classified into 5 categories. The dot type (pit-1) is characterized by small round pits of relatively uniform size and shape. The straight type (pit-2) consists of long straight lines. The long oval and curved type (pit-3) exhibits long extended pits, larger than those of the dot type (pit-1). The tubular type (pit-4) has a complicated and twisted pattern that is similar to a branch or gyrus-like structure. The fifth pattern (pit-5), villous type, has flat, finger-like projections. Methylene blue is applied topically at a concentration of 0.5-1.0% and is absorbed by goblet cells present in metaplastic Barrett's epithelium. Methylene blue stained 0% of the mucosa identified as types 1 and 2. However, intestinal metaplasia was found in 6% of biopsy specimens from mucosa that exhibited the type 1 pattern. The rate of positive methylene blue staining was 23% for type 3, and 40% of biopsy specimens from this type revealed intestinal metaplasia. Intestinal metaplasia was found in 100% of biopsy specimens from mucosa that exhibited either a type 4 or type 5 pattern. However, type 4 and type 5 mucosa were stained by methylene blue in only 60% and 50% of cases, respectively.

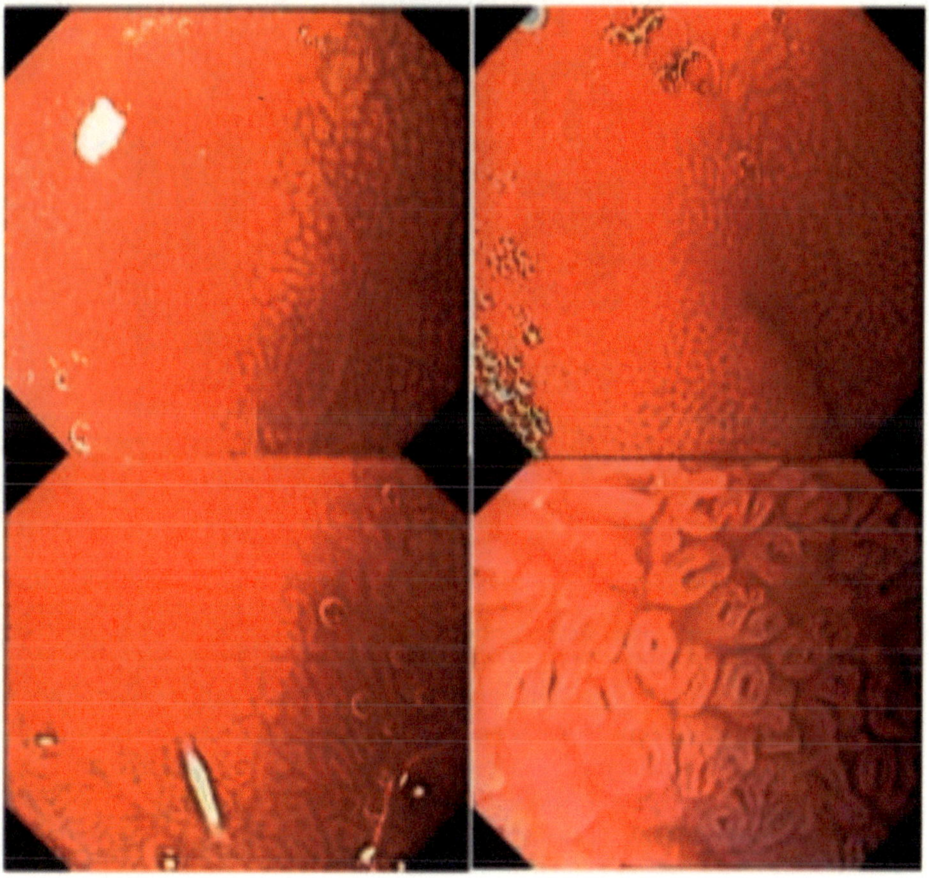

Figure 9. The First Guelrud classification (x35, 1.5% alcohol acetic acid); Pattern I: round pits with a regular and orderly arranged circular dots. Pattern II: reticular pits that are circular or oval and are regular in shape and arrangement. Pattern III: fine villiform appearance with regular shape and arrangement. Pattern IV: thick villous convoluted shape with a cerebriform appearance with regular shape and arrangement. Guelrud et al [36]

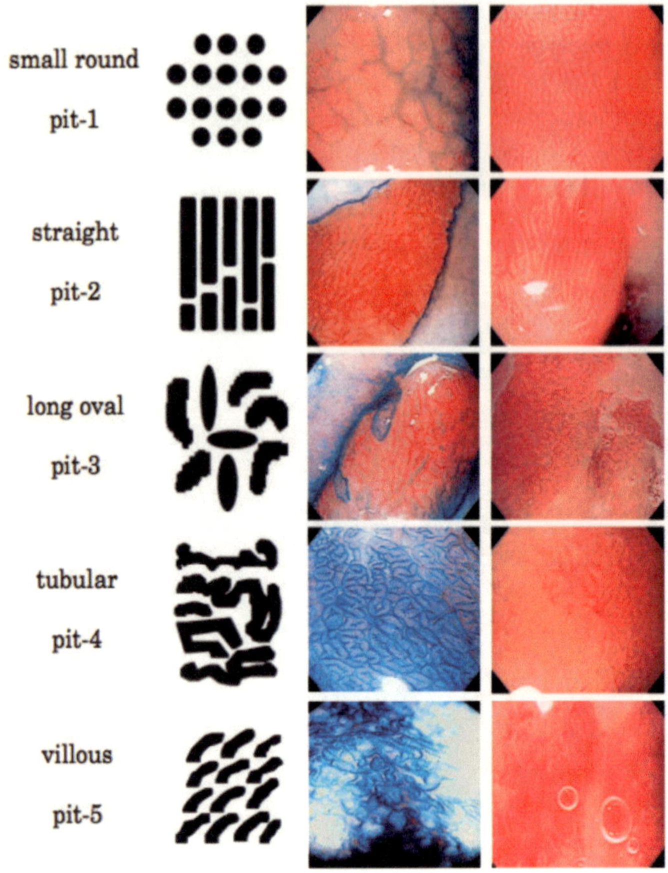

Figure 10. Endo Classification of pit pattern of Barrett's epithelium by magnifying endoscopy. Endoscopic views at right were obtained without methylene blue staining and those at left after application of methylene blue. Note that mucosa with pit-1, pit-2, and pit-3 patterns was not stained by the dye, whereas positive staining is evident within mucosa with pit-4 and pit-5 patterns Endo et al. [37]

Kara *et al.* in 2006 from Amsterdam [38] suggested a further classification system. They used NBI with magnifying endoscopy to image and then biopsy randomly selected areas in 63 patients with BE. Following this there was a formal review process of the images and biopsies. The relationship between mucosal morphology and presence of IM and HGD were evaluated. Areas of intestinal metaplasia were characterized by either villous/gyrus-forming patterns (80%), which were mostly regular and had regular vascular patterns, or a flat mucosa with regular normal-appearing long branching vessels (20%). HGD was characterized by 3 abnormalities: irregular/disrupted mucosal patterns, irregular vascular patterns, and abnormal blood vessels. All areas with HGIN had at least 1 abnormality, and 85% had 2 or more abnormalities. The frequency of abnormalities showed a significant rise with increasing grades of dysplasia. The magnified NBI images had a sensitivity of 94%, a specificity of 76%, a positive predictive value of 64%, and a negative predictive value of 98% for HGIN.

http://dx.doi.org/10.5772/53807

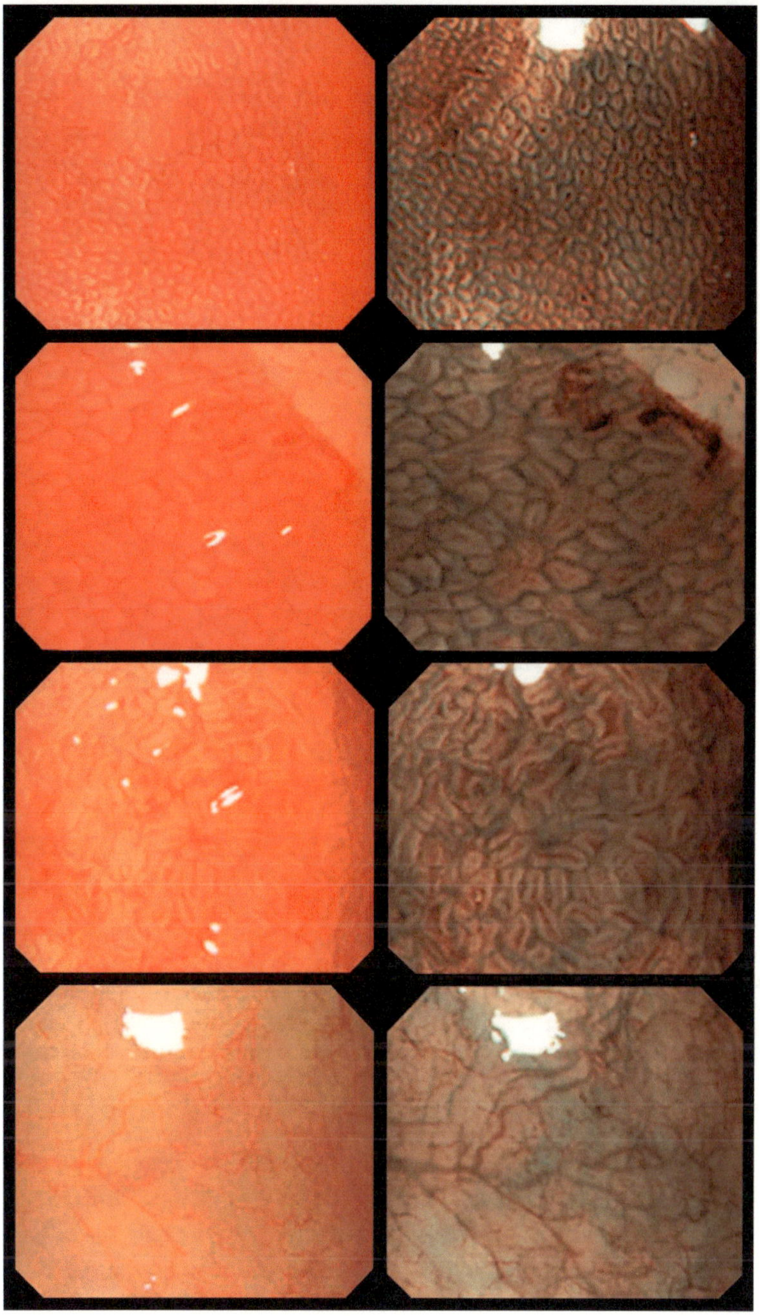

Figure 11. Magnified high-resolution white light (left) and NBI (right) endoscopic photographs of areas with nondysplastic BE (no staining, orig. mag.115). The upper 3 examples have regular villous/gyrus-forming mucosal patterns with regular vascular patterns; the villi are of various sizes and shapes but regular in all areas with blood vessels situated between the mucosal ridges. The lower image has a flat-type mucosa without pits or villi; the vasculature shows regular, normal-appearing long branching vessels. Kara et al. [38]

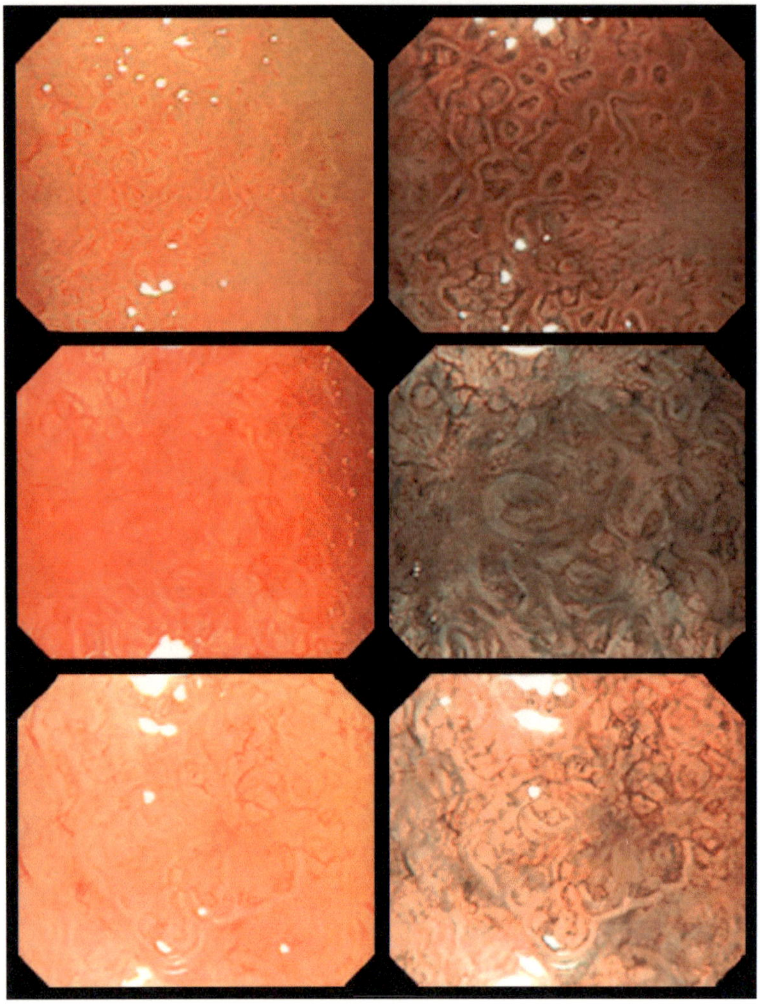

Figure 12. Magnified high-resolution white light (left) and corresponding NBI (right) endoscopic photographs of areas with HGIN in BE (no staining, orig. mag. _115). These examples show irregular/disrupted mucosal patterns, with irregular vascular patterns with remnants of villous/gyrus-forming mucosal patterns. Kara et al. [38]

Singh *et al.* [39] from Nottingham in the United Kingdom have looked at an alternative simplified classification. In a prospective cohort study of 109 patients with Barrett's esophagus, mucosal patterns visualized with NBI were classified into four easily distinguishable types: A, round pits with regular microvasculature; B, villous/ridge pits with regular microvasculature; C, absent pits with regular microvasculature; D, distorted pits with irregular microvasculature. The NBI grading was compared with the final histopathological diagnosis. In 903 out of 1021 distinct areas (87.9%) the NBI grading corresponded to the histological diagnosis. The PPV and NPV for type A pattern (columnar mucosa without intestinal metaplasia) were 100% and 97% respectively; for types B and C (intestinal metaplasia) they were 88% and 91% respectively, and for type D (high grade dysplasia) 81% and 99% respectively.

http://dx.doi.org/10.5772/53807

With respect to inter- and intra-observer agreement, the mean k values in assessing the various patterns were 0.71 and 0.87 in the non-expert group; 0.78 and 0.91 in the expert group.

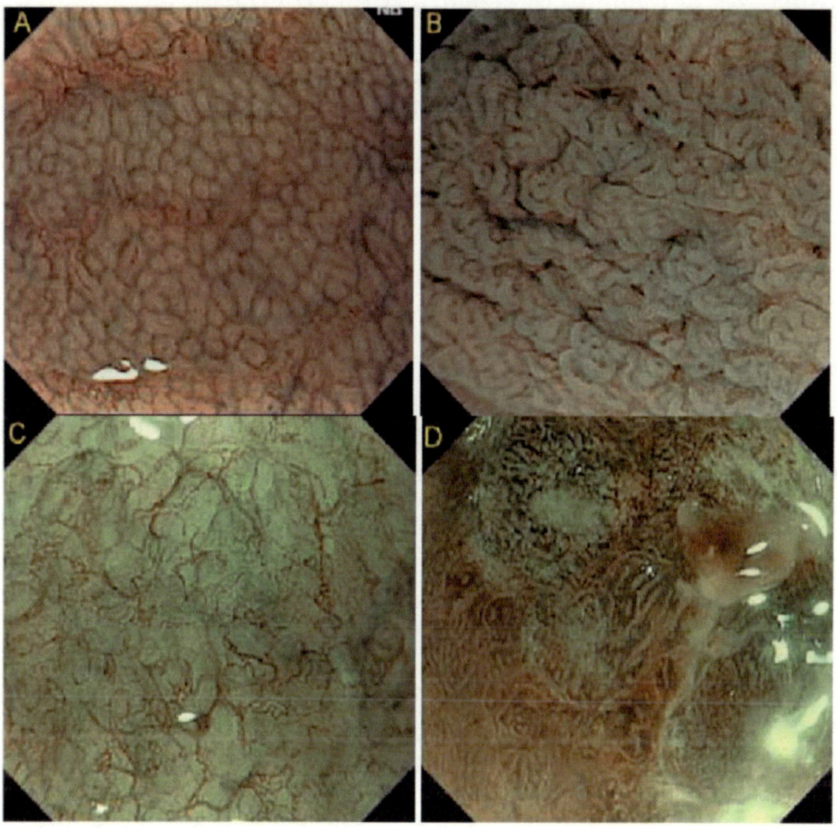

Figure 13. (A) Type A: round pits with regular microvasculature. (B) Type B: villous/ridge pits with regular microvasculature. (C) Type C: absent pits with regular microvasculature. (D) Type D: distorted pits with irregular microvasculature. Singh et al. [39]

A final endoscopic classification system for BE was described by investigators in Kansas again using narrow band imaging [40]. NBI images were graded according to mucosal pattern (ridge/villous, circular and irregular/distorted) and vascular pattern (normal and abnormal), and correlated with histology. Of 51 patients, 28 had IM without dysplasia, 8 had low-grade dysplasia (LGD), 7 had high-grade dysplasia (HGD), and 8 had cardiac-type mucosa. The sensitivity, specificity, and positive predictive value of ridge/villous pattern for diagnosis of IM without HGD were 93.5%, 86.7%, and 94.7%, respectively. The sensitivity, specificity, and positive predictive value of irregular/distorted pattern for HGD were 100%, 98.7%, and 95.3%, respectively. If biopsies were limited to areas with irregular/distorted pattern, no patient with HGD would have been missed. However, NBI was unable to distinguish areas of IM from those with LGD.

6. Interobserver agreement of classification criteria

A potential drawback with all these classification systems has been the lack of intra-observer agreement between endoscopists when using the classification systems described above.

In order to compare the 3 above classification systems from Amsterdam, Nottingham and Kansas a recent comparative study was performed by Silva *et al.* [41]. They examined all 3 classification systems in 84 high quality video recordings collected on cases of BE using HD WLE and NBI. All assessors were blinded to the matched histology form these areas. The global accuracy was 46% and 47% using the Nottingham and Kansa classifications respectively and 51% with the Amsterdam Classification. Accuracy for detecting dysplastic lesions was 75% irrespective of classification system used. The inter-observer agreement ranged from fair (Nottingham κ=0.34) to moderate (Amsterdam and Kansas, κ=0.47 and κ=0.44, respectively). The authors concluded that all three systems revealed substantial limitations when assessed externally and that as a result, NBI could not replace random biopsies for histopathological analysis.

7. Confocal laser endomicrospcopy (CLE)

CLE is a new technology that enables the endoscopist to perform a real time histological assessment of the upper gastrointestinal tract and in particular the esophagus. The most widely used CLE system is the 'endoscope with embedded CLE technology' (eCLE) made by Pentax, Tokyo, Japan and Optiscan, Melbourne, Australia. The eCLE enables visualization of both the epithelium and the subepithelial vascular structures with imaging at variable depths up to 250mm and a magnification power of up to 1000μm. A probe-based endomicroscopy system has been created by Mauna Kea Technologies in which the laser-scanning unit remains outside the patient, and the endomicroscopy probe is passed through the working channel of a standard endoscope. This probe-based CLE (pCLE) provides video sequence imaging at a rate of 12 images per second and allows for the compilation of images from a video sequence to create a composite video mosaic. The depth ranges from 50 to 150mm and is fixed based on the type of probe. These CLE systems use a wavelength of 48nm for excitation. CLE requires the use of contrast agent, most commonly intravenous fluorescein sodium, which is safe for imaging the gastrointestinal tract [42].

CLE classification systems for Barrett's esophagus with and without dysplasia have been described for standard endomicroscopy and probe-based endomicroscopy [43,44]. Signs of non-dysplastic Barrett's epithelium include a regular epithelial lining pattern, regular vascular pattern, presence of goblet cells, and preservation of the villous pattern of glands. Signs of dysplasia in Barrett's esophagus include irregular epithelial lining, fusion of glands, focal accumulation of dark cells with bright lamina propria, irregular vascular pattern, and disruption of the glandular pattern.

Kiesslich *et al.* [43] demonstrated that eCLE could diagnose Barrett's associated dysplasia during endoscopy with a sensitivity of 92.9% and a specificity of 98.4%. Dunbar *et al.* [45] conducted a prospective, double-blind, randomized crossover study comparing four-quadrant random biopsies with eCLE-targeted biopsy in 39 patients. They demonstrated that eCLE improved the diagnostic yield for detecting neoplasia in Barrett's esophagus. The yield of eCLE was 33.7% versus 17.2% with random biopsies (P 1⁄4 0.01). Furthermore, some patients undergoing eCLE would not have needed any random biopsies in order to diagnose neoplasia.

In 2011 Gaddam *et al.* [46] revised and validated a set of criteria for pCLE for dysplasia in BE using video recordings. Of multiple pCLE criteria tested in the first phase of their study, only those with ≥70% sensitivity or specificity were included in the final set. These were epithelial surface: saw-toothed; cells: enlarged; cells: pleomorphic; glands: not equidistant; glands: unequal in size and shape; goblet cells: not easily identified. Using these criteria overall accuracy in diagnosing dysplasia was 81.5% (95% CI: 77.5–81), with no difference between experts vs. non-experts. Accuracy of prediction was significantly higher when endoscopists were "confident" about their diagnosis (98% (95–99) vs. 62% (54–70), P<0.001). Accuracy of dysplasia prediction for the first 30 videos was not different from the last 45 (93 vs. 81%, P=0.51). Overall agreement of the criteria was substantial, $\kappa = 0.61$ (0.53–0.69), with no difference between experts and non-experts.

In a very recent international prospective, multicenter, randomized controlled trial, Sharma *et al.* [47] investigated whether pCLE could allow for real time detection of neoplastic Barrett's esophagus. All patients with BE were examined by HD-WLE, narrow-band imaging (NBI), and pCLE, and the findings were recorded before matched biopsy samples were obtained. The order of HD-WLE and NBI was randomized and performed by 2 independent, blinded endoscopists. All suspicious lesions on HD-WLE or NBI and 4-quadrant random locations were documented. These locations were then examined by pCLE, and a presumptive diagnosis of benign or neoplastic (HGD/EC) tissue was made in real time after which biopsies were taken from all locations and were reviewed by a central pathologist, blinded to endoscopic and pCLE data. The sensitivity and specificity for HD-WLE were 34.2% and 92.7%, respectively, compared with 68.3% and 87.8%, respectively, for HD-WLE or pCLE (P = 0.002 and P < 0.001, respectively). The sensitivity and specificity for HD-WLE or NBI were 45.0% and 88.2%, respectively, compared with 75.8% and 84.2%, respectively, for HD-WLE, NBI, or pCLE (P = 0.01 and P = 0.02, respectively). However with the use of pCLE in conjunction with HD-WLE and NBI enabled the identification of 2 and 1 additional HGD/EC patients compared with HD-WLE and HD-WLE or NBI, respectively, resulting in detection of all HGD/EC patients, although not statistically significant. This may allow better informed decisions to be made for the management and subsequent treatment of BE patients.

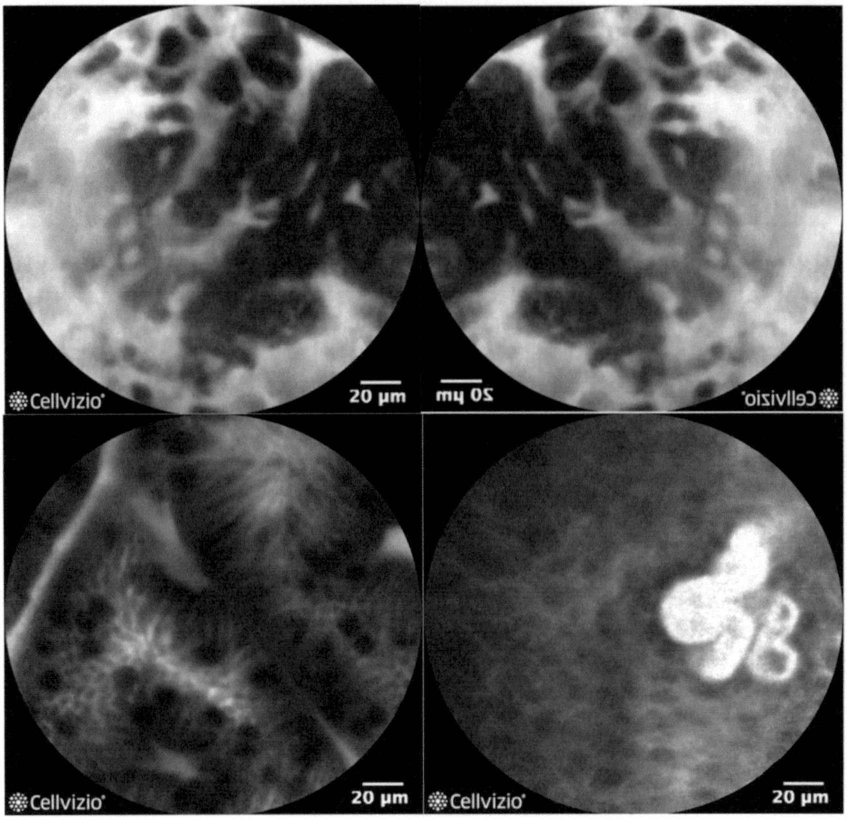

Figure 14. Images of normal, dysplastic and cancer using probe based confocal endomicrosocpy. The presence of goblet cells denoted intestinal metaplasia. (The images are courtesy of the DONT BIOPCE trial)

7.1. OCT – Optical Coherence Tomography

Optical Coherence Tomography (OCT) is an imaging modality that may have the ability to improve the current paradigm for endoscopic screening and surveillance that exists for patients with BE. OCT can be thought of as an analogous technique to ultrasound, however, instead of producing an image from the scattering of sound waves, it utilizes optical scattering based on differences in tissue composition to form a two-dimensional image [48]. The benefit of OCT over ultrasound is that it is capable of generating cross-sectional images of tissues with an axial-resolution of up to 10μm, which is comparable to low-power microscopy.

Original OCT systems or time-domain OCT were limited to discrete locations or 'point' sampling due to slow acquisition rates. However, with the development of second-generation OCT, termed Optical Frequency Domain Imaging (OFDI), it is now possible to perform high-speed acquisition of large luminal surfaces in three-dimensions [49]. Due to its high-resolution and high-acquisition rates, utilizing this technique for screening and surveillance of Barrett's esophagus may provide a means to evaluate pathologic states in long-segments of the esophageal lumen in real-time.

7.2. OCT in Barrett's esophagus

The first clinical application using *in vivo* endoscopic OCT for imaging of the human esophagus and stomach was performed by Bouma *et al.* in 2000 [50]. In this preliminary study, the ability of OCT to image normal esophageal mucosa and stomach, Barrett's esophagus, and adenocarcinoma was investigated. The authors concluded that they were able to differentiate the normal layered structure of the esophagus using OCT, including epithelium, lamina propria, muscularis mucosa, and submucosa. In addition, OCT was capable of differentiating between normal esophageal mucosa and Barrett's esophagus based on the lack of the layered structure found in Barrett's esophagus as well as a disorganized glandular morphology. Finally, esophageal adenocarcinoma was clearly differentiable by the presence of marked architectural disorganization. Several studies immediately followed this landmark study using *in vivo* OCT for the GI tract [51-54]. Similarly, they utilized a non-contact probe, approximately 2.5mm in diameter, introduced through the auxiliary channel of a standard endoscope. These studies all were significant in the contribution of development of OCT for GI imaging and played a major role in the potential clinical utility of OCT, however, they were limited to 'point' sampling and did not address diagnostic information relevant to dysplasia.

Subsequently, diagnostic criteria were developed for endoscopic OCT to diagnose specialized intestinal metaplasia (SIM), high-grade dysplasia (HGD), and intramucosal carcinoma (IMC). In prospective studies performed by Poneros *et al.* and Evans *et al.*, sensitivities from 81%-97% and specificities from 57%-92% for diagnosing SIM were reported [55,56]. Additionally, sensitivities and specificities for detecting HGD and IMC were reported in the ranges of 54%-83% and 72%-75%, respectively [55,57]. Unfortunately, similar to previous investigations, the studies were limited to 'point' sampling where a probe was placed at discrete locations and cross-sectional images were obtained. Although these studies made great strides in the diagnostic potential of OCT, the true clinical utility for Barrett's esophagus was not realized due to the potential for sampling errors analogous to biopsy.

More recently, technological advancements and the development of a second-generation OCT system, OFDI, has provided the ability to image long-segments of tissue with high-resolution and contrast identical to those obtained in OCT but at a rate approximately 100-times faster [58,59]. The first comprehensive imaging of the esophagus in human patients using OFDI was performed by Suter *et al.* In this study, a balloon-centering optical catheter was used to acquire long-segment (6cm) images of the esophagus during an endoscopic procedure (<2 minutes) [60]. During system and catheter development, a total of 32 patients were imaged prior to the design being unchanged. Once the final design had been established, a total of 10 patients out of 12 were successfully imaged using the comprehensive microscopy technique of OFDI, while 2 patients were not imaged due to imaging system malfunction. No adverse events or patient-related complications were reported in the study. Although the study presented promising case findings related to OCT diagnosis of normal esophagus and cardia, ulcerated squamous mucosa, specialized intestinal metaplasia, and dysplasia, it was limited to image criteria established based on a non-contact OCT probe. Additional studies are needed to develop diagnostic criteria, intra-observer and inter-observer variability in diagnosis of OFDI imaging, and an OFDI-histopathologic correlative study using OFDI technology.

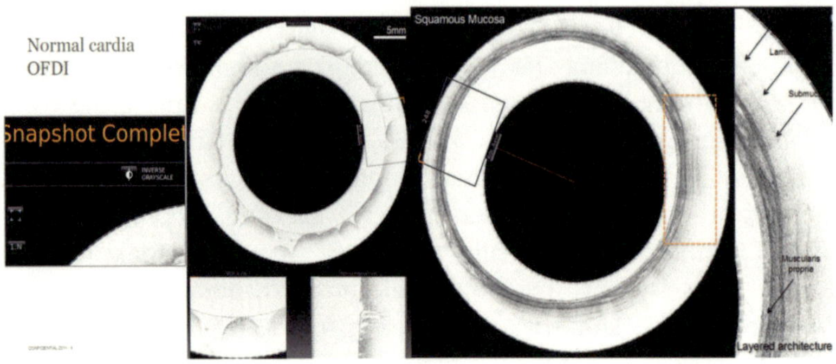

Figure 15. Optical Coherence Tomography images showing normal cardia and a cross sectional image through the squamous oesophagus. (Courtesy of Ninepoint Medical)

7.3. Autofluorescence

When tissues are exposed to a short wave length light, endogenous biological substances (i.e., fluorophores) are excited, leading to emission of fluorescent light of a longer wavelength. This phenomenon is known as autofluorescence. Autofluorescence imaging (AFI) is a technique that can potentially differentiate tissue types based on their differences in fluorescence emission. Normal and neoplastic tissue have different autofluorescence spectra which may enable their distinction. This is due to the various different compositions of the endogenous fluorophores which includes collagen, NADH, aromatic amino acids and porphyrins in these tissues. This phenomenon was first utilized in Barrett's esophagus using spectroscopic point measurements. In brief, low collagen fluorescence and high NAD(P)H fluorescence characterize lesions with high grade dysplasia as opposed to non-dysplastic epithelia. Hence, with progression towards neoplasia one would typically observe a reduction in the intensity of green fluorescence, and a relative increase in red fluorescence.

In a 2006 60 patient study using a standard endoscope with an added AFI component, Kara was able to detect HGD in 22 patients, 14 of which were detected with AFI and WLE, and six of which were detected using AFI alone; thereby increasing the detection rate from 23% to 33% using AFI [61]. Only one of the patients was diagnosed using the standard four-quadrant biopsies alone. Results suggest that AFI may aid in the detection of additional HGD sites; however, it may not exclude the need for the standard four-quadrant biopsies. Sensitivity and specificity based on the 116 samples used for this study were 91% and 43%, respectively. Although no patient was diagnosed without AFI and four-quadrant biopsies, they cite a high rate of false positives using AFI alone, due in part to the loss of autofluorescence associated with acute inflammation.

8. VCE – Video Capsule Endoscopy

Wireless video capsule endoscopy (VCE) was approved by the Food and Drug Administration in 2001 as an adjunctive aid for the detection of small bowel disorders. Because patients ingest the capsule in the standing position and the small bowel VCE captures two frames per second, the traditional VCE often does not capture images of the esophago-gastric junction (EGJ).

Developed in 2004, the Esophageal capsule, or PillCam ESO (Given Imaging, Ltd., Duluth, GA, USA), captures 14 frames per second whereas the patient ingests the capsule in a supine position and then gradually resumes the sitting position during a 5-minute period. Usage of the first generation PillCam ESO demonstrated excellent sensitivity and specificity for the detection of erosive esophagitis and BE in a preliminary study of 106 patients (93 with GERD, 13 with BE). Sixty-six of 106 patients had positive esophageal findings, VCE identified oesophageal abnormalities in 61 (sensitivity, 92%; specificity, 95%). The per-protocol sensitivity, specificity, PPV, and NPV of VCE for Barrett oesophagus were 97%, 99%, 97%, and 99%, respectively, and for esophagitis 89%, 99%, 97%, and 94%, respectively. VCE was preferred over conventional upper GI endoscopy by all patients. There were no adverse events related to VCE. The investigators concluded that VCE is a convenient and sensitive method for visualization of oesophageal mucosal pathology and may provide an effective method to evaluate patients for oesophageal disease.

Following on from this initial landmark study a second generation esophageal capsule, ESO-2, was released by Given Imaging in 2007 with a 30% increase in the frame capture rate from 14 to 18 frames per second, advanced optics with three lenses instead of one lens, and expansion of field of view from 140o to 169o.To maximize visualization of the EGJ and reduce the presence of bubbles, the standardized ingestion protocol (SIP) was published by Gralnek *et al.* [62] and included having the patient lie on his/her right side during capsule ingestion while sipping 5–10 ml of water every 30 seconds. A subsequent clinical trial in 28 subjects using the SIP protocol and ESO-2 demonstrated visualization of the Z-line in 75% of subjects, and sensitivity of 100% with specificity of 74% for BE detection. The agreement between ESO-2 and EGD for description of the Z-line was 86% (k = 0.68).

A 2009 meta-analysis [63] including nine studies with 618 patients undergoing primarily the first generation VCE demonstrated a pooled sensitivity and specificity of VCE for BE detection of 77% and 86% compared to 78% sensitivity and 90% specificity for upper GI endoscopy.

9. ESS - Elastic Scattering Spectroscopy

Elastic scattering spectroscopy (ESS) is based on white light scattering. In ESS, photons hit tissue and are backscattered without a change in wavelength. The relative intensity of this backscattering is influenced by the composition of the interrogated tissue, specifically the relative concentration of scatterers (i.e. nuclei, mitochondria, connective tissue) and absorbers (i.e. hemoglobin). With the transition to dyplasia or neoplasia, tissues typically experience an increase in nuclear crowding and enlargement and a change in biochemical composition. All of these changes lead to characteristic alterations in light scattering, which can be used to delineate different tissue types.

ESS spectra relate to the wavelength-dependence and angular-probability of scattering efficiency of tissue micro-components. The sizes, indices of refraction and structures of the denser sub-cellular components (e.g., the nucleus, nucleolus, mitochondria) are known to change upon transformation to premalignant or malignant conditions. Indeed, histopathologists use these nuclear changes to grade dysplasia, i.e. the sizes and shapes of nuclei and organelles, the ratio of nuclear to cellular volume (nuclear:cytoplasmic ratio) and clustering patterns (nuclear crowding).

ESS is a point measurement. Mourant *et al.* analyzed elastic light scattering from isolated mammalian tumor cells and nuclei [64]. Using cells at different stages of growth in the cell cycle they demonstrated that light scattering at angles greater than about 110° was correlated with the DNA content of these cells. Based on model calculations and the relative size difference of nuclei from cells in different stages of growth, they suggest that this difference in scattering results from changes in the internal structures of the nucleus that are increased in the mitotic states.

In order to take optical measurements a flexible fibre-optic probe is passed down the working channel of an endoscope and normal white light is shone at the underlying tissue for a fraction of a second. The back-scattered light is collected and a spectral analysis performed. This scattering of light is sensitive to changes in the structure of the underlying cells and has already been shown to be able to detect HGD with a high degree of accuracy. Using pattern recognition techniques such as multivariate discriminate analysis, algorithms have been developed to classify spectra as premalignant or benign tissues. Optical measurements require less than a second to collect and during the collection of over 10,000 readings in previous studies no complications have occurred.

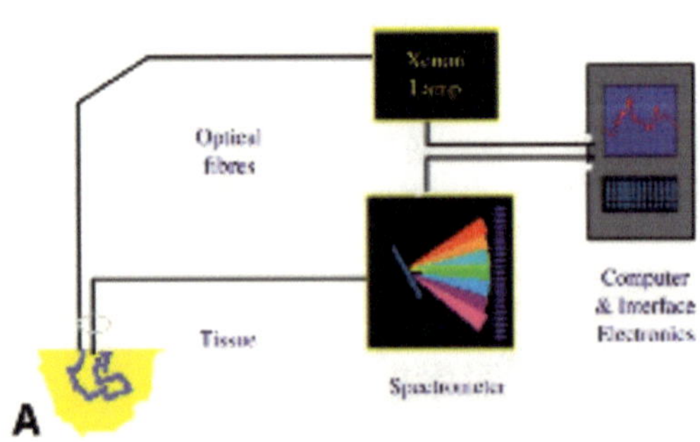

Our group at the National Medical Laser Centre at University College London have performed the largest clinical *in vivo* study of scattering spectroscopy to date, evaluating the value of ESS in discriminating dysplastic and non-dysplastic tissue in Barrett's esophagus

[65]. A total of 181 matched biopsy sites from 81 patients, where histopathological consensus was reached, were analysed. There was good pathologist agreement in differentiating high grade dysplasia and cancer from other pathology (kappa = 0.72). Spectral data was analysed by LDA + PCA to form a model which was then tested by leave one out cross validation (jac-knife analysis). Elastic scattering spectroscopy detected HGD or cancer with 92% sensitivity and 60% specificity. If used to target biopsies during endoscopy, the number of low risk biopsies taken would decrease by 60% with minimal loss of accuracy. ESS had a negative predictive value of 99.5% for high grade dysplasia or cancer. These novel and very promising results show that ESS has the potential to target conventional biopsies in Barrett's surveillance. In order to validate this technique, a prospective study is required.

10. Raman spectroscopy

The Raman effect was first discovered and described in 1928 by Chandrasekhar Venkata Raman, for which he was awarded the Nobel Prize in 1930. It is an optical diagnostic technique that is a very valuable analytical tool. Only recently has it been used for biological and medical research. It exploits the frequency shift, which occurs when a sample is illuminated with laser light, due to the excitation of vibrational states in the constituent molecules. The most significant characteristic of Raman spectra is that the intensity of the individual peaks is linearly proportional to the concentration of the molecular constituents. Thus, a precise molecular fingerprint is obtained. It is a rapid, non-destructive, optical scattering technique that has the ability of objective identification of molecular markers such as protein conformation, nucleic acid and glycogen content. Thus the Raman spectrum is a direct function of the molecular biology of the tissue. Extensive work has identified typical peaks, in the region 900e1800 cm_1, seen in the normal esophageal epithelium that changes during the process of malignant transformation. These may be useful for optical detection of neoplastic transformation during endoscopy.

11. FTIR spectroscopy

FTIR spectroscopy is an analytical technique that is based on the absorption of light in the region that excites molecular vibrations. Most spectrometers operate in the mid-IR range of approximately 4000 to 900 cm^{-1}. Molecular vibrations can be excited to higher levels by the absorption of radiation in this range. Absorption occurs when the energy of the IR radiation matches the energy difference of the 2 vibrational states. In this way, IR spectra gives information about the molecular vibrations in a given sample manifesting themselves in absorbance peaks at variable frequencies.

There is much literature outlining the success of FTIR spectroscopy in the identification of cancerous tissues from normal tissue. Donna *et al.* [66] found specific spectral changes in the Fourier Transform spectrum of esophageal cancers. Such changes were attributed to a range of molecular alterations such as the decrease in glycogen level and the increase in DNA content. Limited work has however been done in the discrimination of the pre-malignant dysplastic states of Barrett's esophagus using FTIR spectroscopy.

In 2009 Wang *et al.* [67] studied the use of FTIR in tissue from patients with BE. In this series, spectra were collected from 98 excised specimens of the distal oesophagus, including 38 squamous, 38 intestinal metaplasia (Barrett's), and 22 gastric, obtained endoscopically from 32 patients. They demonstrated that DNA, protein, glycogen, and glycoprotein comprise the principal sources of infrared absorption in the 950- to 1,800-cm-1 regime. The concentrations of these biomolecules were quantified by using a partial least squares fit and used to classify disease states with high sensitivity, specificity, and accuracy. Moreover, use of FTIR to detect premalignant (dysplastic) mucosa results in a sensitivity, specificity, positive predictive value, and total accuracy of 92%, 80%, 92%, and 89%, respectively, and leads to a better inter-observer agreement between two gastrointestinal pathologists for dysplasia (K 0.72) versus histology alone (K 0.52). This was the first study that demonstrated that the concentration of specific biomolecules can be determined from the FTIR spectra collected in attenuated total reflectance mode and can be used for predicting the underlying histopathology, which will contribute to the early detection and rapid staging of many diseases.

12. Virtual colonoscopy

Virtual colonoscopy (VC) is a diagnostic method enabling the generation of two- dimensional and three-dimensional images of the colon and rectum from the data obtained with relevant imaging modality, usually spiral computed tomography (CT). If CT is used, the method is also called CT colonoscopy, CT colonography, or CT pneumocolon. The main advantages of the VC which support its broader application in medical practice include: limited invasiveness, improved compliance of patients and value for screening for colorectal cancer.

The patient undergoing helical computed tomography with the intent of obtaining VC should undergo complete bowel preparation as for other procedures within abdomen, e.g. endoscopic colonoscopy. The priority is assigned to evacuation of the contents of the colon before CT. For this purpose, many agents are used including ethylene glycol electrolyte solution, magnesium citrate or oral sodium phosphate. Nevertheless, the quality of bowel preparation for VC varies considerably between different centres (Van Uitert et al., 2008). The trend for the optimization of the diagnostic procedures and limitation of the burden to the patient resulted also in a strategy focusing on the performing of the optical colonoscopy just after VC, if it is positive for pathological lesions in the colon, in order to avoid repetition of the bowel preparation procedure. A strategy enabling identification of the artifacts resulting from fecal contents in the bowel in the process of generation of VC images was also proposed. This is achieved by labeling it with some type of contrast agent, e.g. barium or meglumine diatrizoate taken orally before the CT (Iannaccone et al., 2004).

Growing use of the VC is supported by its lower invasiveness in the comparison to other diagnostic procedures and potential for higher compliance from patients. These features increase the value of the techniques as a screening test for disorders of the colon. The main indications for VC include screening for colonic polyps or cancer and failure or inadequate results of optical colonoscopy due to anatomical conditions or pathological lesions, e.g. obstruction of the colon lumen. Furthermore, the VC enables also for examination of extra-colonic structures not accessible during standard colonoscopy. This may be particularly important for these patients in whom pathological lesions were detected inside the colon lumen.

The Guidelines issued in 2008 by American Cancer Society, American College of Radiology and US Multi-Society Task Force on Colorectal Cancer included VC within recommended screening tests for colorectal cancer, which should be performed at 5 years intervals in population of at least 50 years or older (Levin et al., 2008). According to the Guidelines, VC should be performed after complete bowel preparation. The detection of a polyp of size >6 mm in VC necessitates the performance of optical colonoscopy, preferably the same day or second complete bowel preparation is needed

12.1. Patient preparation for VC

The purpose of bowel preparation is to clean out the colon before imaging. Preparations can be the so-called wet preparations, such as polyethylene glycol and sodium phosphate preparations or the drier laxatives including magnesium citrate preparations, fleet enemas, bisacodyl tablets and LoSo Prep. Generally phospho-soda (fleet enema) is recommended for young and healthy patients while the polyethylene glycol preparation is preferable for the elderly.

Prepless techniques are currently also being investigated, requiring faecal tagging methods. This is achieved by the use of orally ingested agents, usually dilute barium or iodinated contrast medium that 'tag' or 'label' residual fluid or faecal matter.

A single dose of laxative together with three doses of 250 ml 2.1 % w/v barium sulphate the day before the scan may equal diagnostic performance in fully pre- pared patients. Image analysis requires a dedicated CT colonographic software package to 'subtract' the high attenuation labelled faecal residue from the colonic lumen, i.e. CT colonographic software package with a subtraction capability.

12.2. Data acquisition

Thin-slice acquisition protocols with multi-detractor row CT to cover the entire abdomen in a single breath hold should be used; 2.5 mm or 1.25 mm collimation is recommended.

12.3. Positioning

Scanning usually begins in the supine position and is subsequently performed in the prone position if fluid is present in the colon. The second acquisition is to ensure that fluid-filled segments can be interpreted later.

12.4. Premedication

The efficacy of administering Buscopan or glucagon before scanning to improve colonic distension is con- troversial. In a study of 240 patients who underwent virtual colonoscopy, Rogalla and colleagues found that glucagon improved distension significantly only when the results were analysed per segment; however Buscopan provided better volume distension and sig- nificantly reduced the number of collapsed colonic segments.

12.5. Insufflation

Automated insufflation with carbon dioxide (CO_2) using an automatic insufflation device is recommended as this maintains a constant CO_2 pressure during scan- ning. Where an automatic insufflator is not available, a hand pump may be used with insufflation of room air.

12.6. Low-dose CT

Intrinsic high contrast between the colonic wall and insufflated gas allows dose-saving low MA protocols (e.g. 50 mAs). Recent data suggest that excellent sen- sitivity for cancer and polyps of over 6 mm can be achieved using a collimation of 2.5 mm and tube cur- rent of 10 mAs giving an effective dose of 2.15 mSV in men and 2.75 mSV in women.

12.7. Intravenous contrast for problem solving

The use of contrast is also controversial in virtual colo- noscopy. A study performed by Martina Morrin and colleagues foundthatsensitivityimprovedfrom58%to 75% with the use of IV contrast. Intravenous contrast is helpful if there is poor preparation of the patient and should be used as a problem-solving tool.

12.8. Interpretation of data

Interpretation of data can be performed by a 3D fly- through endoluminal approach, with simultaneous cor- relation with 2D axial images and 2D MPR images, soft- ware packages which include multiple imaging layout formats for adequate visualisation of the entire colon.

As CT colonography becomes more widespread, there is increasing inter-observer variation in interpretation. Computer-aided diagnosis (CAD) plays an important role in this regard. When applied to the colon, CAD relies on three main steps: (*i*) extraction of the colon from the 3D CT volume; (*ii*) identification of potential polyp candidates; and (*iii*) eliminating false positives as far as possible.

12.9. Detection of lesions

In a study performed by Pickhardt *et al.* polyps greater than 6 mm were detectable using 1.25 – 2.5 mm col- limitation with multi-detector row CT. Sensitivity and specificity of CT colonography decreases as lesion size decreases below 5 mm.

The gastroenterological literature emphasizes the advanced adenoma as an appropriate target for screening. The advanced adenoma is classified by size or histology, with lesions greater than 10 mm or with villous histology being significant.

There has been debate about significance of small lesions in CT colonography screening or surveillance programmes; however practically this is not an issue for endoscopic screening techniques, as all lesions seen are removed. However with radiological screening, Pickhardt *et al.* have considered a cut-off size of 8 mm or greater as a recommendation for conventional colonoscopy, and recommend repeat follow-up scans for smaller lesions after 2 – 3 years.

13. Endoscopic ultrasound (EUS)

EUS combines 2 modalities: endoscopic visualization and high-frequency US. The ability to image the wall of the GI tract as a series of definable layers corresponding to histology, rather than as a single entity, is the basis for most indications for EUS. Other indications have emerged from the ability of EUS to provide detailed images of areas in immediate proximity to the GI tract and to guide needles precisely through the gut wall into surrounding structures.

The addition of endoluminal US offers a unique advantage over traditional endoscopy, allowing precise differentiation of the individual layers of the GI tract, and direct imaging of the surrounding organs and tissue. EUS allows assessment of submucosal GI lesions, loco regional staging of GI malignancy, tissue diagnosis, and staging of pancreaticobiliary lesions, non small-cell lung carcinoma, and mediastinal disease. In prospective trials, EUS has consistently been shown to have a significant impact on diagnosis and management. EUS-guided FNA has emerged as an adjunctive modality during standard endosonography, allowing tissue diagnosis of submucosal lesions, extraluminal lesions, and/or lymph nodes. Further- more, therapeutic uses for EUS have been described and are used on a limited basis in some institutions.

EUS has become firmly established as an adjunctive endoscopic imaging study for patients with previously identified lesions of the GI tract and surrounding organs. Multiple studies suggest that EUS is superior to CT for tumor (T) and lymph node (N) staging of luminal and pancreaticobiliary malignancies. The ultimate choice of staging modalities is largely dependent upon patient selection and local expertise.

13.1. The role of endoscopic ultrasound in staging of oesophageal cancer

Following on from a histological diagnosis of OAC it is imperative to complete a clinical TNM staging. This has recently been changed in the American Joint Committee on Cancer (AJCC) Seventh Edition.

TNM staging of esophagogastric junction (EGJ) adenocarcinoma

Primary tumor (T)*	
TX	Primary tumor cannot be assessed
T0	No evidence of primary tumor
Tis	High-grade dysplasia•
T1	Tumor invades lamina propria, muscularis mucosae, or submucosa
T1a	Tumor invades lamina propria or muscularis mucosae
T1b	Tumor invades submucosa
T2	Tumor invades muscularis propria
T3	Tumor invades adventitia
T4	Tumor invades adjacent structures
T4a	Resectable tumor invading pleura, pericardium, or diaphragm
T4b	Unresectable tumor invading other adjacent structures, such as aorta, vertebral body, trachea, etc.
Regional lymph nodes (N)Δ	
NX	Regional lymph node(s) cannot be assessed
N0	No regional lymph node metastasis
N1	Metastasis in 1-2 regional lymph nodes
N2	Metastasis in 3-6 regional lymph nodes
N3	Metastasis in seven or more regional lymph nodes
Distant metastasis (M)	
M0	No distant metastasis
M1	Distant metastasis
Histologic grade (G)	
GX	Grade cannot be assessed - stage grouping as G1
G1	Well differentiated
G2	Moderately differentiated
G3	Poorly differentiated
G4	Undifferentiated - stage grouping as G3 squamous

Table 1. 2011 AJCC 7th Edition TNM staging guidelines

The evidence suggests that EUS can successfully differentiate early (T1) from advanced intramucosal disease but it is poor at differentiating mucosal from submucosal lesions. Its role in managing patients with early disease therefore appears to be limited, although it does appear valuable for detecting associated malignant lymphadenpathy. Although the quality of computed tomography (CT) and magnetic resonance imaging (MRI) images has improved dramatically, EUS remains part of the standard algorithm for staging tumours [66;67].

Studies with small cohorts of cases have demonstrated that EUS can accurately predict submucosal invasion, especially when lesions are examined with high frequency EYS probes (20MHz) as this modality helps to delineate all 9 layers of the oesophagus compared to just the conventional 5 layers as seen by normal resolution EUS. Furthermore the role of EUS staging is limited by operator experience, location of the neoplasia and morphology of the lesion (flat versus elevated versus depressed).

In the last few years, endoscopic assessment of patients with early oesophageal cancers has come increasingly to rely on EMR to assess for submucosal invasion. In a prospective study of 64 patients by the Wiesbaden group, all subjects were carefully screened with conventional radial EUS at a frequency of 7.5 MHz and with HFPUS if a visible lesion was present [68]. Pre-EMR staging was in agreement with the histological findings in 58 of the 64 patients (91%) evaluated. Two cases of EUS tumor over stage and 4 cases of EUS tumor downstage occurred.

In the largest trial to date, a prospective blinded trial by the same group compared staging of early oesophageal carcinoma using high resolution endoscopy (HR-E) with HFPUS [69]. There was no significant difference in diagnostic accuracy between the two techniques (83% for HR-E and 80% for HFPUS). Sensitivity for mucosal tumours was more than 90% for both modalities while sensitivity for submucosal tumours was lower, at 56% for HR-E and 48% for HFPUS. HFPUS was significantly more accurate at staging submucosal tumours in the tubular oesophagus (10/11; 91%) than those located at the oesophagogastric junction (2/14, 14%).

In a large study of 50 patients from Notingham by Thomas et al. [70] the role of EUS in detecting depth of invasion and nodal involvement was investigated in patients with early Barrett's associated neoplasia of the oesophagus. Visible lesions in the Barrett's segment were described as Paris types 0-1 (n = 9), 0-IIb (n = 12), 0-IIa (n = 12), 0-IIa + IIc (n = 6), and 0-IIc (n = 5). Of the 50 patients, 46 (92%) had either EMR (n = 17), oesophagectomy (n = 23), or both (n = 6). All 12 patients (100%) with Paris 0-IIb lesions had T0/T1 m staging on EUS confirmed with resection histology. The sensitivity for EUS T-staging for Paris classification was 71.4% for type 0-I, 100% for type 0-IIb, 83% for type 0-IIa, 66.7% for type 0-IIa + IIc, and 66.7% for type IIc. Overall, 8 (17%) of the 46 patients were under staged and 2 (4%) were over staged. This study demonstrated that for detecting submucosal invasion, EUS has a sensitivity of 66%, a specificity of 93%, a negative predictive value of 85%, and a diagnostic accuracy of 84.4%.

14. Comparing EUS to CT and PET CT

EUS is also an important tool for evaluating malignant lymph nodes with a high sensitivity and specificity. The ability of EUS to detect lymph node involvement has been compared to computerised tomography (CT) in several studies. In a prospective study of 100 patients with confirmed early cancer in BE, Pech *et al.* compared the two modalities for accuracy of lymph node staging [71]. For the purposes of this study lymph nodes were considered as non-malignant when the pathological assessment was negative or the long-term follow-up showed no progression. EUS had a sensitivity of lymph node involvement of 75% and specificity of 97%, compared to 38% sensitivity and 100% specificity for CT.

In a more recent series by Choi et al. [72] where a total of 109 patients with respectable OAC were prospectively enrolled and retrospectively reviewed for evaluation of pre-operative EUS,PET and CT. The study showed that the overall accuracy of EUS for T-staging was 72%, and importantly it was the only method of delineating the oesophageal wall layers. The sensitivities for N staging were 42% for EUS, 49% for PET, and 35% for CT, and their specificities were respectively, 9187 and 93%. The accuracy for N staging was 66% for EUS, 68% for PET and 63% for CT, and it did not differ across the 3 diagnostic modalities. This series shows that for loco-regional staging, EUS provides excellent T staging accuracy and similar accuracy for N staging compared with PET and CT scanning.

15. Conclusion

There have been significant efforts in recent years towards improving the ability to make real-time pathological diagnoses during endoscopy of the upper gastrointestinal tract. Decision making with respect to endoscopic treatment has been informed greatly as a result, meaning therapy can be delivered without delay obviating the need for repeated endoscopic procedures.

Practices have evolved greatly from the traditional approach of WLE and non-targeted biopsy. Today many more additional techniques are available, from chromoendoscopy and NBI to improved post- processing technology, through to the potential of OCT and ESS. These have prospective roles not only in detecting dysplasia in Barrett's esophagus, but also in the diagnosis and management of early esophageal squamous cell carcinoma and adenocarcinoma. The introduction of virtual colonoscopy with high sensitivity and specificity will allow skilled endoscopists to focus their time on interventional procedure and remove some of the growing burden of routine diagnostic colonoscopy. EUS continues to use the established radiological modalities in the GI tract to define tissue layers and stage neoplastic diseases accurately.

The challenge remains to clarify the exact roles of these techniques in clinical practice, to standardize their use (particularly with respect to classification systems) and to appropriately incorporate them into clinical practice on a large scale.

Author details

Rehan Haidry[1,2*] and Laurence Lovat[1,2]

*Address all correspondence to: r.haidry@ucl.ac.uk

1 University College Hospital, London, UK

2 National Medical Laser Centre, University College London, UK

References

[1] Guelrud M, Herrera I, Essenfeld H *et al*. Enhanced magnification endoscopy: a new technique to identify specialized intestinal metaplasia in Barrett's esophagus. Gastrointestinal Endoscopy 2001;53(6) 559-65.

[2] Kara MA, Peters FP, Rosmolen WD *et al*. High-resolution endoscopy plus chromoendoscopy or narrow-band imaging in Barrett's esophagus: a prospective randomized crossover study. Endoscopy 2005;37(10) 929-36.

[3] Kara MA, Smits ME, Rosmolen WD *et al.* A randomized crossover study comparing light-induced fluorescence endoscopy with standard videoendoscopy for the detection of early neoplasia in Barrett's esophagus. Gastrointestinal Endoscopy 2005;61(6) 671-8.

[4] Reid BJ, Blount PL, Feng Z *et al.* Optimizing endoscopic biopsy detection of early cancers in Barrett's high-grade dysplasia. American Journal of Gastroenterology 2000;95(11) 3089-96.

[5] Falk GW, Rice TW, Goldblum JR *et al.* Jumbo biopsy forceps protocol still misses unsuspected cancer in Barrett's esophagus with high-grade dysplasia. Gastrointestinal Endoscopy 1999;49(2) 170-6.

[6] Tada M, Katoh S, Kohli Y *et al.* On the dye spraying method in colonofiberscopy. Endoscopy 1977;8(2) 70-4.

[7] Acosta MM, Boyce HW, Jr. Chromoendoscopy--where is it useful? Journal of Clinical Gastroenterology 1998;27(1) 13-20.

[8] Canto MI. Staining in gastrointestinal endoscopy: the basics. Endoscopy 1999;31(6) 479-86.

[9] Canto MI, Yoshida T, Gossner L. Chromoscopy of intestinal metaplasia in Barrett's esophagus. Endoscopy 2002;34(4) 330-6.

[10] Canto MI, Setrakian S, Petras RE *et al.* Methylene blue selectively stains intestinal metaplasia in Barrett's esophagus. Gastrointestinal Endoscopy 1996;44(1) 1-7.

[11] Canto MI, Setrakian S, Willis J *et al.* Methylene blue-directed biopsies improve detection of intestinal metaplasia and dysplasia in Barrett's esophagus. Gastrointestinal Endoscopy 2000;51(5) 560-8.

[12] Canto MI, Setrakian S, Petras RE *et al.* Methylene blue selectively stains intestinal metaplasia in Barrett's esophagus. Gastrointestinal Endoscopy 1996;44(1) 1-7.

[13] Canto MI, Setrakian S, Willis J *et al.* Methylene blue-directed biopsies improve detection of intestinal metaplasia and dysplasia in Barrett's esophagus. Gastrointestinal Endoscopy 2000;51(5) 560-8.

[14] Horwhat JD, Maydonovitch CL, Ramos F *et al.* A randomized comparison of methylene blue-directed biopsy versus conventional four-quadrant biopsy for the detection of intestinal metaplasia and dysplasia in patients with long-segment Barrett's esophagus. American Journal of Gastroenterology 2008;103(3) 546-54.

[15] Canto MI, Setrakian S, Willis JE *et al.* Methylene blue staining of dysplastic and nondysplastic Barrett's esophagus: an in vivo and ex vivo study. Endoscopy 2001;33(5) 391-400.

[16] Wo JM, Ray MB, Mayfield-Stokes S *et al.* Comparison of methylene blue-directed biopsies and conventional biopsies in the detection of intestinal metaplasia and dyspla-

sia in Barrett's esophagus: a preliminary study. Gastrointestinal Endoscopy 2001;54(3) 294-301.

[17] Sharma P, Topalovski M, Mayo MS *et al*. Methylene blue chromoendoscopy for detection of short-segment Barrett's esophagus. Gastrointestinal Endoscopy 2001;54(3) 289-93.

[18] Kiesslich R, Hahn M, Herrmann G *et al*. Screening for specialized columnar epithelium with methylene blue: chromoendoscopy in patients with Barrett's esophagus and a normal control group. Gastrointestinal Endoscopy 2001;53(1) 47-52.

[19] Ngamruengphong S, Sharma VK, Das A. Diagnostic yield of methylene blue chromoendoscopy for detecting specialized intestinal metaplasia and dysplasia in Barrett's esophagus: a meta-analysis. Gastrointestinal Endoscopy 2009;69(6) 1021-8.

[20] Lambert R, Rey JF, Sankaranarayanan R. Magnification and Chromoscopy with the Acetic Acid Test. Endoscopy 2003;35(05) 437-45.

[21] Guelrud M, Herrera I, Essenfeld H *et al*. Enhanced magnification endoscopy: a new technique to identify specialized intestinal metaplasia in Barrett's esophagus. Gastrointestinal Endoscopy 2001;53(6) 559-65.

[22] Toyoda H, Rubio C, Befrits R *et al*. Detection of intestinal metaplasia in distal esophagus and esophagogastric junction by enhanced-magnification endoscopy. Gastrointestinal Endoscopy 2004;59(1) 15-21.

[23] Reaud S, Croue A, Boyer J. Diagnostic accuracy of magnifying chromoendoscopy with detection of intestinal metaplasia and dysplasia using acetic acid in Barrett's esophagus. Gastroenterologie Clinique et Biologique 2006;30(2) 217-23.

[24] Hoffman A, Kiesslich R, Bender A *et al*. Acetic acid-guided biopsies after magnifying endoscopy compared with random biopsies in the detection of Barrett's esophagus: a prospective randomized trial with crossover design. Gastrointestinal Endoscopy 2006;64(1) 1-8.

[25] Longcroft-Wheaton G, Duku M, Mead R *et al*. Acetic acid spray is an effective tool for the endoscopic detection of neoplasia in patients with Barrett's esophagus. Clinical Gastroenterology and Hepatology 2010;8(10) 843-7.

[26] Curvers WL, van den Broek FJ, Reitsma JB *et al*. Systematic review of narrow-band imaging for the detection and differentiation of abnormalities in the esophagus and stomach (with video). Gastrointestinal Endoscopy 2009;69(2) 307-17.

[27] Kara MA, Peters FP, Rosmolen WD *et al*. High-resolution endoscopy plus chromoendoscopy or narrow-band imaging in Barrett's esophagus: a prospective randomized crossover study. Endoscopy 2005;37(10) 929-36.

[28] Wolfsen HC, Crook JE, Krishna M *et al*. Prospective, controlled tandem endoscopy study of narrow band imaging for dysplasia detection in Barrett's Esophagus. Gastroenterology 2008;135(1) 24-31.

[29] Kara MA, Bergman JJ. Autofluorescence Imaging and Narrow-Band Imaging for the Detection of Early Neoplasia in Patients with Barrett's Esophagus. Endoscopy 2006;38(6) 627-31.

[30] Curvers WL, Bohmer CJ, Mallant-Hent RC *et al*. Mucosal morphology in BarrettΓ Ms esophagus: interobserver agreement and role of narrow band imaging. Endoscopy 2008;40(10) 799-805.

[31] Curvers WL, van den Broek FJ, Reitsma JB *et al*. Systematic review of narrow-band imaging for the detection and differentiation of abnormalities in the esophagus and stomach (with video). Gastrointestinal Endoscopy 2009;69(2) 307-17.

[32] Sharma P, Hawes RH, Bansal A *et al*. Standard endoscopy with random biopsies versus narrow band imaging targeted biopsies in Barrett's oesophagus: a prospective, international, randomised controlled trial. Gut 2012; Feb 7 [Epub ahead of print] doi: 10.1136/gutjnl-2011-300962.

[33] Banks MR, Haidry R, Butt MA *et al*. High resolution colonoscopy in a bowel cancer screening program improves polyp detection. World Journal of Gastroenterology 2011;17(38) 4308-13.

[34] Osawa H, Yamamoto H, Yamada N *et al*. Diagnosis of endoscopic Barrett's esophagus by transnasal flexible spectral imaging color enhancement. Journal of Gastroenterology 2009;44(11) 1125-32.

[35] Pohl J, May A, Rabenstein T *et al*. Comparison of computed virtual chromoendoscopy and conventional chromoendoscopy with acetic acid for detection of neoplasia in Barrett's esophagus. Endoscopy 2007;39(7) 594-8.

[36] Pohl J, Pech O, May A *et al*. Incidence of Macroscopically Occult Neoplasias in Barrett's Esophagus: Are Random Biopsies Dispensable in the Era of Advanced Endoscopic Imaging? American Journal of Gastroenterology 2010;105(11) 2350-6

[37] Endo T, Awakawa T, Takahashi H *et al*. Classification of Barrett's epithelium by magnifying endoscopy. Gastrointestinal Endoscopy 2002;55(6) 641-7.

[38] Kara MA, Ennahachi M, Fockens P *et al*. Detection and classification of the mucosal and vascular patterns (mucosal morphology) in Barrett's esophagus by using narrow band imaging. Gastrointestinal Endoscopy 2006;64(2) 155-66.

[39] Singh R, Anagnostopoulos GK, Yao K *et al*. Narrow-band imaging with magnification in Barrett's esophagus: validation of a simplified grading system of mucosal morphology patterns against histology. Endoscopy 2008;40(6) 457-63.

[40] Sharma P, Bansal A, Mathur S *et al*. The utility of a novel narrow band imaging endoscopy system in patients with Barrett's esophagus. Gastrointestinal Endoscopy 2006;64(2) 167-75.

[41] Silva FB, Dinis-Ribeiro M, Vieth M *et al*. Endoscopic assessment and grading of Barrett's esophagus using magnification endoscopy and narrow-band imaging: accuracy

and interobserver agreement of different classification systems (with videos). Gastrointestinal Endoscopy 2011;73(1) 7-14.

[42] Wallace MB, Meining A, Canto MI *et al*. The safety of intravenous fluorescein for confocal laser endomicroscopy in the gastrointestinal tract. Alimentary Pharmacology and Therapeutics 2010;31(5) 548-52.

[43] Kiesslich R, Gossner L, Goetz M *et al*. In vivo histology of Barrett's esophagus and associated neoplasia by confocal laser endomicroscopy. Clinical Gastroenterology and Hepatology 2006;4(8) 979-87.

[44] Pohl H, Rosch T, Vieth M *et al*. Miniprobe confocal laser microscopy for the detection of invisible neoplasia in patients with Barrett's oesophagus. Gut 2008;57(12) 1648-53.

[45] Dunbar KB, Okolo P, III, Montgomery E *et al*. Confocal laser endomicroscopy in Barrett's esophagus and endoscopically inapparent Barrett's neoplasia: a prospective, randomized, double-blind, controlled, crossover trial. Gastrointestinal Endoscopy 2009;70(4) 645-54.

[46] Gaddam S, Mathur SC, Singh M *et al*. Novel probe-based confocal laser endomicroscopy criteria and interobserver agreement for the detection of dysplasia in Barrett's esophagus. American Journal of Gastroenterology 2011;106(11) 1961-9.

[47] Sharma P, Meining AR, Coron E *et al*. Real-time increased detection of neoplastic tissue in Barrett's esophagus with probe-based confocal laser endomicroscopy: final results of an international multicenter, prospective, randomized, controlled trial. Gastrointestinal Endoscopy 2011;74(3) 465-72.

[48] Huang D, Swanson EA, Lin CP *et al*. Optical coherence tomography. Science 1991;254(5035) 1178-81.

[49] Bouma BE, Yun SH, Vakoc BJ *et al*. Fourier-domain optical coherence tomography: recent advances toward clinical utility. Current Opinions in Biotechnology 2009;20(1) 111-8.

[50] Bouma BE, Tearney GJ, Compton CC *et al*. High-resolution imaging of the human esophagus and stomach in vivo using optical coherence tomography. Gastrointestinal Endoscopy 2000;51(4 Pt 1) 467-74.

[51] Jackle S, Gladkova N, Feldchtein F *et al*. In vivo endoscopic optical coherence tomography of the human gastrointestinal tract--toward optical biopsy. Endoscopy 2000;32(10) 743-9.

[52] Li XD, Boppart SA, Van DJ *et al*. Optical coherence tomography: advanced technology for the endoscopic imaging of Barrett's esophagus. Endoscopy 2000;32(12) 921-30.

[53] Sivak MV, Jr., Kobayashi K, Izatt JA *et al*. High-resolution endoscopic imaging of the GI tract using optical coherence tomography. Gastrointestinal Endoscopy 2000;51(4 Pt 1) 474-9.

[54] [54] Yang VX, Gordon M, Tang SJ *et al.* High speed, wide velocity dynamic range Doppler optical coherence tomography (Part III): in vivo endoscopic imaging of blood flow in the rat and human gastrointestinal tracts. Optics Express 2003;11(19) 2416-24.

[55] Evans JA, Poneros JM, Bouma BE *et al.* Optical coherence tomography to identify intramucosal carcinoma and high-grade dysplasia in Barrett's esophagus. Clinical Gastroenterology and Hepatology 2006;4(1) 38-43.

[56] Poneros JM, Nishioka NS. Diagnosis of Barrett's esophagus using optical coherence tomography. Gastrointestinal Endoscopy Clinics of North America 2003;13(2) 309-23.

[57] Isenberg G, Sivak MV, Jr., Chak A *et al.* Accuracy of endoscopic optical coherence tomography in the detection of dysplasia in Barrett's esophagus: a prospective, double-blinded study. Gastrointestinal Endoscopy 2005;62(6) 825-31.

[58] Vakoc BJ, Shishko M, Yun SH *et al.* Comprehensive esophageal microscopy by using optical frequency-domain imaging (with video). Gastrointestinal Endoscopy 2007;65(6) 898-905.

[59] Yun S, Tearney G, de BJ *et al.* High-speed optical frequency-domain imaging. Optics Express 2003;11(22) 2953-63.

[60] Vakoc BJ, Shishko M, Yun SH *et al.* Comprehensive esophageal microscopy by using optical frequency-domain imaging (with video). Gastrointestinal Endoscopy 2007;65(6) 898-905.

[61] Kara MA, Peters FP, ten Kate FJ *et al.* Endoscopic video autofluorescence imaging may improve the detection of early neoplasia in patients with Barrett's esophagus. Gastrointestinal Endoscopy 2005;61(6) 679-85.

[62] Gralnek IM, Adler SN, Yassin K *et al.* Detecting esophageal disease with second-generation capsule endoscopy: initial evaluation of the PillCam ESO 2. Endoscopy 2008;40(4) 275-9.

[63] Bhardwaj A, Hollenbeak CS, Pooran N *et al.* A meta-analysis of the diagnostic accuracy of esophageal capsule endoscopy for Barrett's esophagus in patients with gastroesophageal reflux disease. American Journal of Gastroenterology 2009;104(6) 1533-9.

[64] Mourant JR, Canpolat M, Brocker C *et al.* Light scattering from cells: the contribution of the nucleus and the effects of proliferative status. Journal of Biomedical Optics 2000;5(2) 131-7.

[65] Lovat L, Bown S. Elastic scattering spectroscopy for detection of dysplasia in Barrett's esophagus. Gastrointestinal Endoscopy Clinics of North America 2004;14(3) 507-17, ix.

[66] Maziak DE, Do MT, Shamji FM *et al*. Fourier-transform infrared spectroscopic study of characteristic molecular structure in cancer cells of esophagus: an exploratory study. Cancer Detection and Prevention 2007;31(3) 244-53.

[67] Wang TD, Triadafilopoulos G, Crawford JM *et al*. Detection of endogenous biomolecules in Barrett's esophagus by Fourier transform infrared spectroscopy. Proceedings of the National Acadademy of Sciences of the U S A 2007;104(40) 15864-9.

Chapter 8

Vocal Folds Stroboscopic Image Processing for Otolaryngology

A. Méndez Zorrilla and B. García Zapirain

Additional information is available at the end of the chapter

http://dx.doi.org/10.5772/55343

1. Introduction

Nowadays it is very common to go to a specialist's surgery because of voice disorders. Voice pathologies are characterized by the abnormal production and/or absence of vocal quality, pitch, loudness or resonance. Approximately 28 million workers in the U.S. experience daily voice problems [1][2] and the statistics indicate that voice pathologies affect almost five percent of the population [3].

Daily life sometimes affects our voice and our vocal cords. Talking too much (in the case of occupational voice users, such as singers, teachers, lawyers, telephonists…), screaming, constantly clearing your throat or smoking can make you hoarse. For example, teachers have missed many workdays due to voice problems and are more likely to consider changing occupations because of their voice [4].

Other psychosocial factors, such as stress and anxiety involve voice problems as well [5]. All the causes mentioned above. All the aforementioned causes can also lead to pathologies such as nodules, polyps and sores on the vocal cords [6].

The vocal folds (or vocal cords) are composed of twin infoldings of mucous membrane stretched horizontally across the larynx. Their vibration produces each person's voice [7].

The most common benign pathologies are the following (all of them analysed in this study):

- Nodules. This disorder prevents the vocal folds from meeting in the midline, which produces an hourglass deformity on closure resulting in a harsh/rough/coarse…, breathy voice. Nodules are most common in children and females.

- Polyps. This pathology is a benign lesion of the larynx, occurring mostly in adult males, usually located on the phonating margin of the vocal folds and preventing the vocal folds from meeting in the midline.
- Cysts. A cyst is a firm mass of organic material contained within a membrane. Cysts can be located near the surface of the vocal fold or deeper, near the ligament of the vocal fold.
- Paralysis. Paralysis occurs when only one side is paralyzed in the paramedian position or has very limited movement. It is more common than bilateral involvement.

All previously mentioned morphological path morphological pathologies disturb the phonation process resulting into a hoarse voice signal, and the hoarse is the main reason To go to the specialist. Usually, patients can recover their voice with rehabilitation, and only sometimes the surgery is necessary.

The most widely used clinical voice disorder assessment tools for capturing vocal fold videos are digital videostroboscopies [8] and high speed recordings [9]. The vocal folds can be examined by inserting an endoscope through the nose or mouth. The examiner uses the endoscope light to view the folds and their movement patterns during phonation (producing sound) and when at rest. This test is invasive and very uncomfortable for the patient and in some cases the process has to be/ needs to be repeated in order to view the vocal folds correctly.

In this research, only low-speed recordings illuminated with a stroboscopic light are used. We employ low-speed recorded images since there are intensively used among othorhinolaryngologists and voice specialists [10].

These recordings are usually very problematic because of the different level… the different level of illumination inside the video, the patient's movements while the doctor is recording, or the zoom. Figure 1.a and 1.b shows two very poor-quality frames. Figure 1.a represents a low level of illumination and Figure 1.b illustrates patient movement because both frames are consecutive.

Due to recording difficulties… difficulties, segmentation without initialization (other related works with user interaction or initialization are supported in [11][12]) is more difficult to obtain than in high-speed recordings.

However, the problem lies in the fact that a specialist delivers a diagnosis in a subjective way and it depends on his experience in this area. The study of glottal space (illustrated in Figure 1) in a video sequence can be very useful and decisive when it comes to obtaining an accurate diagnosis. Figure 1.c shows a very good quality image of healthy vocal folds and in Figure 1.d vocal folds with one of the studied pathologies –polyps- can be seen.

The main goal is to find a methodology to parameterize vocal folds, obtaining glottal space segmentation without user interaction, a pre-diagnosis support based on a classification stage and some objective measurements to support the doctors' final diagnosis and it allows (the doctor) to do comparatives and control the patients' evolution after rehabilitation or surgery. This chapter has been drawn up taking into account specially the context of development in clinical medicine and telemedicine applications in the otolaryngology field.

http://dx.doi.org/10.5772/55343

In this process we consider that the following specific objectives have to be taken into account:

- To work and analyze the commercial database "Laryngeal Videostroboscopic Images (Dr. Wendy LeBorgne; Plural Publishing)" and some recordings given by the otolaryngologist Dr. Agustín Pérez Izquierdo from Basurto Hospital.
- To segment vocal fold glottal space correctly and reduce a significant amount of image data
- To classify the images to carry out a pre-diagnosis
- To apply block matching techniques to have information about vocal folds movement
- To define and measure objective parameters to help the diagnosis

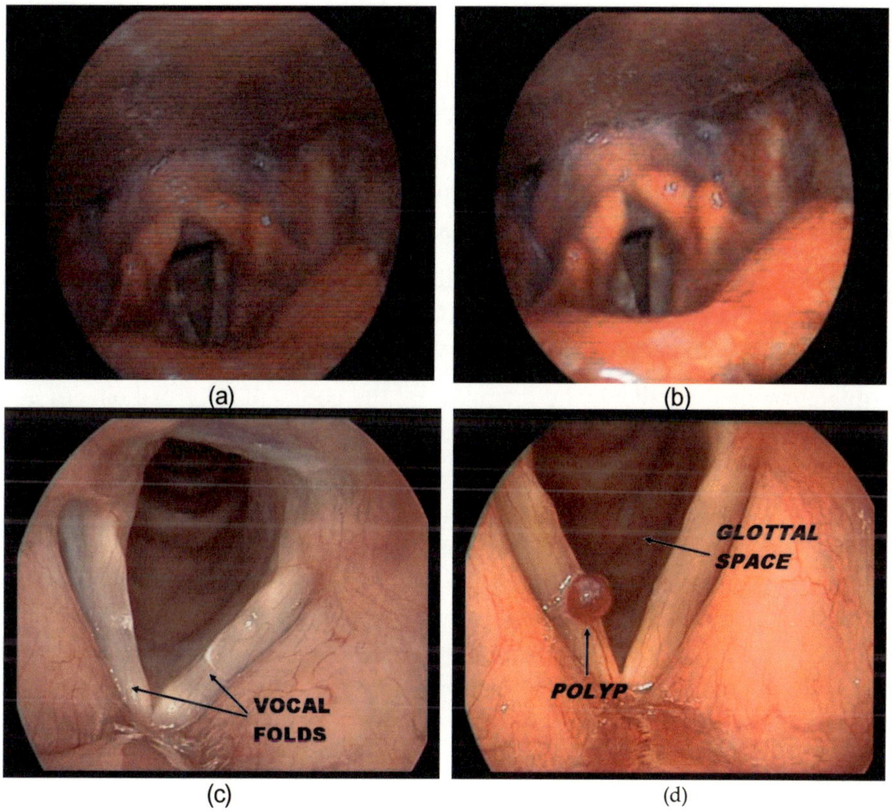

Figure 1. Vocal folds Images. a) and b) Poor quality frames with different illumination. c) and d) Good quality vocal folds images. c) Healthy folds and b) Pathological folds.

2. State of the art in image processing for otolaryngology

This section is divides into 3 subsections to describe the state of the art in otolaryngology field.

2.1. Image capture techniques and software analysis

Given that this research is focused on the study of images (and videos) of vocal cords, It is also object of this study the analysis of different methods of image digital capture of them,.

Nowadays, the scientific and medical community accepts mainly two capture techniques whose results can help to determine the diagnosis of different vocal fold pathologies. On the one hand there is **videostroboscopy**, and, on the other hand, de **videoquimiography** or high speed image capture.

The way to visualize and study the vocal cords has been object of study for many centuries.

Manuel García is considered as the the first discoverer of the indirect laryngoscopy with the speculum. It was in 1854 [13]. At the beginning he was considered an intruder, since he was a composer, a tenor and a singing teacher, but not a doctor, as might have been expected. But his idea of placing a dentist speculum in the throat and going on illuminating the larynx with the sun light reflected in a mirror he holds in her hands, examining the vocal cords [14] was subsequently recognized by all the laryngological societies.

Later on, it was Johan Nepomuk Czermal from Budapest [15] who improved that technique using artificial light and speculums of different sizes and it is precisely him who achieved to introduce the indirect laryngoscopy as the main exploratory method.

In 1975, Stuckrad and Lakatos [16] developed this technique with amplification, that is to say, with a magnifier. But it is not until 1978 when Oertel [17] developed the laryngostroboscope, which permits the examination of vocal cords vibration.

This exploratory method allows the diagnosis by the observation of pathologies in initial stages, or else, those ones which do not affect the morphology of the vocal fold, but its movement.

In the nineties, the high speed digital videoquimiography of the larynx emerged [18]. This technique wishes to give a solution to the problems in the speed of the image capture in the videostroboscopy. The human eye is only capable of capturing 5 or 6 images per second, whereas the videostroboscopy captures between 25 and 30 frames per second [8] but it continues to be insufficient to observe the dynamic movements that take place in the larynx during the phonation. That is why the videoquimiography is currently being an appraised tool, mostly in the research field.

From the point of view of clinical examination, the digital videostroboscopy is the essential and routine method in the diagnosis of voice disorders, since it provides an extraordinary amount of information about the behavior of the vibratory cycle and its alterations.

And it is here where the next sections of this chapter are framed, and precisely in the diagnosis of the vocal cord alterations within the objective parameterization of stroboscopic videos.

2.2. Software analysis

Recently, international research groups, in collaboration with specialist medical staff are showing their interest in the development of the characteristics of the vocal fold images' software analysis, though, habitually, they don't reach the market. Given that the VKG images are of better quality, the development of this application typology use to be developed for its analysis, as it can be observed in the literature [19-20].

Kay owns software named KIPS (Kay's Image Processing Software). KAY oriented to the vocal fold digital image processing, coming from stroboscopic captures or from high quality. It includes a multitude of tools for the image editing and processing, providing the specialist with a very valuable information in support of the diagnostic, but it neither issues a diagnosis nor it automates the process % 100.

Habitually, the softwares used by the otolaryngologists/ otolaryngologists, or any voice specialist have only into account the voice analysis, and take part of a unit or voice laboratory [21].

It is important to remember that the measurement of the acoustic parameters does not issue the diagnosis of the injury, but it may indicate the level of alteration of the dysphonia. The objective parameters accepted by the scientific community in the acoustic analysis are: pitch, jitter, shimmer and HNR (and its variants) and are indicative of a good or low vocal quality [22].

2.3. Image processing techniques to process vocal fold images

In this subsection, the authors describe come techniques which could be applied to this kind of images.

2.3.1. Active contours

These contours [23] model the boundaries between the object, the background/the bottom, and the remaining objects of the image. They allow to extract the contours of the object of interest based on models or forms that use previous information about the form of the objects. The active contours, or, also named Snakes [24] are much more robust against the presence of noise and other elements, and allow to segment much more complex images, like the medical images which are the object of this study, for instance.

The segmentation results, provided by this technique, applied to the vocal cords images are fairly positive, as it can be seen, but no previous initialization is required.

2.3.2. Wavelet transform

The Wavelet transforms [25] and other multiscale analysis functions are widely used in the digital image processing for the applications of noise elimination/reduction, compression and feature extraction.

Its application in bioengineering is very extended [26], and more specifically in applications of medical images like: ultrasound images, tomography images or magnetic resonance images. The capture methods of these images and, therefore, its characteristics are very different to the vocal cord images that are object of study in this chapter.

2.3.3. *Kalman filter*

Within the digital image processing field, the Kalman filter is a recursive algorithm that is used to estimate the position of a moving point or characteristic, and the measurement uncertainty in the following image. It is about to reach the feature (point, edge, corner, region, and so on), in a particular area of the following image around the aforesaid position, in which we are sure to find the feature within a certain degree of confidence.

The aim of the filter is the acquiring of an optimal estimator of the state variables of a dynamic system, based on noisy observations and on an uncertainty model of the dynamics of the system [27-28].

It is more appropriate to conduct the study of the vocal cord movements through high-speed captured images, and in this study stroboscopic images were used. Thus, in this case, the Kalman filter has not been applied

3. Parameterization system proposal

The developed algorithms, belonging to the Middleware layer, normalize process, analyze and extract the features of different vocal fold pathologies. Mainly those pathologies which affect to the morphology of the vocal fold, and which, at least lead to dysphonia, and, in other cases, pathologies caused by an abnormal function in the movement and vibration of the vocal folds, as it can be the paralysis of the vocal fold.

The application layer is responsible for the representation of the data to the user in a friendly graphic interface.

Thus, a sequential order for the implementation of the study and the application of the algorithms, it is considered 0 stage, to the capture of the image by the specialist. Once the images are available, we focus in the extraction of all the parameters/features of the sequences of images that will give us some information about the pathology suffering by the patient or the absence of it. Subsequently, we try to classify/identify the image comparing withe the database (with previously classified and diagnosed images) that is available. Finally, with all the information a diagnosis to the specialist can be offered, supported by all the objective parameters extracted during the process.

The methodology followed during the whole design process has been constant, defining in each case the entrance and output requirements and variables of each of the blocks of the defined stages, as it can be described in the following point.

3.1. Design

The high level design establishes the form and substance of the system considering it as a whole, as a set of functions that constitute the structure or architecture of the system without going into detail of each one, since this will be made in the low level detailed Design.

In all the applications, except by the smallest ones, the first step to design a complete system consist on dividing it in a small number of components, blocks or stages. Each of the main blocks of a system covers some aspects of the system that share any common property. Each one of the blocks or stages contains/comprises a package of functions and interconnected events that share a common purpose, which have a well-defined interface with the remaining blocks or stages (and they habitually can be reused in various systems or applications).

The general bock diagram proposed to reach the established objectives can be observed in Figure 2.

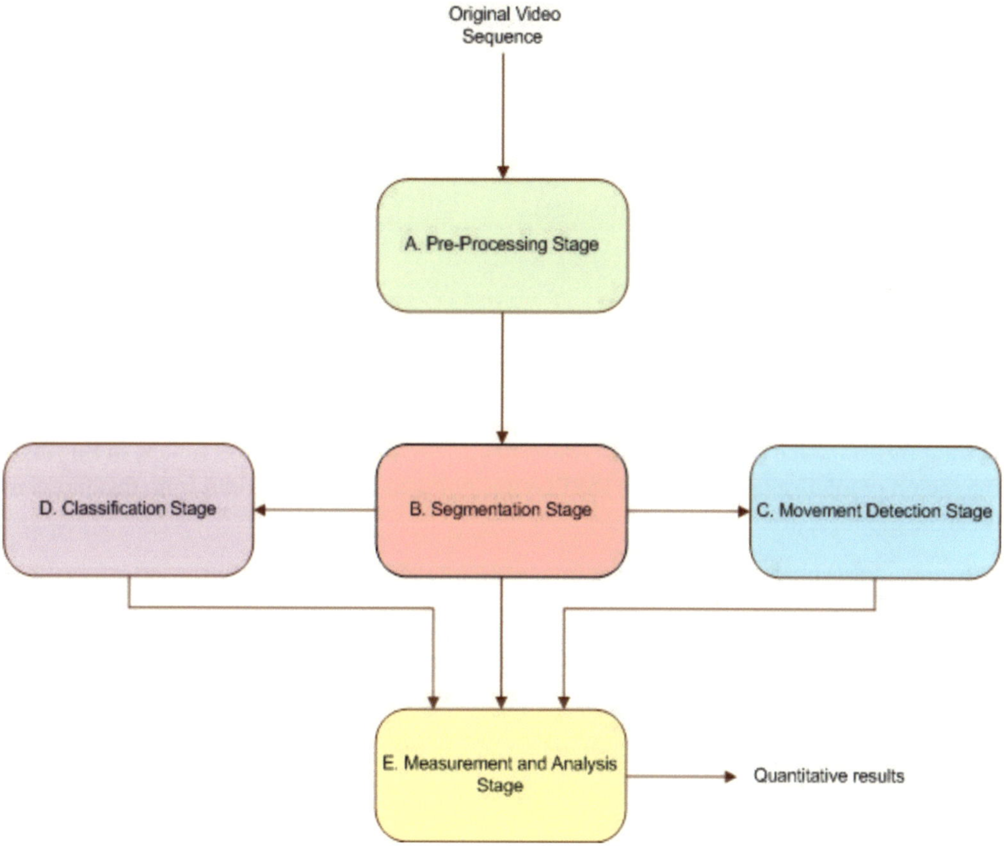

Figure 2. High Level Diagram

The entrance of the systems are the frames of each of the sequences in original format (In colour, and with the quality and resolution acquired by the camera). Each one of the blocks apply the necessary transformations to obtain as a final result a report with those objective data which may help and support the otolaryngologist with the diagnoses, and to evaluate rehabilitation processes or the evolution after a surgical intervention.

Next, the five main blocks which compose/contain the low level design are described (Each one identified with a colour coding which will be maintained throughout the chapter (As it can be seen in Figure 2).

3.1.1. *Pre-processing stage*

This first block carries out the necessary functions like the unification, normalization and standardization of the characteristics of the stroboscopic videos of the vocal folds, or vocal fold images, so they can be treated more easily and efficiently in the subsequent blocks.

The *input* of this block is the original recording provided by the otolaryngologist. An isolated image can also be analyzed, but the results in some of the stages have a low reliability. In some stages the comparison/study of certain parameter between frames within the same sequence is necessary. It has to be taken into account the variability of the intraframe recording. Thus, the comparison is a utility that provides much information,

The *Output* of this block is a sequence of frames in JPG format normalized in characteristics and transformed into a grayscale whose gradient has been calculated (to facilitate the application of the filters of the subsequent stage).

3.1.2. *Segmentation stage*

Due to its level of criticality this is the main stage of the system. The validity of the system and the error rate obtained in subsequent stages depend, in part of its success. The three subsequent stages are based (even are used as Input) in the result of the segmentation stage.

During this stage the necessary transformations are used to segment and isolate, in this case, the region of interest. In this system the ROI it is going to be working with from this moment on is the glottal space.

The *input* of this block are the gradient images result of the normalization carried out in the A block.

The *output* of this block is the sequence of frames where the glottal space has been segmented. From the block B, the attention is paid mainly to this part of the image and to the study of the features of the glottal space perimeter.

3.1.3. *Movement detection stage*

In this stage Block Matching algorithms are applied, habitually used for the image compression MPEG standards, and widely extended in a multitude of applications [29]. The aim is to detect and study the interframe movement of the vocal folds. Always assuming that the stroboscopic images are not the most adequate ones to evaluate neither the movement nor the vibrations of the folds, since the frame rate is between 25 and 30 frames per second, far lower the vocal fold vibration speed.

For this reason, the results of this stage are relative and have to be complemented with the E stage measures, or even with other studies.

The *input* of this block is the frame sequence whose glottal space has been segmented in the block B.

The *Output* of this block are all the motion vectors calculated as a result of the application of the Block Matching algorithms.

3.1.4. Classification stage

With the stages described hitherto it has not been obtained any result which can guide us in the diagnosis. It only has been extracted the region of interest and movement measures. It is in this stage where a pre-diagnosis of the data obtained in the stages B and C is carried out. A classification of the entrance images is made through various algorithms, to discern between morphological and non-morphological pathologies, comparing the entrance of this stage with a previously classified and studied images database. The results of this stage, partially, depend on the choice and the size of that database to compare the inputs of this stage.

The D block has various inputs unlike the previous blocks. For the execution of this blocks three inputs are needed: the original frame sequence, the sequence of frames with the segmented glottal space (result of the B block), and the motion vectors calculated in Block C (Output of Block C).

The output of this block is a pre diagnosis/classification, according to the identification/classification algorithms applied.

3.1.5. Analysis and measurement stage

It is in this stage where finally, the necessary calculations are made to achieve some objective results which allow us to carry out an evaluation and a possible diagnosis, and even to discern which is the morphological pathology of the vocal folds the patient suffers. As far as the pathologies related to the vocal fold movements are concerned, some parameters which may guide the specialist to a more deep study will be provided, but bearing in mind that the results provided may not be 100% consistent, due to the frame rate of the available capture.

Once the necessary transformations are made, to achieve those results, some objective measures over the vocal fold images are made, and it is on their representation in which the evaluation and/or the diagnosis and the value of this contribution will be based.

The *input* of this block is multiple, as in Block D. To calculate the objective parameters which will be the final result of this thesis it is necessary to make calculations and transformations over the results in blocks B, C and D.

The *output* of this block will be the set of objective measures supporting the final diagnosis proposed to the specialist, which may become part of the final report given to the patient.

The novelty, complexity and main feature of the proposed system is that it does not **require** any type of neither **initialization** nor interaction with the user during its execution for the achieving of the diagnosis, evaluation and/or the measurement of the effectiveness of the treatment (computer-aided pre-diagnosis).

4. Results

As it has been reflected in the "Design" section, to illustrate de experimentation carried out, it would be taken into account that the system has 5 differentiated stages, and the results for each stage will be showed.

Special emphasis will be placed in the results of the pathologies related to the morphology of the vocal folds against those related to the movement, because of the type of the images studied and because of the sample available in the database, and finally the results obtained in different formats will be presented.

4.1. Segmentation stage tests

The segmentation stage is the first and the most important one in the whole process, since from its results it depends on the success in the subsequent stages. The obtaining of objective results for the characterization of the vocal folds and the emission of the diagnosis depend also on this stage.

In this stage we can observe graphic and numerical results. Those later ones are used to express the success percentage in the segmentation within the sequence.

If we analyze the results grouping the sequences into pathologies they can be further improved:

- *Healthy vocal fold Sequences*. The average frames in these sequences is 22,1, having obtained a correctly segmented frames average of 95,95%.
- *Sequences of Vocal Folds with Nodules*. The average frames in these sequences is 26, having obtained an average of correctly segmented frames average of 95,34%. Although the mean number of frames in the sequences is slightly higher, and this does not affect considerably to the percentage value of the correctly segmented frames.
- *Sequences of Vocal Folds with polyps*. The average frames in these sequences is 33,44, having obtained a correctly segmented frames average of 94,96%.
- *Sequences of Vocal Folds with Oedema*. The average frames in these 4 sequences is 31,75, having obtained a correctly segmented frames average of 89,82%.
- *Sequences of Vocal Folds with Cyst*. The average frames in these 5 sequences is 28,6, having obtained a correctly segmented frames average of 94,96%.
- *Sequences of Vocal Fold with Paralysis*. For the segmentation and the subsequent classification, these images are not differentiated each other in an independent way, from the frames of the healthy vocal folds. The average frames in these 7 sequences is 30, having obtained a correctly segmented frames average of 96,88%.

4.2. Classification stage tests

The classification stage is the third stage in the system, and it is applied to provide the doctor with a reference pre-diagnosis. It is also used as an entrance in subsequent stages, and,

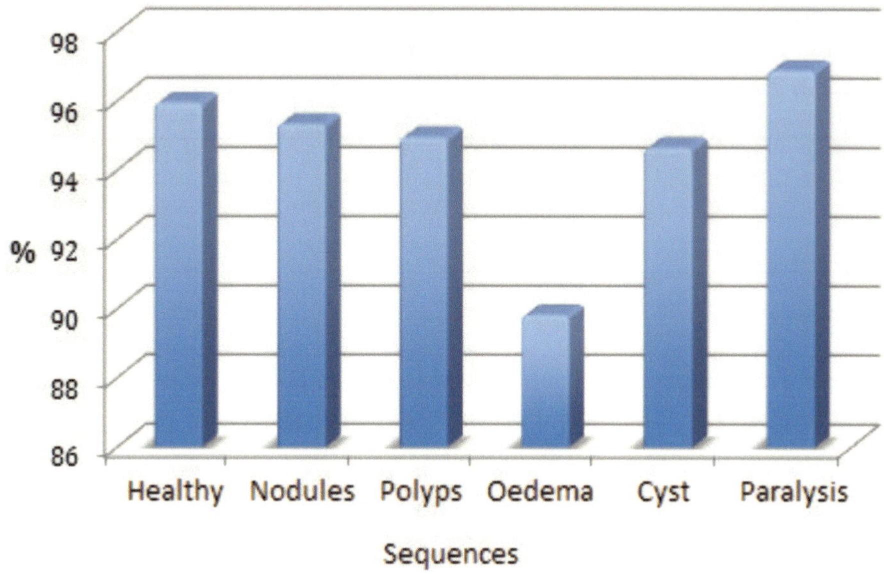

Figure 3. Graphic representation of the segmentation results

depending on the results in this stage, either one or other transformations are applied in the "Analysis and measurement" stage.

The critic element in the validation and the success of this stage is the choice of the Training Set and to establish which ones have to be those images are the most important decisions that was to be taken in this stage. Indeed, the success rate and the processing time in this stage, which it can be considerable, also depend on that decision. This whole system is a post processing in itself, and it is assumed that it is not carried out in real time.

During the experimentation some tests have been made with different Training Sets of 16,18, 25 and 100 images, being the definitive/final one that Set composed by 100 images.

The results obtained can be seen in Table 1. The percentage of correctly classified images with the exact pathology (nodules, polyp, oedema, cyst..) is 71,8%, whereas if we simply focus on the correctly classified ones as healthy or pathological the percentage is 92,1%. The latter is the result that matters to us, since the success of the final parameterization depends, in part, on it.

It is demonstrated that to change the Training Set makes the results to be completely different, see the Training Set of 25 images tested with 330 images, where the percentage of the images correctly classified with the exact pathology varies from 67,23% to 71,20%. 4% of difference, which, depending on the images of the Training Set can be wider.

In Table 1 is demonstrated that as we go by raising the number of images of the Training Set the results improve, from 85% of a Training Set with 16 images to 92,09 % of the Training Set of 25 Images.

Number of images in Training Set	Number of test images	% of images classified with the correct pathology	% of images correctly classified (healthy or pathological)
25	330	67,23	92,09
25	330	71,20	87,65
18	330	69,98	86,34
16	330	68,51	85,00

Table 1. Classification Experiment. Eigenfolds results in %

Up to now, the tests were made with frames containing both Vocal Folds, but, in reality, each Vocal fold separately can be classified as healthy or pathological.

In the following tests each of the vocal folds were treated independently though the same Training Sets were maintained but, this time with the double of images, as Table 2 shows.

Number of images in Training Set	Number of test images	% of images classified with the correct pathology	% of images correctly classified (healthy or pathological)
25 *2	330 *2	65,10%	95,04%
18*2	330*2	64,23%	90,56%
16*2	330*2	37,41%	80,21%

Table 2. Eigenfolds Results using a Vocal Fold Training Set treated the right Fold and the Left Fold independently

Observing Table 2, It can be seen how, analyzing each fold separately, the results improve up to obtaining 95,04%of success differentiating between those folds that suffer any pathology related to the morphology or not.

Number of images in Training Set	Number of test images	% of images classified with the correct pathology	% of images correctly classified (healthy or pathological)
100*2	900*2	71,80%	92,10%

Table 3. Eigenfolds Results Treating Independently the Right Fold and the Left Fold

Finally, in Table 3 the result considered as final is shown, using a Training Set of 100 images (200 since each vocal fold is studied separately) tested with 900 test images (1800 in reality). The final result of this stage is that 92,1% of the images are correctly classified. Hence, the Analysis and Measurement stage will follow the process correctly.

The Movement detection stage is applied only to those images or sequences of images previously classified as "Morphologically healthy" and which are really healthy or have a vocal Fold paralysis. At this point in the system, the movement in some points of the lower third of each of the vocal fold is measured.

Statistical measures are made, mainly mean, variance, standard deviation, paying special attention to the measure of the variance.

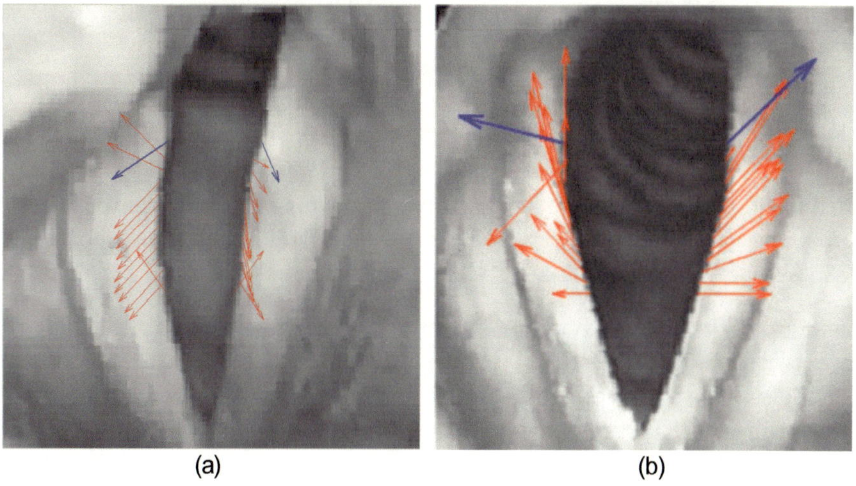

Figure 4. Motion vectors in a) a sequence of vocal Folds with paralysis b) a sequence of Healthy Vocal Folds

In Figure 4 two examples with studied frames are showed, with and without paralysis. In red appear all the studied vectors in the Vocal Fold contour and calculated through block matching techniques and in blue the mean vector for all of them.

Observing the vectors in Figure 4a it can be seen, how, one of the folds has less movement, and, what is more, the quantity of motion represented by the vector is unequal. However in Figure 4b the motion represented is more synchronous between both vocal folds.

4.3. Analysis and measurement stage tests

This is the stage where the last tests of the system are made and it might be suggested a diagnosis supported by the objective results obtained over the sequence of images captured by the doctor.

The objective measurements made of the first 15 sequences studied can be appreciated in Table 4. The measurements carried out are intended to identify the morphological pathologies and quantify the size of the previously classified polyp, cyst, nodule or edema.

The measurements are made in pixels and per vocal cord, as that is the only way of doing it. The "0" means that nothing significant was found to measure and therefore confirms that there is no morphological pathology. When intervals appear, this means that there is some kind of irregularity on the inside edge of the vocal cord, and the area comprising this pathology is measured.

Interval is the term used for the measured area because the vibration of the cords and the image captured by the camera mean that the measurement can vary from one frame to another. The final column in Table 4 provides the algorithm's final decision; that is, when the image analyzed has some kind of morphological pathology and when it does not. There were sequences where quantifying the measurement was scrapped due to its being practically imperceptible: areas below 10 pixels were not taken into account.

5. Conclusions

In this section the compliance of the foreseen objectives will be checked, and the lines that open as a continuation of this research work, whose contributions were demonstrated in the "Proposed System" Chapter will be proposed.

As a summary of the above exposed, a series of conclusions can be obtained, from which a very important one is underscored. It is possible to provide with help to the diagnosis of vocal fold pathologies through the vocal fold digital image processing, and the extracting of objective measures. Furthermore, it has been demonstrated that the interaction with the user it is not necessary (in this case, the doctor specialist in otolaryngology) during the analysis process and the vocal fold digital image processing. An algorithm has been developed and it is divided mainly in two parts: One to carry out the segmentation of the glottal space of the vocal folds and other one to discern between healthy vocal folds, with morphological pathologies, as could be those ones related to the movement.

In connection with the segmentation topic, in chapter for it can be observed how, the 95,07% of the images containing the database were correctly segmented, after the applying of the proposed algorithm. This ratio was calculated without taking into account the small segmentation errors which not affect neither to the subsequent stages of the algorithm nor to the diagnosis (taking into account that the location of this small deviations in the segmentation is the higher part of the glottal space). The results of the segmentation by sequences grouped by pathologies were presented, and in all of the 95% ratio is exceeded, except for those sequences of vocal folds with oedema, where this ratio is below 90%.To differentiate and optimize the processing concerning the detected pathology, the statistic PCA algorithm was developed/applied, to carry out a first classification between vocal folds with a morphological pathology and with the absence of it. It has been demonstrated that the Principal Component Analysis gives good results using a Training Set of significant images of each pathology. In this block, results of 92,1% were obtained with a Training set of 100 images (200 in reality, since the right fold and the left fold were separated).The tests with greater Training Sets are not included, since the processing time increased exponentially, reaching to be of various minutes.

The objective measures carried out allow the specialist to quantify the size of the pathology which is describing/visualizing, being able, this way to provide the patient with more infor-

Sequence number	Otolaryngologist's Diagnosis	Pathology size of right-hand cord (in pixels) Average Size	Standard Deviation	Pathology size of left-hand cord (in pixels) Average Size	Standard Deviation	Final Decision
1	Healthy	0,2	0,0	2,4	1,1	Morphologically Healthy
2	Healthy	0,1	0,0	0,0	0,0	Morphologically Healthy
3	Healthy	0,1	0,0	0,0	0,0	Morphologically Healthy
4	Healthy	5,2	2,9	0,0	0,0	Morphologically Healthy
5	Healthy	0,0	0,0	0,0	0,0	Morphologically Healthy
6	Healthy	0,0	0,0	0,0	0,0	Morphologically Healthy
7	Nodules	95,5	0,8	120	0,4	Nodules
8	Nodules	32,5	1,8	36,3	0,5	Nodules
9	Healthy	0,0	0,0	0,0	0,0	Morphologically Healthy
10	Polyps	97,9	0,8	0,0	0,0	Pathological Right cord
11	Nodules	157	1,1	156	0,7	Nodules
12	Paralysis	0,0	0,0	0,0	0,0	Morphologically Healthy
13	Paralysis	0,0	0,0	0,0	0,0	Morphologically Healthy
14	Edema	0,0	0,0	925	0,6	Pathological Left cord
15	Cyst	0,0	0,0	90,9	1,1	Pathological Left cord

Table 4. Measurements results

mation, to **refine the treatment** or even **measure the evolution** in post-operative processes or in **vocal rehabilitation processes**. The system, without foregoing the doctor, can suggest a diagnosis supported by the results obtained.

From these results we can conclude that the designed algorithm operates properly, and, which is more important, avoiding to the maximum the interaction with the user.

And it is precisely in this interaction with the user where the few commercial softwares which are in the market about the subject-matter before us.

Attending to clinical benefits, the proposed system is based mainly on providing the otolaryngologist with the most sophisticated technological means for the diagnosis, quantification of the extent of the pathology, on measuring the efficiency of the treatment of a surgery, and in a collateral way, on reducing the health costs in this service.

Author details

A. Méndez Zorrilla* and B. García Zapirain

*Address all correspondence to: amaia.mendez@deusto.es, mbgarciazapi@deusto.es

DeustoTech Life Unit, DeustoTech Institute of Techology, University of Deusto, Bilbao, Spain

References

[1] Roy, N, Merrill, R. N, Gray, S. D, & Smith, E. M. Voice disorders in the general population: Prevalence, risk factors, and occupational impact. *Laryngoscope, 1151119881995*November, (2005).

[2] Verdolini, K, & Ramig, L. O. Review: occupational risks for voice problems. *Logopedics, Phoniatrics, Vocology, 2613746* (2001).

[3] Becker, W, Naumann, H. H, & Faltz, C. R. Ear, Nose and Throat Diseases. Thieme Medical Publishers, 2nd Edition. (1994).

[4] Roy, N, Merrill, R. N, Thibeault, S, Gray, S. D, & Smith, E. M. Voice disorders in teachers and the general population: effects on work performance, attendance, and future career choices. *Journal of Speech, Language, Hearing Research, 473542551*June, (2004).

[5] Goldman, S, Hargrave, J, Hillman, R, & Holmberg, E. Stress, Anxiety, Somatic Complaints, and Voice Use in Women With Vocal Nodules. *American Journal of Speech-Language Pathology* February (1996). , 5

[6] Cogwell AndersonR., Rusch, M., Pitt, S., Stacy, S., Franke, K. Observed Similarities in Four Adolescents with Paradoxical Vocal Fold Disorder. *The Internet Journal of Pulmonary Medicine.* (2005). , 5(1)

[7] Titze, I. The physics of small-amplitude oscillation of the vocal folds. *J. Acoust. Soc. Am.* 83, 1536, DOI:10.1121/1.395910. (1998).

[8] Poburka, B. A New Stroboscopy Rating Form. *Journal of Voice*, (1999). , 13(3), 403-413.

[9] Švec, J, & Schutte, H. Videokymography: High-speed line scanning of vocal fold vibration. *Journal of Voice*, (1996). (2), 201-205.

[10] Hess, M. M, Ludwigs, M, Kobler, J. B, & Schade, G. Imaging of the larynx-extending the use of stroboscopy-related techniques. *Journal of Logopedics Phoniatrics Vocology*, May (2002). , 27, 50-58.

[11] Allin, S, Galeotti, J, Stetten, G. D, & Dailey, S. H. Enhanced snake based segmentation of vocal folds. *Proc. of IEEE International Symposium on Biomedical Imaging: Macro to Nano*, April, (2004). , 1, 812-815.

[12] Manfredi, C, Bocchi, L, Bianchi, S, Migali, N, & Cantarella, G. Objective vocal fold vibration assessment from videokymographic images. *Biomedical Signal Processing and Control*. April (2006). , 1(2), 129-136.

[13] Fernández GonzálezS., Vázquez de la Iglesia, F., Marqués Girbau, M., & García-Tapia Urrutia, R. Manuel P. García. *Revista Medica Univ. Navarra, 50* (3), 14-18. (2006).

[14] García, M. *Traité complet du chant.* Paris. (1847).

[15] Nepomuk CzermakJ. *Du laryngoscope.* Paris. (1860).

[16] Stuckrad, H, & Lakatos, I. A new magnifying laryngoscope (epipharyngoscope). *Laryngol Rhinol Otol, 54* (4), 336-40. (1975).

[17] Oertel, M. Das laryngokospiche untersuchung. *Arch Laryngol Rhinol, 3116* (1985).

[18] Švec, J, & Schutte, H. Videokymography: High-speed line scanning. *Journal of Voice*, 10 (2), 201-205. (1996).

[19] Manfredi, C, Bocchi, L, Cantarella, G, Peretti, G, Guidi, G, & Mezzatesta, C. Objective parameters from videokymographic images: a user-friendly interface. *Proceedings of INTERSPEECH 2007200712221225*

[20] Manfredi, C, Bocchi, L, Cantarella, G, & Peretti, G. Videokymographic image processing: Objective parameters and user-friendly interface. *Biomedical Signal Processing and Control*, (2012). , 7, 192-201.

[21] González, J, Cervera, T, & Miralles, J. L. Análisis Acústico de la voz: Fiabilidad de un conjunto de parámetros multidimensionales. *Acta Otorrinolaringol Esp,53256268* (2002).

[22] Baken, P, & Orlikoff, R. *Clinical Measurement of Speech and Voice* (2 nd ed.). San Diego: Singular Publishing Group. (2000).

[23] Kass, M, Witkin, A, & Terzopoulos, D. Snakes: Active contour models. *International Journal of Computer Vision.* (1988)., 1(4)

[24] Allin, S, Galeotti, J, Stetten, G, & Dailey, S. H. Enhanced snake based segmentation of vocal folds. *In proc. ISBI 2004.* 812- 815 (2004)., 1

[25] Cavalcanti, N, Silva, S, Bresolin, A, Bezerra, H, & Guerreiro, A. Comparative analysis between wavelets for the identification of pathological voices. *Proceedings of the 15th Iberoamerican congress conference on Progress in pattern recognition, image analysis, computer vision, and applications.* Sao Paulo. Brasil. (2010).

[26] Rees, J. M, Regunath, G, Whiteside, S. P, Wadnerkar, M. B, Cowell, P. E, et al. Adaptation of Wavelet Transform analysis to the investigation of biological variations in speech signals. *Medical Engineering & Physics,* 30 (7), 865-871. (2008).

[27] Ertürk, S. Real-Time Digital Image Stabilization Using Kalman Filters. *Real-Time Imaging,* 8 (4), 317-328. (2002).

[28] Di, M, Joo, E. M, & Beng, L. H. A comprehensive study of Kalman filter and extended Kalman filter for target tracking in Wireless Sensor Networks. *Proceedings of International Conference on System, Man and Cibernetics.* (2008)., 2792-2797.

[29] Goffredo, M, Schmid, M, Conforto, S, & Alessio, D. T. A markerless sub-pixel motion estimation technique to reconstruct kinematics and estimate the centre of mass in posturography". *Medical Engineering & Physics,* 28 (7), 719-726. (2006).

Chapter 9

Infectious Foci Imaging with Targeting Radiopharmaceuticals in Nuclear Medicine

Mojtaba Salouti and Akram Fazli

Additional information is available at the end of the chapter

http://dx.doi.org/10.5772/52882

1. Introduction

Despite the advances in public health during the 18th and 19th centuries and the introduction of immunization and antibiotics in the 20th century, bacterial infection is among the most frequently encountered and costly causes of diseases and one of the major causes of morbidity and mortality especially in developing countries (El-Ghany et al., 2005). Localizing and distinguishing the "infection foci" in body sites are very important and life saving processes. The identification of an infection at early stage of disease is critical for a favorable outcome. The diagnosis of deep seated infections such as osteomyelitis, endocarditis and intra-abdominal abscesses is still a challenging problem. Although imaging techniques such as x-ray, computerized tomography (CT-scan), magnetic resonance imaging (MRI) and ultrasonography (US) might be helpful, but none of these techniques are specific for infection diagnosis because of their limitations due to insignificant anatomical changes in the early stages of the infection process. In addition, these techniques are not capable of differentiating between inflammatory and infectious processes. In contrast, nuclear medicine procedures can determine the location and the degree of disease activity in infectious processes based on physiologic and/or metabolic changes that are associated with these diseases rather than gross changes in the structure (Hall et al., 1998). This method requires a reliable radiopharmaceutical that can selectively concentrate in sites of infection. Various ^{99m}Tc-labeled compounds have been developed for the scintigraphic detection of infection and sterile inflammation in humans. Unfortunately, these radiopharmaceuticals do not discriminate between infection and sterile inflammatory process, which is often of clinical importance (Welling et al., 2001). In recent years, the development of radiolabeled antimicrobial agents for specific diagnosis of infection has received considerable attention, sparking a lively debate about the infection specificity of these radiopharmaceuticals (Oyen et al., 2005). Direct targeting of the locally present microorganisms is a new approach for improving the selectivity of radiopharmaceuticals for infection detection in nuclear medicine (Kyprianidou et al., 2011). The use of radiolabeled antibiotics and antimicrobial peptides are fast emerging as promising targeted diagnostic tests for detection of infective lesions because of their specific binding to the bacterial component. These targeting molecules reliably locate sites of infection and make a differential diagnosis between infection and sterile inflammation. In this chapter, the new approaches to scintigraphic imaging of infection and inflammation by radiolabeled antibiotics and antimicrobial peptides are thoroughly discussed in order to assess their diagnostic value as targeting imaging radiopharmaceuticals.

2. Inflammation and infection

Inflammation and infection are different processes. Inflammation is merely a nonspecific immune response-one which does not require the presence of microorganisms to occur. Inflammation can occur from trauma, ischemia, neoplasm, autoimmune attack or invasion by microorganisms (Petruzzi et al., 2009). Infection can be considered as a special subcategory of inflammatory disease, i.e. an inflammatory reaction of the host in response to invasion by microorganisms (Oyen et al., 2005). All inflammatory processes develop along a known sequence: locally increased blood supply, leakage of a fluid, small molecules and proteins and infiltration of cells (Rennen et al., 2002). In response to tissue damage, powerful defense mechanisms are activated, consisting of leukocytes and plasma proteins. Furthermore, a complex of variety of chemical mediators is involved. The migration of leukocytes from the blood stream is facilitated by chemical mediators which up regulated the expression of adhesion molecules on endothelial cells and leukocytes. This process starts within minutes from the injury and resolves in hours or days. It causes the classical symptoms of acute inflammation; rubor (redness), calor (warmth), tumor (edema), dolor (pain) and fastio laesa (impaired function) (Bleeker-Rovers, 2004). The ability to identify focal sites of infection in patients who do not present with localizing symptoms is a key step in delivering appropriate medical treatment. This is particularly critical in immune compromised patients, since signs and symptoms of infection may be minimized in patients with neutropenia (Babich & Fischman, 1999). There are several reasons why imaging of infection and inflammation and distinguishing between them becomes increasingly important in the next decade. The population is ageing; the application of implants and transplants is increasing. The number of immune compromised patients is growing, mainly because of frequent use of chemotherapeutic agents leading to neutropenia. Furthermore, the increased use of antibiotics leads to insensitivity for some of these pharmaceuticals (Larverman et al., 2008).

3. Types of infection

The most common infections are: (1) *Pneumocystis carinii* pneumonia (PCP) which, the large number of patients receiving chemotherapy or harboring the HIV (human immunodeficiency virus) are susceptible to opportunistic infection, (2) protozoal infections include cryto-sporidiosis and toxoplasmosis (abscess, encephalitis), (3) viral infections include cytomegalovirus (retinitis, adrenalitis, lung, neurological, disseminated) and herpes viruses (simplex and zoster), (4) fungal infections include *Cryptococcos neoformans* (meningitis, pneumonitis, disseminated) and (5) bacterial infections (specially *Stereptococcos* and *Haemophilus*) are being seen more frequently in children and intravenously drug users. Other bacterial infections include *Listera monocytogenes, Salmonella, Nocardia* and *Mycobacteria* both *toberclusis* and *avium* intracellular (Roohi, 2006).

Infections can also be classified according to the type of pathogens including: (1) opportunistic infections: infections caused by microbes belonging to the normal host flora and that initiate an infective process consequently to environmental changes, antimicrobial treatment, traumas and injuries, the reduction of the host immune defenses, or the migration to a new body-compartment, (2) exogenous infections: caused by pathogen organisms, which do not belong to the normal flora but are transmitted to healthy hosts from a contaminated environment (food and water) or from infected carriers (humans or animals). The main routes of transmission of exogenous pathogens from an infected carrier are the air and aerosol, sexual intercourse, blood transfusions or animal bites. Exogenous infections can be classified according to the site of acquirement in: (1) community-acquired infections: when the transmission occurs within the community, (2) healthcare-acquired infections: when the pathogen is transmitted within a hospital or a health-care institution; Finally, iatrogenic infections are those developed consequently to a medical procedure such as pharmaceutical treatment or surgery, and could be caused either by endogenous or exogenous pathogens (Baldoni, 2009).

4. Infection diagnosis techniques

The identification of infection at early stage of the disease is critical for a favorable outcome. Conventional methods of diagnosis, relying on examination and culture of organisms from infected foci have continued to advance embracing new technologies and automation. Despite this, these methods are still time consuming, insensitive and the results often obtain too late to guide clinical decision making (Wareham et al., 2005). Clinicians usually use a variety of laboratory tests, clinical and radiological tests, to aid diagnosis and make a decision (Yurt Lambrecht et al., 2008a).

4.1. Laboratory tests

Many current laboratory tests used to guide the diagnostic process rely on factors in the inflammatory response: erythrocyte sedimentation rate, white-blood cell count, acute-phase proteins and cytokines, but the tests are not specific enough to discriminate between infection and inflammation. New techniques, especially within immunology and molecular biology, are yielding new insights into the discrimination of infection and inflammation (Yurt Lambrecht et al., 2008b).

4.2. Imaging techniques

Imaging techniques can be classified as either structural or functional. Structural imaging procedures are used to evaluate macroscopic morphological changes and implant loosening. Differently, functional imaging procedures aim to visualize the specific accumulation of an injected gamma-emitter radiotracer at the site of infection (Baldoni, 2009). Structural imaging methods like x-ray, US, CT-scan and MRI are based on important anatomic alterations and the possibility of a precocious diagnosis is limited. These are not the best of methods for the localization of infection at early stages (Diniz et al., 2005). These procedures detect the morphologic alterations of the tissues after significant process has taken place in the infective site leading to abscess formation (Motaleb, 2007a). The results of these techniques are unsatisfactory in the early stages of the diseases (Shah & Khan, 2011a), while nuclear medicine images are functional and can therefore identify the infection at the early stages (Mora et al., 2010).

4.2.1. X-ray

X-ray provides a powerful tool in medicine for mapping internal structures of the human body. Relatively inexpensive and readily available, radiographs should routinely be the initial imaging procedure performed in all patients suspected of having musculoskeletal infection. But, the earliest radiographic changes of osteomyelitis are soft-tissue swelling and blurring of adjacent fat planes, which may take several days to become apparent after the onset of infection. Approximately 10 days after the onset of infection, radiographs may demonstrate lysis of medullary trabeculae, focal loss of cortex, and periosteal reaction The sensitivity of plain radiography ranges from 43% to 75%, and the specificity from 75% to 83%. Though helpful when positive, a negative study does not exclude osteomyelitis (Palestro et al., 2006). Despite its limitations, radiographs remain the best initial examination in cases of symptomatic postoperative patients and may depict findings associated with postoperative infection (Peterson, 2006).

4.2.2. Ultrasonography

Musculoskeletal tissues are, for the most part, accessible to examination by ultrasound, allowing its deployment as a first-line investigation in a wide range of musculoskeletal infections. In addition, ultrasound is noninvasive, portable, and versatile. Further, it does not use ionizing radiation, and it is relatively lower in cost. However, ultrasound images have a major disadvantage: poor quality because of multiplicative speckle noise that results in artifacts. Segmentation of lesions in ultrasound images is therefore a challenging task that remains an open problem despite many past research efforts (Yap et al., 2008). On the other hand, ultrasonography is very commonly used during the initial work-ups of children with urinary tract infection (UTI) because it gives a rapid anatomical overview of the kidneys, especially with regard to the dilatation of the collecting system (Wu et al., 2003). The disadvantages are that the results are highly operator-dependent, penetration and reflection of the sound waves in tissue may be hindered by gas (bowel) or dense structures (bone), and structures deep within the body may be difficult to visualize because the image quality suf-

http://dx.doi.org/10.5772/52882

fers from the longer wavelengths used for deep imaging (Gotthardt et al., 2010). Ultrasonography is useful technique for diagnosing and localizing fluid collections, but it often cannot determine whether a particular fluid collection is infected or not (Fortner et al., 1986).

4.2.3. Computed Tomography (CT)

CT-scan is an x-ray imaging technique that produces three dimensions (3D) images of an object by using a series of two-dimensional (2D) set of images data to mathematically reconstruct a cross-section of it. CT is unique because it provides imaging of a combination of soft tissues, bone and vessels, and many studies have confirmed CT to be a valid complement to conventional imaging methods (Cotti & Campisi, 2004). CT is highly reproducible, has an excellent spatial resolution, and although more expensive than ultrasonography, is still relatively inexpensive. The disadvantages are exposure of the patient to radiation and lack of functional information (Gotthardt, 2010). It is also limited by a lack of specificity of many of the imaging findings that are noted in the setting of infection or inflammation (Kumar et al., 2008).

4.2.4. Magnetic Resonance Imaging (MRI)

While MRI provides very high resolution (up to 10 μm) and unlimited depth of penetration, it is, however, limited by low sensitivity, with detectabilities in the milli to micromolar (10^{-3} to 10^{-6}) range. Therefore, amplification techniques are often needed to image molecular processes *in vivo* (Bonekamp et al., 2010). Advantages of MRI are the superb anatomic details it reveals (including the ability to evaluate both bone and adjacent soft tissue), its lack of ionizing radiation, and its rapid completion. Disadvantages of MRI are occasional inability to distinguish infectious from reactive inflammation, and difficulty in imaging sites with metallic instrumentation such as joint prostheses (Palestro et al., 2006). It is also limited by a lack of specificity of many of the imaging findings that are noted in the setting of infection or inflammation (Kumar et al., 2008). Because of the long imaging times and the considerable exposure to noise, MRI is not convenient for patients. Furthermore, there are limitations to the scanning of patients with pacemakers, implants, and other devices, and the procedure is relatively expensive (Gotthardt et al., 2010).

5. Nuclear medicine

Nuclear medicine is a highly multi-disciplinary specialty that develops and uses instrumentation and radiopharmaceuticals to study physiological processes and non-invasively diagnose, treat and identifying the staging of a disease (Hricak, 2007). The radiopharmaceuticals are molecular and cellular structures labeled with a specific radionuclide and are applied to patients after appropriate quality control (Bernardo-Filho et al., 2008). A radiopharmaceutical is usually made up of two components: a basic substance for localization in a desired tissue or organ, and a radionuclide for tagging to the basic substance to emit the gamma rays that can be detected and imaged with a gamma camera. The efficacy of the radiopharmaceutical is therefore determined by these components (Korkmaz & Ozer., 2006). Radiopharmaceuticals localize in inflamed or infected tissue in the body. The radiopharmaceuticals emit gamma rays that can be detected and imaged when a patient is placed in a gamma camera (Truluck, 2007). Radionuclide emission-based nuclear medicine modality is a noninvasive technique, which is a quick, sensitive, and specific method to detect as well as locate the lesion at any anatomical site at early stage of the disease (Singh & Bhatnagar, 2010).

5.1. Advantages of nuclear medicine technique

Nuclear medicine has an important role in adding the diagnosis of particularly deep seated infections such as abscesses, osteomylitis, septic arthritis, endocarditis and infections of prosthetic devices (Das et al., 2002). It provides information on pathophysiological and pathobiochemical processes. In this respect it differs from other current imaging procedures such as x-ray, CT and MRI, which supply information with high resolution on the morphological changes that occur in a specific disease. In addition, nuclear medicine technique permits whole-body imaging, whereas CT and MRI routinely focus on just a part of the body (Becker & Meller, 2001). Nuclear medical imaging has an important role in discriminating infections from inflammation. Inflammatory processes can be visualized in their early phases, when anatomical changes are not yet apparent (Yurt Lambrecht et al., 2008a). The early detection of the infectious focus by radionuclide imaging helps both patient and physician to reduce the cost and the length of hospitalization (El-Ghany et al., 2005).

5.2. Current radionuclides for infection imaging

The radionuclide is a substance which continuously emits the radiation. Generally this radiation consists of alpha-rays, beta-rays and gamma-rays (Patei Riddhi et al., 2011). Radiopharmaceuticals can be labeled with various radionuclides such as ^{67}Ga, ^{99m}Tc, ^{111}In, ^{18}F, ^{131}I, etc. (Oyen et al., 2001). Technetium-99m is one of the most desirable radionuclides that is used in clinical nuclear medicine, due to the emission of gamma ray of optimal energy (140 keV), a suitable half-life (6 h), availability from ^{99}Mo-^{99m}Tc generator systems and low cost (Arano, 2002, & Oyen et al., 2001).

5.3. Imaging systems in nuclear medicine for infection diagnosis

Gamma camera, single photon emission tomography (SPECT) and positron emission tomography (PET) are current imaging systems in nuclear medicine for infection diagnosis.

5.3.1. Gamma camera

In nuclear medicine, the most common imaging systems are general-purpose systems, which allow a wide variety of morphological and physiological studies. While dedicated x-ray equipments for specific examinations are largely found in diagnostic radiology, this is not the case for nuclear medicine, where general purpose gamma cameras are commonly used (Sanchez et al., 2004). Tools like portable gamma cameras make it possible to quickly and simply perform the gamma mapping of an area to be processed, with the advantage of remote measurements of hot spots, not necessarily on contact. However, the use of such

http://dx.doi.org/10.5772/52882

cameras on site sometimes comes up against an insufficient sensitivity or space resolution, or against their excessive bulk (Gal et al., 2006).

5.3.2. Single photon emission tomography

Single photon emission computed tomography (SPECT) is a functional and molecular imaging modality, which is being used clinically to localize targets prior to biopsy and surgery (Roper et al., 2012). SPECT shows function by means of a three dimensional activity distribution of a radioactive tracer, which was injected prior to the measurement (Changizi et al., 2008). The principal values of SPECT are, as the result of the disposability of numerous single-photon radiopharmaceuticals, its broad clinical availability and its versatility for the everyday management of patients affected by several different conditions. Moreover, it is able to increase contrast and to allow better delineation of pathologies than planar imaging. However, the main limitation of SPECT imaging is its poor anatomical information; in fact, it yields essentially functional or molecular information that therefore are very suitable to be integrated with imaging modalities such as CT or magnetic resonance imaging (MRI), which provide morphological details (Schillaci et al., 2007). The hybrid SPECT/CT system delivers the high sensitivity of scinitigraphic technology with the high specificity of CT. This reduces the disadvantage of the SPECT's low spatial resolution (Bruni et al., 2008).

5.3.3. Positron emission tomography

Positron emission tomography is an improving technology and it is a promising field for the diagnosis of the diseases in relatively early stages. β^+ emitting radioactive isotopes are used in PET imaging (Silindir & Ozer, 2008). The most commonly used PET radionuclides are ^{11}C (half-life ≈ 20 min) and ^{18}F (half-life ≈110 min) (Bonekamp et al., 2010). FDG (flourodeoxyglocose) has proven to be an excellent tracer to detect inflammation in the setting of either infectious or noninfectious processes. The potential of FDG-PET for detecting inflammatory processes in disorders such as regional ileitis, sarcoidosis, rheumatologic disease, and vasculitis and any other disorders is also vast (Alavi et al., 2004). The major shortcomings of this modality include (1) limited availability in most parts of the world, (2) relatively high cost, and (3) difficulty in differentiating malignant tissue from infection or inflammation, although delayed imaging and dual-time-point PET is of considerable help in this regard (Basu et al., 2009). A newer technique that has recently gained favor in clinical use is PET-CT imaging for the rapid detection and localization of occult infection (Petruzzi et al., 2009).

6. Conventional nuclear medicine techniques for infection/inflammation imaging

Conventional nuclear medicine techniques make the use of the following radiopharmaceuticals for infection/inflammation imaging: ^{67}Ga-citrate, ^{99m}Tc or ^{111}In-labeled leukocytes, ^{99m}Tc-labeled granulocyte antibodies, radiolabeled chemotactic peptides, ^{99m}Tc or ^{111}In-labeled human immunoglobulin (HIG), ^{99m}Tc-nanocolloids, radiolabeled liposomes, cytokines, streptavidin-biotin and ^{18}F-flourodeoxyglocose (^{18}F-FDG).

6.1. ^{67}Ga-citrate

Gallium-67 (^{67}Ga) citrate has been used for detecting infection and inflammation ever since its discovery in 1971 (Kuo et al., 2002). Gallium-67 is a bioisoester of ferric iron with physical half-life of 3.3 days (78 hr) and biologic half-life of 2-3 weeks that binds to serum via transferrin, haptoglobin, albumin and globulins. Gallium attaches to tissues mediated by lactoferrin, as well as lymphocytes and macrophages (Jallilian et al., 2009). Gallium citrate is a radiopharmaceutical used for the detection and staging of some cancers and for identifying inflammation and infection. In the second category, typical indications for ^{67}Ga scanning include sarcoidosis, pneumonia, pyelonephritis, fibrosis, AIDS-related inflammations, osteomyelitis, and fevers of unknown origin (Truluck, 2007). However, this radiopharmaceutical has long physical half-life and high energy gamma radiations, which are unfavourable characteristics for gamma camera imaging and cause high radiation absorbed dose in the patients (Malviya et al., 2007). The specificity of the technique is low, due to physiologic al bowel excretion and accumulation in malignant tissues and areas of bone modeling (Rennen et al., 2002).

6.2. ^{99m}Tc- or ^{111}In-labeled leukocytes

Since the 1970s, scintigraphic imaging with labeled white blood cells has been the most frequently used nuclear imaging method for clinical diagnosis of infection and inflammation worldwide. The success of white blood cell scintigraphy is primarily due to its superb diagnostic accuracy (Signore et al., 2009). Of many radioisotopes used to label leucocytes, Indium-l11 tropolonate (^{111}In) and Technetium-99m hexamethyl propylene amine oxime (^{99m}Tc HMPAO) are the most widely used (Giaffer, 1996). The principal clinical indications for radiolabeled leukocytes include inflammatory bowel disease, osteomyelitis, follow-up of patients with infections of vascular or orthopedic prostheses and soft tissue infections. There has always been concern that chronic infections could be missed using radiolabeled leukocytes, because these infections generate a smaller granulocyte response compared to acute infections (Larverman et al., 2008). Radiolabeled white blood cell (WBC) scintigraphy, enables detection of areas of general inflammation but cannot be used to distinguish between bacterial and nonbacterial inflammatory processes (Sonmezoglou et al., 2001). Although, the radiolabeled leucocytes can be considered as "gold standard" that can visualize a majority of infectious and inflammatory lesions, but it is labor-intensive and the *in vitro* labeling carries risks of handling potentially contaminated blood and also requires specialized equipment, taking approximately three hours (Mirshojaei et al., 2011).

6.3. ^{99m}Tc-labeled granulocyte antibodies

Ever since it became clear that labeled leukocytes could visualise infectious foci, investigators have been developing a method that could label leukocytes *in vivo* (Larikka, 2003). For *in vivo* labeling, immunoscintigraphy with ^{99m}Tc labeled monoclonal anti-granulocyte antibodies (AGAb) is used (Gyork et al., 2000). The accumulation mechanism involves nonspecific related uptake of free antibody because of an increased capillary permeability at the focus, with subsequent binding to granulocytes (Lyra et al., 1998). The first approach regarding *in vivo* labeling was the murine IgG1k antibody BW 250/183 (^{99m}Tc-besilesomab, Scintimun®) which recognized the nonspecific cross reacting antigen 95 (NCA-95; also referred to as CD66b and CEACAM8) in the cytoplasm and on the cell membranes of granulocytes and granulocyte precursor cells (Ritcher et al., 2011). Three antigranulocyte antibodies have been tested for infection imaging: anti-NCA-95 immunoglobulin G (IgG) (BW250/183), anti-NCA-90 Fab (Immu-MN3, Leukoscan: anti-CD66), and anti-CD15 (LeuTech). Each of these antigranulocyte antibodies labeled with ^{99m}Tc were determined to accurately delineate infection and inflammation. None of these compounds, however, were specific for infection only (Petruzzi et al., 2009). Fanolesomab is a monoclonal murine M class immunoglobulin that binds to CD15 receptors present on leukocytes. Antibody fragments are appealing because, unlike the whole antibody, they do not induce a human antimouse antibodies (HAMA) response. Sulesomab is a murine monoclonal antibody fragment of the IgG1 class that binds to normal cross-reactive antigen-90 present on leukocytes (Palestro & Love, 2009). Disadvantages of the use of monoclonal antibodies, however, are the high molecular weight, resulting in slow diffusion into sites of inflammation, a long plasma half life and uptake in the liver due to clearance by the reticulo-endothelial system. Use of monoclonal antibodies of murine origin sometimes induces generation of HAMA, which can lead to allergic reactions and altered pharmacokinetics when repeated injections are given. This is, of course, a major limitation for follow-up studies (Larverman et al., 2008). Some radiolabeled mAbs (such as anti-E-selectin and anti-CD4) demonstrated their excellent capability for the localization of inflammatory regions, but lack of their use for the therapeutic purposes, thus limiting their further development and (Malviya et al., 2011).

6.4. ^{99m}Tc- or ^{111}In-labeled chemotactic peptides

Radiolabeled chemotactic peptides are promising tools for the imaging of inflammation and infection. Chemotactic peptides are naturally released by bacteria and initiate leukocyte chemotaxis by binding to high-affinity receptors on the white blood cell membrane. These receptors are present on polymorphonuclear neutrophils and monocytes (Hartwig et al., 1999). The tripeptide, formyl-methionyl-leucyl phenylalanine (f-MLF), is a bacterial product which the initial studies for the design of infection imaging agents focused on the conjugation of f-MLF peptide analogs with the cyclic anhydride of DTPA and radiolabeling with ^{111}In (Babich et al., 2000). The results of radiolabeling of four DTPA derivatized chemotactic peptides analogs established that they are effective agents for imaging sites of infection (Fischman et al., 1991). Small radiolabeled synthetic peptides are currently preferred over proteins and antibodies for imaging applications, since they present several distinct advantages over these biomolecules. Small peptides can be readily synthesized chemically. They can withstand harsher chemical conditions for modification or radiolabeling. They are less likely to induce an immunogenic response. Their plasma clearance is more rapid, yet they often reach a high concentration in the target tissues (Okarvi, 2001). Although ^{111}In and ^{99m}Tc-labeled chemotactic peptides accumulate at sites of infection with high target-to-background ratios, receptor specificity has not been completely established and a significant amount of localization could be due to nonspecific processes, such as increased tissue permeability, blood pool or blood flow characteristics of inflammatory lesions, or characteristics of the peptides that are not related to For-MLF receptor binding (Babich et al., 1997). However, their development as radiopharmaceuticals has been curtailed because they cause significant leucopenia at physiological concentration (Das et al., 2002).

6.5. ^{99m}Tc- or ^{111}In-labeled Human Immunoglobulin (HIG)

Investigations with monoclonal antibodies by the research group of Rubin et al. led to the discovery of the usefulness of In-IgG scintigraphy for imaging infectious and inflammatory foci (Oyen et al., 1992). Nonspecific polyclonal human immunoglobulins have been shown to localize to sites of infection/inflammation by extravasations from the bloodstream due to the induced local hyperemia and this agent is, thus, nonspecific for infection (Petruzzi et al., 2009). ^{111}In or ^{99m}Tc-labeled HIG has been extensively tested in a large number of clinical studies. It has shown excellent performance in the localization of musculoskeletal infection and inflammation, in pulmonary infection, particularly in immunocompromised patients and abdominal Inflammation. Poor sensitivity of radiolabeled HIG is found in the diagnosis of endocarditis and vascular lesions in general, due to long lasting high levels of circulating activity. A general limitation is the long time span between injection and final diagnosis (24-48 h) (Rennen et al., 2002).

6.6. ^{99m}Tc-nanocolloids

Nanocolloids are colloids of human serum albumin (HAS) less than 50 nm in size, which localize at sites of inflammatory foci through increased capillary permeability (Das et al., 2002). Nanocolloids are good carriers for drugs or radionuclides, the latter can be used for diagnosis or for therapy. Radiolabeled nanocolloids have been widely used in diagnostic nuclear medicine (Lin et al., 2003). Uptake of the tracer is presumably caused by extravasation through the capillary basement membrane, followed by phagocytosis or adsorption of the particles by granulocytes and macrophages (Palestro & Love, 2009). ^{99m}Tc labeled nanocolloids have been most commonly used for marrow and lymphatic imaging and for patient with musculoskeletal infection. The greatest disadvantage is their inability to image infections outside the musculoskeletal system and, as with most of the currently available radiopharmaceuticals, distinguishing infection from inflammation (Das et al., 2002).

6.7. Radiolabeled liposomes

Liposomes are small vesicles consisting of one or more concentric lipid bilayers enclosing discrete aqueous spaces. Liposomes are formed spontaneously when (phospho) lipids are suspended in aqueous media (Larverman et al., 1999). Liposomes have been extensively used as potential delivery systems for a variety of compounds primarily due to their high degree of biocompatibility and the enormous diversity of structures and compositions (Mufamadi et al., 2011). A formulation of liposomes, which is capable of being labeled by both ^{99m}Tc and ^{111}In, simultaneously would have many advantages. This formulation would ena-

http://dx.doi.org/10.5772/52882

ble the acquisition of good early images in the ^{99m}Tc window of the gamma camera and acceptable delayed images in the ^{111}In window (Awasthi et al., 1998). Preliminary studies have shown uptake in sterile and non sterile inflammation (Turpin & Lambert, 2001). Liposomes continue to be very promising carriers for delivery of drugs to inflamed regions of the body, although, to date, no clinical products have specifically taken advantage of the inflammatory targeting of liposomes (Phillips et al., 2009).

6.8. Cytokines

Cytokines are proteins and glicoproteins, members of a family of overlapping and interdependent molecules with important roles in the homeostatic control of the immune system and of pathophysiology of different organs (Signore et al., 2000). Cytokine receptors, usually of high affinity, are normally present at low levels on non-activated cells, but expression is up-regulated during the cell activation and therefore these receptors on the affected tissue are suitable targets for the detection of infection/inflammation (Malviya et al., 2007). Labeled cytokines such as interleukin-1, interleukin-2 and interleukin-8 are a promising class of protein radiopharmaceuticals of small molecular weight (<20 kDa) (Rennen et al., 2001). IL-1, IL-1ra, IL-2, IL-6, IL-8, IL-10, IL-12, p40, interferon γ IFN-γ and epidermal growth factor (EGF) have been radiolabeled for *in vivo* targetting of different leukocyte subsets with promising results for their clinical use. Radiolabeled cytokines, therefore, have the potential for use in the study of the pathophysiology of several diseases and have been used for the diagnosis of inflammation and tumours (Signore et al., 2000). Cytokines and receptor antagonists are specific for inflammation but not for infection (Das et al., 2002).

6.9. Streptavidin-biotin

The biotin-straptavidin system has been used for many years in a varity of different applications (Diamandis & Christopoulos, 1991). Streptavidin is a protein extracted from the bacterium *Streptomyces avidinii* with a molecular weight of 60 kDa and has four binding sites with high affinity (K_D=10^{-15} M) for biotin, which is a water soluble vitamin with a molecular weight of 244 kDa (Kittigul et al., 1998). Avidin/indium-111 biotin scintigraphy is based on the non-specific accumulation of avidin at sites of inflammation or infection, linked to increased transcapillary leakage of macromolecules and to interstitial oedema at these sites. Due to its extremely high affinity for and low dissociation constant with biotin, sites of infection can be imaged using avidin as a pre-target, followed by ^{111}In-labeled biotin (Lazzeri et al., 1999). The potential of radiolabeled biotin as an infection imaging agent has already been shown in an experimental animal model of infection using biotin labeled with fluorine-18 as well as in a small group of patients with osteomyelitis using ^{111}In-labeled biotin (Lazzeri et al., 2008). Because, the mechanism of localization is nonspecifically, based on the increasing vascular permeability, this radiopharmaceutical is not specific for infection imaging.

6.10. ^{18}F-flourodeoxyglocose (^{18}F-FDG)

A number of positron emitting radioisotopes are available for clinical use but the one most commonly used is 18 Fluorine fluorodeoxyglucose. FDG is an analogue of glucose which concentrates in areas of high glycolytic activity such as rapidly dividing cells. Neutrophils and macrophages have increased FDG uptake allowing localization of infection and inflammation (Robinson & Scarsbrook, 2009). PET with fluorine-18 fluorodeoxyglucose is a powerful molecular imaging technique that allows areas with different pathologies such as malignant neoplasias and active inflammation in clinical human studies to be assessed (Wyss et al., 2004). Numerous reports have demonstrated increased FDG uptake at the sites of infection and inflammation. FDG-PET is very helpful in the evaluation of chronic osteomyelitis, sarcoidosis, fever of unknown origin (FUO), and differentiating toxoplasmosis from lymphoma in the central nervous system in HIV-positive patients. Despite all of these findings, however, FDG-PET has not been fully accepted as an effective way to evaluate infection and inflammation (Zhuang et al., 2005). This is nonspecific since ^{18}F-FDG is also taken up at non-specific sites of inflammation as well as sites of tumor (Petruzzi et al., 2009).

7. Properties of an ideal infection imaging agent

The ideal radiopharmaceutical should enable early diagnostic imaging, a low absorbed radiation dose and make a distinction between inflammation and infection, which is of paramount importance in the field of various infections including musculoskeletal, soft-tissue and parenchymal infections. Furthermore, it should be nontoxic, inexpensive, readily available, and rapidly cleared from the blood and the body (Gemmel et al., 2009). The preparation of the radiopharmaceutical should be quick and easy, preferably with technetium-99m as the radionuclide (Larverman et al., 2008). Low levels of accumulation in bowel and blood pool are particularly important characteristics of such an agent. Focal accumulation or transient activity in the bowel would make detection of infections in this area very difficult. Similarly, high blood pool activity increases background and complicates the imaging of vascular infections (Babich & Fischman, 1999). These properties for an ideal infection imaging agent are shown in Table 1 (Gemmel et al., 2009).

1. Rapid localization and good retention at the site of infection
2. Rapid clearance from non infected tissues (high target to background ratio)
3. Uptake in infection not in sterile inflammation, identifyingbacterial, viral and fungal infections.
4. The uptake of radiotracer should be proportional to the degree of infection. Therapy response can be monitored.
5. No pharmacological effect/immunological response, saferepeated injection.
6. Labeling should be simple and uncomplicated and wellcharacterized
7. ^{99m}Tc labeling is preferable, positron labeling is still experimental
8. Not depending on host leukocyte function
9. Less expensive than other combined modalities

Table 1. The requirements for an ideal radiopharmaceutical for infection imaging

http://dx.doi.org/10.5772/52882

Considering these criteria for an ideal radiopharmaceutical for infection imaging, the best techniques which fit this criteria better, are following by next topic.

8. Targeting nuclear medicine techniques in microorganisms imaging

The theoretical advantage of using an antimicrobial agent as the localizing agent for infective foci is the selective toxicity of the compound for microbes rather than human targets. Such agents should therefore be able to distinguish between inflammation due to infection with microbial pathogens, and inflammation due to immune activity i.e. autoimmune disease where microbes are not involved (Wareham et al., 2005). There is now a wide range of radiolabeled antimicrobial agents that are undergoing evaluation. The first group consists of radiolabeled antibiotics such as ^{99m}Tc- or 18F-ciprofloxacin, ^{99m}Tc-sparfloxacin, ^{99m}Tc-ceftizoxime and anti-fungal agents such as ^{99m}Tc-fluconazole and ^{99m}Tc-isoniazid and the anti-*Mycobacterium tuberculosis* agent ^{99m}Tc-ethambutol. The second group of radiopharmaceuticals for imaging infections is derived from the array of human antimicrobial peptides/proteins that binds to specific bacterial antigens, e.g. peptides derived from human lactoferrin, ubiciquidin and human neutrophil peptide 1–3 (^{99m}Tc-HNP1–3; members of the α-defensins) (Signore et al., 2008).

8.1. Antibiotics

In 1945, Selman Waksman proposed that the word antibiotic can be defined as "a chemical substance of microbial origin that possesses antibiotic powers" (Davies, 2006). Antibiotics are drugs of natural or synthetic origin that have the capacity to kill or inhibit the growth of micro-organisms. Antibiotics are sufficiently non-toxic to the host are used as chemotherapeutic agents in the treatment of infectious diseases of humans, animals and plants (Hernandez Serrano, 2005). Antibiotics are designed to support host defense in controlling infection (Kristian et al., 2007). Most antibiotics used in human treatment were originated from natu ral templates produced by particular species of bacteria or fungi as a mechanism of competition to ensure their own survival (e.g., to gain a larger share of environmental food supplies by killing competitors (Hancock, 2005).

8.1.1. Types of antibiotics

Antimicrobial drugs are classified according to their mechanism of action, for example, cell wall inhibiting, cell membrane inhibiting, protein synthesis inhibiting and nucleic acid inhibiting (Riaz et al., 2011). The major targets for the main classes of antibiotics include cell membranes (e.g., mupirocin), cell-wall biosynthesis enzymes and substrates (e.g., beta-lactams, vancomycin, and bacitracin), bacterial protein synthesis (e.g., chloramphenicol, tetracyclines, macrolides, clindamycin, aminoglycosides, linezolid, mupirocin, and fusidic acid), and bacterial nucleic acid replication and repair (e.g., co-trimoxazole [trimethoprim/sulfamethoxazole], which acts via an anti-metabolite mechanism, rifampicin, and quinolones) (Hancock, 2005).

8.1.2. Mechanisms of antibiotics action

Antibiotics interfere with the growth of bacteria by undermining the integrity of their cell wall or by interfering with bacterial protein synthesis or common metabolic pathways. The terms bactericidal and bacteriostatic are broad categorizations, and may not apply for a given agent against all organisms, with certain antimicrobials being bactericidal for one bacterial pathogen but bacteriostatic for another (Niederman, 2009). Bacteriostatic agents inhibit the growth of bacterial cells but do not kill them, whereas bactericidal agents kill the bacteria. However, these categories are not absolute, since the killing effect of the drug varies with the test method and the species being tested. Agents may be bactericidal against one group of organisms and bacteriostatic against another) (French, 2006). Bactericidal antibiotics, such as the beta-lactams (including the cephalosporins, carbapenems, and cephems), glycopeptides (including vancomycin), fluoroquinolones, polymyxins, and the lipopeptide daptomycin, are often preferred for treatment of these diseases, particularly for cases of febrile neutropenia, meningitis, and endocarditis (Hancock, 2005). The importance of bactericidal drugs versus bacteriostatic drugs in the treatment of infections has been debated for many years. Although the advantages of bactericidal agents appear obvious (e.g., rapid elimination of bacteria and a decreased possibility of resistance development or infection recurrence), bactericidal activity could be undesirable in some clinical settings. In CNS (central nervous system) infection, for example, the sudden lysis of bacteria by a bactericidal agent leads to a sudden increase in bacterial products (e.g., lipopolysaccharide in gram-negative organisms or peptidoglycans in gram-positive organisms) that may stimulate cytokine production, causing potentially harmful inflammation (Finberg et al., 2004).

8.1.3. Review on radiolabeled antibiotics

Agents that specifically target the infectious organisms (e.g., bacteria, fungi or viruses) have potential to distinguish microbial from non microbial inflammation (Boerman & Nijmegen, 2008). The first and most intensively studied agent in this category is ^{99m}Tc-ciprofloxacin (^{99m}Tc-infecton), a member of fluoroquinolone group that was introduced by Solanki et al. as a new class of radiopharmaceutical for infection imaging in 1993 (Solanki et al., 1993). The results of 99mTc-infecton clinical application in imaging patients with various infections are shown in Table 2.

Moreover, radiolabeling of some other quinolone antibiotics, cephalosporines, antifungal agents, anti *mycobacterium tuberculosis* and also antiviral radiopharmaceuticals for targeting diagnosis of infectious foci, were investigated up to now.

8.1.3.1. Radiolabeled antibacterial agents

The use of radiolabeled antibiotics is fast emerging as a promising diagnostic test for the detection of infective lesions, because of their specific binding to the bacterial component (Singh et al., 2005). The first clinical application of ^{99m}Tc-ciprofloxacin was performed by Vinjamuri et al. in 1996 and the ability of ^{99m}Tc infecton imaging in comparison with radiolabeled white blood cell imaging for evaluating of bacterial infection, were investigated (Vin-

http://dx.doi.org/10.5772/52882

Type of infection	Number of patients	Sensitivity (%)	Specificity (%)	Reference
Known or suspected sites of infection	56	84	96	Vinjamuri et al., 1996
Various infections with proven microbiological tests	99	83	91	Britton et al., 1997
Suspected of a variety of infections	90	70.3	93.1	Hall et al., 1998
Suspected orthopaedic infection	15	85	92	Yapar et al., 2001
Clinically suspected chronic skeletal infection	51	63	96	Sonmezoglo et al., 2001
Suspected bacterial infection	879 (in 8 country under the auspices of the IAEA)	85.4	81.7	Britton et al., 2002
Proven or suspected bone infection	45	97.2	80	Malamitsi et al., 2003
Suspected septic arthritis or osteomyelitis	27	100	37.5	Sarda et al., 2003
Postoperative spinal infection	48	52	79	De Winter, et al., 2004
Acute or chronic cholecystitis based on the clinical and ultrasonographic findings	60	91.7	75	Cho et al., 2007

Table 2. Some reported clinical applications of ^{99m}Tc-ciprofloxacin (infecton).

jamuri et al., 1996). The results showed 84% sensitivity and 96% specificity of ^{99m}Tc ciprofloxacin in contrast to 81% sensitivity and 77% specificity of white blood cell imaging. Ciprofloxacin has several advantages over radiolabeled leucocytes, and other methods for imaging infection, which include the following: (1) specificity for infection, (2) lack of bone marrow uptake, which is a significant advantage in imaging bone and joint and orthopedic prostheses infections, (3) ease and cost of preparation of the agent, (4) *ex vivo* labeling, which avoids contact with blood and hence the risk of acquiring blood borne infections such as HIV and hepatitis B and C, (5) independence of the host inflammatory response and neutrophil count and hence it can be used to image infections in immunocompromised patients, including those who are neutropaenic, where culture is often negative and white blood cell imaging unreliable and (6) availability in a kit format with long shelf-life, making it user friendly and more widely available (Akhtar et al., 2012). However, the low binding affinity of ^{99m}Tc-ciprofloxacin to bacteria and the risk of emerging antibiotic-resistant microorganisms make this radiopharmaceutical unattractive for imaging bacterial infections (Welling et al., 1999). The majority of other fluoroquinolone antibiotics, some of the cephalosporins and also other antibacterial agents were radiolabeled up to now for bacterial infection imaging with promising results (Table 3).

Antibiotic	**Antimicrobial group**	**Radio-nuclide**	**Microorganisms**	**Target to non target ratio (T/NT)**	**Reference**
Ceftizoxime	Cephalosporine- third generation	Tc-99m	*Escherichia coli*	3.24	Gomes Barreto et al., 2000, 2005
Floclunazol	Antifungal	Tc-99m	*Candida albicans -Aspergillus fumigates*	3.6	Lupetti et al., 2002
Isoniazid	Antituberclosis	Tc-99m	*Mycobacterium tuberculosis*	-	Singh et al., 2003
Enrofloxacin	Fluoroquinolone- second generation	Tc-99m	*Staphylococcos aureus* and *Candida albicans*	4.25	Siaens et al., 2004
Vancomycin	Glycopeptide antibiotic	Tc-99m	*Staphylococcos aureus 25923*	5	Roohi et al., 2005
Pefloxacin	Fluoroquinolone- second generation	Tc-99m	*Escherichia coli*	5.6	El Ghany et al., 2005
Ethambutol	Antituberclosis	Tc-99m	*Mycobacterium tuberculosis*	-	Verma et al., 2005
Kanamycin	Aminoglycoside	Tc-99m	*Staphylococcos aureus 25923*	2.5	Roohi et al., 2006
Cefoperazone	Cephalosporin-forth generation	Tc-99m	*Staphylococcus aureus*	4.5	Motaleb, 2007a
Lomefloxacin	Fluoroquinolone- second generation	Tc-99m	*Staphylococcus aureus*	6.5	Motaleb, 2007b
Ofloxacin	Fluoroquinolone- second generation	Tc-99m	*Staphylococcus aureus*	4.3	Motaleb, 2007b
Sparafloxacin	Fluoroquinolone- third generation	Tc-99m	*Staphylococcus aureus*	5.9	Motaleb, 2009
Cefuroxime axetil	Cephalosporin-second generation	Tc-99m	*Staphylococcus aureus*	2.5	Yurt Lmbrecht et al., 2008a
Linezolid	Oxazolidinone	I-131	*Staphylococcus aureus*	5.5	Yurt Lmbrecht et al., 2009

Antibiotic	Antimicrobial group	Radio-nuclide	Microorganisms	Target to non target ratio (T/NT)	Reference
Moxifloxacin	Fluoroquinolone-forth generation	Tc-99m	*Escherichia coli*	6.8	Chattopadhyay et al., 2010
Norfloxacin	Fluoroquinolone-second generation	Tc-99m	*Staphylococcus aureus*	6.9	Ibrahim et al., 2010
Rifampicin	Rifamycin group	Tc-99m	Methicillin-resistant *Staphylococcus aureus*	7.34	Shah et al., 2010
Ceftriaxone	Cephalosporin- third generation	Tc-99m	*Escherichia coli*	5.6	Mostafa et al., 2010
Gemifloxacin	Fluoroquinolone-forth generation	Tc-99m	*Streptococcus pneumoniae*	4.88	Shah & Khan, 2011a
Rufloxacin	Fluoroquinolone-second generation	Tc-99m	*Staphylococcus aureus*	6.04	Shah & Khan, 2011b
Clinafloxacin	Fluoroquinolone-forth generation	Tc-99m	*Staphylococcus aureus*	4.96	Shah & Khan, 2011c
Nitrofurantoin	Nitrofuran derivatives-DNAinhibitors	Tc-99m	*Escherichia coli*	4.84	Shah et al., 2011a
Garenoxacin	Fluoroquinolone-forth generation	Tc-99m	multi resistant *Staphylococcus aureus* (MRSA) --penicillin-resistant *Streptococci* (PRSC)	5.2 5.4	Shah et al., 2011b
Cefotaxime	Cephalosporin- third generation	Tc-99m	*Staphylococcus aureus*	2.98	Mirshojaei et al., 2011
Gatifloxacin	Fluoroquinolone-forth generation	Tc-99m	*Escherichia coli*	4.5	Motaleb et al., 2011
Cefepime	Cephalosporin- forth generation	Tc-99m	*Escherichia coli*	8.4	Motaleb et al., 2011
Levofloxacin	Fluoroquinolone-third generation	Tc-99m	*Staphylococcus aureus*	17.2	Naqvi et al., 2012

Table 3. The history of radiolabeled antibiotics applied in infection imaging.

8.1.3.2. Radiolabeled antituberculous agents

Mycobacterial infections have been shown to be increasing in number worldwide, mainly due to a global increase in developing countries, the increased number of patients with HIV infection and AIDS disease worldwide, an increasing the number of elderly patients and the emergence of multidrug resistant tuberculosis (De Backer et al., 2006). Tuberculosis is an ancient infectious disease that remains a threat for public health around the world. Although the etiological agent as well as tuberculosis pathogenesis is well known, the molecular mechanisms underlying the host defense to the bacilli remain elusive (Jordao & Vieira, 2011). A suitable ligand, ethambutol (EMB) that is, specific first line antitubercular drug was chosen for detection as well as localization of the lesion using nuclear medicine modality. ^{99m}Tc-EMB was used in humans for tubercular imaging. The mycobacterial lesion uptake study carried out so far in humans suggested that ^{99m}Tc-EMB is specific and sensitive radiopharmaceutical for sensitive as well as resistant tubercular lesion detection and localization (Singh & Batnagar, 2010). Isoniazid is another antituberculous agent that binds to mycolic acid in the cell walls of living mycobacteria. Successful imaging of *Mycobacterium tuberculosis* cold abscesses in rabbits was reported along with rapid washout from *Staphylococcos aureus* infected abcesses suggesting the agent my be very useful for the detection and follow up of tuberculous lesions in humans (Wareham et al., 2005). Ethambutol was successfully labeled with ^{99m}Tc followed by studies on mice and rabbits for labeling efficiency, *in vitro* and *in vivo* stability, blood kinetics, and organ distribution (Table 3). Therefore it was concluded that this radiolabeled agent can be used for detection and follow up of tuberculous lesions in patients especially to determine the treatment endpoint of antituberculous drugs (Akhtar et al., 2012).

8.1.3.3. Radiolabeled antifungal agents

During the past two decades, invasive fungal infections have emerged as a major threat to immunocompromised hosts. Patients with neoplastic diseases are at significant risk for such infections as a result of their underlying illness and its therapy (Shoham & Levitz, 2005). *Candida albicans* is the most common fungal pathogen, and is the organism responsible for the majority of localized fungal infections in humans (De Assis et al., 2008). Fluconazole is the most frequently employed among the triazole antifungal agents in treating *Candida* infections in individuals with severe immunodeficiency (Lupetti et al., 2011). It was successfully labeled with ^{99m}Tc by Lupetti et al., in 2002. This labeled compound successfully detected infections with *Candida albicans* but not bacterial infections or sterile inflammatory sites in animals (Table 3) (Lupetti et al., 2002). In the attempt to develop new tracers that specifically detect fungal infections, components of fungal cell wall have been considered highly selective targets. Since chitin is a component of fungal cell wall, which is absent in mammalian cells, a radiolabeled marker for chitine, ^{123}I-chitinase was developed in order to bind specifically to fungal cells (Lupetti et al., 2011). It was tested for specificity in a mouse model to localize fungal infections with both *Candida* and *Aspergillus* species. Furthermore, the chitinase uptake appeared to correlate well with the number of viable fungal cells (Gemmel et al., 2009). The results revealed that this radioiodine labeled enzyme accumulates in *Candida albicans* and *Aspergillus fumigatus* infections in mice; these infections can be visualized at 24 h after injection of the tracer and its accumulation, correlates with the number of viable fungal cells without visualizing bacterial infections or sterile inflammations (Lupetti et al., 2011).

8.1.3.4. Radiolabeled antiviral agents

Antiviral therapeutics deals specifically with the treatment of viral infections and refers to the use of drugs and the methods of the execution in the treatment of life-threatening viral diseases (Saxena et al., 2009). Development of a suitable radiolabeled antiviral drug probe must take into account the specificity of metabolism of the drug by virus-infected cells, the capability and convenience of labeling the drug without altering that specificity, and the biodistribution of the drug (Price et al., 1983). The possibility of using a naturally occurring virus-encoded molecule as an imaging reporter was first explored in the early 1980s, when acyclovir was approved as an antiviral drug for the treatment of HSV (herpes simplex virus) infections. The ability of this and other nucleoside analogues to selectively inhibit HSV replication is based on their ability to undergo phosphorylation by the viral thymidine kinase (TK), but not by corresponding host enzymes (Bray et al., 2010). Ideally, the drug to be used should be phosphorylated exclusively by viral TK and, therefore, label only infected cells (Price et al., 1983). Among various substrates, radiolabeled 2′-fluoro-2′-deoxy-5-iodo-1-β-D-arabinofuranosyluracil (FIAU) demonstrated high sensitivity and selectivity for the detection of HSV1-tk expression. FIAU is trapped intracellularly only in the presence of HSV1-tk (Bengel et al., 2000). Another antiviral drug, 2'-fluoro-5-methyl-1-beta-D-arabinosyluracil labeled with carbon 14 ([^{14}C]FMAU), was used as a probe for selectively imaging brain infection in a rat model to diagnosis of herpes simplex encephalitis by quantitative autoradiography (Saito et al., 1984). Stavudine, 2′, 3′ didehydro-3′-deoxythymidine (d4T), is a synthetic thymidine nucleoside analog that is effective in the treatment of human immunodeficiency virus (HIV) infection. Stavudine enters cells rapidly by nonfacilitated diffusion, with the rate of influx being linear with respect to concentration. This potent antiviral agent was radiolabeled with ^{11}C and the results showed that future PET studies with this radiopharmaceutical will allow in vivo measurements of the pharmacokinetics of stavudine in both animal models and human subjects (Livni et al., 2004). The replication cycles of various DNA and RNA viruses offer a variety of targets for drugs and probes that interact specifically with virus-encoded molecules which made candidate tracers of different virus families for virus-specific imaging (Bray et al., 2010).

8.2. Antimicrobial peptides

Antimicrobial peptides are widespread in living organisms constitute an important component of innate immunity to microbial infections. By the early 1980s, more than 800 different antimicrobial peptides had been isolated from mammals, amphibians, fish, insects, plants and bacterial species. In humans, they are produced by granulocytes, macrophages and most epithelial and endothelial cells (Kamysz, 2005). Antimicrobial peptides usually contain hydrophobic and cationic amino acids, which are able to organize in an amphipatic structure (Lupetti et al., 2003a). They can be expressed constitutively or induced during inflammation or microbial challenge. Antimicrobial peptides displayed antibacterial, antiviral and antifungal activities *in vitro* and were effective in experimental infections with multidrug resistant *Staphylococcus aureus* and *Mycobacterium tuberculosis* (Lupetti et al., 2003b). Due to the development of microorganisms' resistant to the most widely used antibiotics and antifungal agents, antimicrobial peptides have gained renewed attention as possible therapeutic candidates (Lupetti et al., 2003c). Difficulties arising in purifying natural antimicrobial peptides from various sources have prompted the recombinant production of antimicrobial peptides by genetically engineered bacteria or by peptide synthesis. Such methods result in sufficient amounts of antimicrobial peptides produced under good laboratory practice conditions, which is essential for future approval to use the peptides in clinical trials. Peptide synthesis also allows the production of chemical variants, such as denantiomers, peptides that have amino acid substitutions at various positions, and peptide libraries (Lupetti et al., 2003b). Synthetic peptides are usually small, rapidly removed from the circulation and other body compartments, and flexible, because they do not hold a particular structure in a hydrophilic environment, and display a favorable adverse effect profile (Akhtar et al., 2012).

8.2.1. Types of antimicrobial peptides

Antimicrobial peptides usually contain less than 50 amino acids with a net positive charge due to an excess of basic residues, such as lysine and arginine, and approximately 50% hydrophobic amino acid (Lupetti et al., 2003c). According to combination of sequence homologies, three dimensional structures and functional similarities classification, antimicrobial peptides can be divided into 5 main classes: (1) linear, mostly α-helical peptides without cysteine residue, with or without hinge region (bombinins, cecropins, magainins), (2) antimicrobial peptides with one disulfide bond that form a loop structure with a tail (bactenecins, esculentins), (3) antimicrobial peptides with two or more disulfide bonds giving mainly or only β-sheet structure (defensins, protegrins), (4) linear peptides without cysteine residue and with an unusual composition of regular amino acids (histatins, indolicidin, temporins) and (5) antimicrobial peptides derived from larger peptides or proteins with other known functions (lactoferricins, MUC7). Despite differences in structure, all the peptides display a similar motif: an amphiphilic structure, with one surface being highly positive and the other hydrophobic (Kamysz, 2005). Ubiquicidin 29-41 (UBI) is a fragment of the cationic antimicrobial peptide that is present in various species including humans (Melendez-Alafort et al., 2003). Short peptides from lactoferrin (a 692-amino acid iron-binding protein found in body fluids, secretary granules of neutrophils and mucosal epithelium), consist of HLF (human lactoferrin peptide) 1-11 and 2-11, were tested for their ability to target infections (Knight, 2003). One of the best-studied antimicrobial peptides is human neutrophil peptide (HNP)-1, which is a member of the family of defensins. This antimicrobial peptide, which is stored in the granules of human neutrophils, contributes to bacterial killing during phagocytosis. HNP-1 displays antimicrobial activity against gram-positive and gram-negative bacteria, many fungi and some enveloped viruses (Welling et al., 1999). Bacteriocins are ribosomally synthetized antimicrobial peptides produced by bacteria (Oscariz & Pisabarra, 2001). Bacteriocins are peptides secreted by cells to inhibit or kill closely related species. They are divided into two basic types. The first group comprises peptides which have been subjected to post-translatory treatment (modified bacteriocins-lantibiotics). The second group includes unmodified bacteriocins. Furthermore, bacteriocins comprise colicins and microcins, i.e. peptides produced by Gram-negative bacteria (e.g., *Escherichia coli*) (Kamysz, 2005).

http://dx.doi.org/10.5772/52882

8.2.2. Mechanisms of antibacterial peptides action

Although the exact mechanism of action of antimicrobial peptides (AMPs) remains a matter of controversy, there is a consensus that these peptides selectively disrupt the cell membranes and the amphipathic structural arrangement of the peptides is believed to play an important role in this mechanism (Peddy et al., 2004). Based on the available data, all proposed modes of action have implicated the cationic and hydrophobic nature of the AMPs in its initial interaction with the negatively charged lipids in bacterial membranes while some variations are expected in non-bacterial targets. Due to their cationic nature, AMPs are electrostatically attracted to negatively charge microbial surfaces such as lipopolysaccharide (LPS) in Gram-negative bacteria and teichoic and teichuronic acids in Gram-positive bacteria (Rotem & Mor, 2009). Insertion of the peptides into the bacterial cytoplasmic membrane under the influence of the transmembrane electrical potential gradient results in transient permeability of membranes and leakage of cellular constituents, such as potassium ions, thus destroying the proton gradient across the membrane, resulting in bacterial cell death (Lupetti et al., 2003c).

8.2.3. Review on radiolabeled antibacterial peptides

Because antimicrobial peptides preferentially bind to bacterial membranes, radiolabeling of these peptides would offer the medical community the novel candidates for the development of bacteria-seeking radiopharmaceuticals (Welling et al., 1999). A number of radiolabeled peptides have been evaluated for the scintigraphic detection of infections (Table 4). Among the most specific ones are technetium-99m labeled cationic antimicrobial peptides derived from ubiquicidin (UBI) that preferentially bind to microorganisms (Welling et al., 2004). ^{99m}Tc-labeled ubiquicidin 29-41 (^{99m}Tc-UBI 29-41) is a highly sensitive and specific agent for the scintigraphic detection of bacterial and fungal infections in animals and humans. ^{99m}Tc-UBI 29-41 allows rapid visualization of Gram-positive and Gram-negative bacterial infections with little or no accumulation in sterile inflammatory processes, indicating that this peptide directly tags the microorganisms at the site of infection (Vallejo et al., 2008). Tc-99m labeled antimicrobial peptides UBI 29-41, UBI 18-35, UBI 31-38, hLF 1-11, and defensins accumulate significantly in tissues infected with Gram-positive and Gram-negative bacteria and *Candida albicans*. Significantly lower accumulation of these peptides occurs in sterile inflamed tissues (Fard-Esfahani et al., 2010). The peptides hLF 1-11 and 2-11, when labeled with ^{99m}Tc by a direct reduction technique, bound well to bacterial cells *in vitro*. Unlike ^{99m}Tc-UBI peptides, however, the labeled hLF peptides also bound to human leukocytes. This makes them less useful for infection imaging, because they cannot adequately discriminate between bacterial infection and sterile inflammation. Furthermore, the peptides had a relatively high degree of hepatobiliary clearance (Knight, 2003). There are limitations attributed to synthesis/isolation of antimicrobial peptides, labeling with isotopes, minimum detection limit of 10^3 Colony-Forming Unit (CFU) of bacteria, and inability to distinguish between bacterial and fungal infections. In addition, different bacterial types reveal different tracer accumulation (*Staphylococcus aureus* versus *Escherichia coli*). Currently no evidence regarding resistance against antimicrobial peptides has been reported. Considering the merits and demerits of radiolabeled peptides and radiolabeled antibiotics, it can currently be concluded that radiolabeled peptides are better specific infection localizing agents than radiolabeled antibiotics (Akhtar et al., 2012).

Antimicrobial Peptides	Radionuclide	Microorganisms	Experimental model	Reference
Human neutrophil peptide (HNP) -1	Tc-99m	*Staphylococcus aureus* -*Klebsiella pneumoniae*	Swiss mice	Welling et al., 1999
Ubiquicidin (UBI) 29–41 -UBI 18–35 -UBI 31–38 -Human lactoferrin (hLF) 1–11 -Defensins	Tc-99m	Multidrug-resistant *Staphylococcus aureus (MRSA)* -*Klebsiella pneumonia* -Fluconazole resistant *Candida albicans*	Swiss mice -New Zealand White rabbits	Welling et al., 2001
UBI 29-41	Tc-99m (HYNIC- or N2S2-chelate conjugated)	*Staphylococcus aureus* -*Klebsiella pneumonia*	Swiss mice	Welling et al., 2003
UBI 29-41 hLF 1-11	Tc-99m	*Staphylococcus aureus* -MRSA	Swiss mice -Wistar rats	Nibbering et al., 2004
UBI 29-41 (in a kit formulation)	Tc-99m	*Staphylococcus aureus* -*Escherichia coli*	Rabbits	Akhtar et al., 2004
UBI 29-41	Tc-99m	Various bacterial microorganisms	Human (with suspected bone infection)	Melendez-Alafort et al., 2004
UBI 29-41	Tc-99m	Various bacterial microorganisms	Human (with soft tissue infection and osteomyelitis)	Akhtar et al., 2005
UBI 29-41	Tc-99m	*Staphylococcus aureus* (prosthetic joint infection)	New Zealand rabbits	Sarda-Mantel et al., 2007
hLF 1–11	Tc-99m	MRSA	Swiss mice	Brouwer & Welling, 2008
UBI 29-41	^{99m}Tc/Tricine/ HYNIC^{0} from lyophilized kits	Various bacterial microorganisms	Human (with suspected bone or soft-tissue infections)	Gandomkar et al., 2009
UBI 29-41	Tc-99m	Various bacterial microorganisms	Human (with diabetic foot infection)	Fard-Esfahani et al., 2010

Table 4. Some reported applications of antimicrobial peptides as infection imaging agents.

http://dx.doi.org/10.5772/52882

9. Antibiotics and antimicrobial peptides radiolabeling

A simple, efficient and reproducible radiolabeling procedure is essential to develop radiopharmaceuticals for routine clinical use (Gandomkar et al., 2009). The various methods of radiolabeling with ^{99m}Tc, including the direct labeling methods for antibiotics and peptides and indirect labeling of peptides using the bifunctional chelating agents have been discussed. The radionuclide should be firmly attached or incorporated into the peptide to allow the visualization of the target and reliable assessment of its pharmacokinetics after its intravenous administration. Moreover, the labeling conditions should not affect the binding activity of the peptide to the microorganism (Lupetti et al., 2003c).

Quality assurance is the sum of all parameters concerning the preparation and control of a finished product. Biological quality control of pharmaceutical products becomes essential as they are ultimately to be consumed by living organisms, in particular the humans (Patei Riddhi et al., 2011). Radiochemical purity and labeling efficiency analyses techniques are performed by high performance liquid chromatography (HPLC), C18-Sep-pak, instant thin layer chromatography (ITLC) and paper chromatography (IAEA-TECDOC-1414, 2004). Optimum condition of labeling are required for maximum labeling of ^{99m}Tc-conjugates by optimizing the affecting factors on radiolabeling such as: pH, the amount of reducing agent and incubation time of reaction mixture. Moreover, the stability of radiolabeled complex in human blood serum and room temperature are determined. The biodistribution study of labeled complex is done by percent uptake calculation of the tracer at various organs of experimental animal, after intravenous administration of the radiopharmaceutical at different intervals to monitor the distribution style of radio complex at different organs, localization and high uptake at target site without any accumulation in vital organs.

9.1. Direct labeling

The direct labeling method is a simple procedure in which the peptide is labeled in absence of an exogenous chelator (Lupetti et al., 2003b). The direct approach is characterized by poorly defined chemical structures, and it is generally thought that the 99mTc binds to the sulfhydryl groups produced by reduction of the peptide disulfide bridge. Therefore, peptides containing cysteine seem to be a basic requirement for this labeling approach (Melendez-Alafort et al., 2009). The various complexes of ^{99m}Tc may be formed by interaction between electron donor atoms and reduced technetium. In the case of antibiotics radiolabeling, in order to form bonds with technetium, the structure must contain electron donors such as oxygen, nitrogen and sulfur. The labeled complex may be formed electron pairs of these atoms with reduced technetium that is +1 or +3 in the reduced states similar to other studies (Yurt Lambrechtet al., 2008b).The mechanism underlying the direct labeling method is not fully elucidated, but it probably involves the reduction of ^{99m}Tc-pertechnetate by stannous ions and KBH_4, the production of a TcO (pyrophosphate) intermediate, and the substitution reaction transferring the reduced technetium from this intermediate to the amino groups of cationic peptides. The end-product from this reaction could be a reduced metal (N4) complex, as reported for many tetrapeptides (Lupetti et al., 2003c).

9.2. Indirect labeling

Indirect method of labeling is used mostly for radiolabeling of peptides and it is not common for antibiotics labeling. A widely used method for labeling of small peptides is by conjugation of bifunctional chelators to the peptide and several attampts have been made using hydrazinonicotinamid (HYNIC) and N_3S compounds (S-benzoyl MAG3) (IAEA-TEC-DOC-1414, 2004). Among the various bifunctional chelating agents developed to date, HYNIC constitutes a representative agent for ^{99m}Tc radiolabeling. Since HYNIC serves as a monodentate or bidentate ligand, a coligand is necessary to complete the coordination sphere of the technetium core. Tricine is often used as the coligand because of the production of ^{99m}Tc-HYNIC-labeled peptides and polypeptides with high radiochemical yields and high specific activities in a short reaction time (Ono et al., 2001). Moreover, the indirect labeling method permits post conjugation labeling, whereby the peptide is first conjugated to the BFCA and then stored and labeled when required for clinical use. Furthermore, this approach is the only choice for peptides containing disulfide bridges essential for receptor recognition (Melendez-Alafort et al., 2009).

10. Conclusion

Nuclear medicine technology offers an attractive option for diagnosis of focal infections due to its sensitivity based on pathophysiological and pathobiochemical processes. This approach needs a reliable radiopharmaceutical that can concentrate in site of infection with high specificity. As reviewed in this chapter, various conventional radiopharmaceuticals which are basically on the uptake mechanism of targeting host inflammatory response are not specific for infection imaging. In contrast, the use of radiopharmaceuticals for specific targeting of microorganisms responsible for infection, have been proposed. In this respect, radiolabeled antibiotics and antimicrobial peptides, by specific binding to the bacterial component, have the potential to distinguish microbial from non infectious inflammation at the early stage of diseases. However, according to the irregular usage of antibiotics and increasing antibiotic-resistant microorganisms, it seems that antimicrobial peptides have more advantages over antibiotics. We suggest that, antimicrobial peptides with wide promising properties as the infection imaging agents have the ability to be used in clinical usages in patients with suspected infections for more accurate diagnosis.

Author details

Mojtaba Salouti and Akram Fazli

Biology Research Center, Zanjan Branch, Islamic Azad University, Zanjan, Iran

References

[1] Alavi, A., Kung, J. W., & Zhuang, H. (2004). Implications of PET based molecular imaging on the current and future practice of medicine. *Seminars in Nuclear Medicine,* 34, 56-69.

[2] Akhtar, M. S., Iqbal, J., Khan, M. A., Irfanullah, J., Jehangir, M., Khan, B., Ul-Haq, I., Muhammad, G., Nadeem, M. A., Afzal, M. S., & Imran, M. B. (2004). ^{99m}Tc-Labeled antimicrobial peptide ubiquicidin (29-41) accumulates less in Escherichia coli infection than in Staphlococcus aureus infection. *Journal of Nuclear Medicine*, 45, 849–856.

[3] Akhtar, M. S., Qaisar, A., Irfanullah, J., Iqbal, J., Khan, B., Jehangir, M., Nadeem, M. A., Khan, M. A., Afzal, M. S., Ul-Haq, I., & Imran, M. B. (2005). Antimicrobial peptide ^{99m}Tc-Ubiquicidin 29–41 as human infection-imaging agent: Clinical trial. *Journal of Nuclear Medicine*, 46, 567–573.

[4] Akhtar, M. S., Imran, M. B., Nadeem, M. A., & Shahid, A. (2012). Antimicrobial peptides as infection imaging agents: better than radiolabeled antibiotics. *International Journal of Peptides*, 1-19.

[5] Arano, Y. (2002). Recent advances in ^{99m}Tc radiopharmaceuticals. *Annals of Nuclear Medicine*, 16, 79–93.

[6] Artiko, V., Davidovic, B., Nikolic, N., Petrovic, M., Valajkovic, M., & Pesko, p. (2005). Detection of gastrointestinal and abdominal infections by ^{99m}Tc-ciprofloxacin. *Hepato-gastroenterology*, 52, 491-5.

[7] Awasthi, V. D., Goins, B., Klipper, R., & Phillips, W. T. (1998). Dual radiolabeled liposomes: biodistribution studies and localization of focal sites of infection in rats. *Nuclear Medicine & Biology*, 25, 155–160.

[8] Babich, J. W., Tompkins, R. G., Graham, W., Sandra A. Barrow, S. A., & Fischman, A. J. (1997). Localization of radiolabeled chemotactic peptide at focal Sites of Escherichia coli infection in rabbits: Evidence for a receptor-specific mechanism. *Journal of Nuclear Medicine*, 38, 1316-1322.

[9] Babich, J. W., & Fischman, A. J. (1999). Targeted imaging of infection. *Advanced Drug Delivery Reviews*, 37, 237–252.

[10] Babich , J. W., Coco, W. G., Barrow, S., Fischman, A. J., Frank J. Femia, F. J., & Zubieta, J. (2000). ^{99m}Tc-labeled chemotactic peptides: influence of coligand on distribution of molecular species and infection imaging properties. Synthesis and structural characterization of model complexes with the {Re (h^2HNNC5H4N)(h^1-NNC5H4N)} core. *Inorganica Chimica Acta*, 309, 123–136.

[11] Baldoni, D. (2009). *Innovative methods for the diagnosis and treatment of implant-associated infections*. Basel University, Italy, pp. 16-17.

[12] Basu, S., Chryssikos, T., Moghadam-Kia, S., Zhuang, H., Torigian, D. A., & Alavi, A. (2009). Positron emission tomography as a diagnostic tool in infection: Present role and future possibilities. *Seminars in Nuclear Medicine*, 39, 36-51.

[13] Becker, W., & Meller, J. (2001). The role of nuclear medicine in infection and inflammation. *Lancet Infectious Diseases*, 1, 326–33.

[14] Bengel, F. M., Anton, M., Avril, N., Brill, T., Nguyen, N., Haubner, R., Gleiter, E., Bernd Gansbacher, B., & Schwaiger, M. (2000). Uptake of radiolabeled 2′-Fluoro-2′-Deoxy-5-Iodo-1--arabinofuranosyluracil in cardiac cells after adenoviral transfer of the herpesvirus thymidine kinase gene : The cellular basis for cardiac gene imaging. *Circulation*, 102, 948-950.

[15] Bernardo-Filho, M., Santos-Filho, S. D., Fonseca, A. S., Carter, K., & Missailidis, S. (2008). Nuclear medicine procedures for the evaluation of male sexual organs: A brief review. *Brazilian Archives of Biology and Technology*, 51, 13-21.

[16] Bleeker-Rovers, C. P., Boerman, O. C., Rennen, H. J. J. M., Corstens, F. H. M., & Oyen, W. J. G. (2004). Radiolabeled compounds in diagnosis of infectious and inflammatory disease. *Current Pharmaceutical Design*, 10, 2935-2950.

[17] Boerman, O. C., & Nijmegen, N. L. (2008). The uptake mechanisms of infection and inflammation imaging agents. *Annual Congress of the Europian Association of Nuclear Medicine*, pp. 39-42.

[18] Bonekamp, D., Hammoud, D. A., Martin, G., & Pomper, M. G. (2010). Molecular imaging: Techniques and current clinical applications. *Applied Radiology*, 10-21.

[19] Bray, M., Di Mascio, M., De Kok-Mercado, F., Mollura, D. J., & Jagoda, E. (2010).Radiolabeled antiviral drugs and antibodies as virus-specific imaging probes. *Antiviral Research*, 88, 129–142.

[20] Britton, K. E., Vinjamury, S., Hall, A. V., Solanki, K., Siraj, Q. H., Bomanji, J., & Das, S. (1997). Clinical evaluation of technetium-99m infecton for the localization of bacterial infections. *Europian Journal of Nuclear Medicine*, 24, 553-556.

[21] Britton, K. E., Wareham, D. W., Das, S. S., Solanki, K. K., H Amaral, H., Bhatnagar, A., Katamihardja, A. H. S., Malamitsi, J., Moustafa, H. M., Soroa, V. E., Sundram,F. X., & Padhy, A. K. (2002). Imaging bacterial infection with ^{99m}Tc-ciprofloxacin (Infecton). *Journal of Clinical Pathology*, 55, 817–823.

[22] Brouwer, C. P. J. M., & Welling, M. M. (2008). Various routes of administration of ^{99m}Tc-labeled synthetic lactoferrin antimicrobial peptide hLF 1–11 enables monitoring and effective killing of multidrug-resistant Staphylococcus aureus infections in mice. *Peptides*, 29, 1109 – 1117.

[23] Bruni, C., Padovano, F., Travascio, L., Schillaci, O., & Simonetti, G. (2008). Usefulness of hybrid SPECT/CT for the ^{99m}Tc-HMPAO-labeled leukocyte scintigraphy in a case of cranial osteomyelitis. *The Brazilian Journal of Infectious Diseases*, 12, 558-560.

[24] Chattopadhyay, S., Das, S. S., Chandra, S., Mirsha, M., Sarkar, BR., Sinha, S., & Ganguly, S. (2010). Synthesis and evaluation of ^{99m}Tc-moxifloxacin, a potential specific imaging agent. *Applied Radiation and Isotopes*, 68, 314-316.

[25] Changizi, V., Takavar, A., Babakhani, A., & Sohrabi, M. (2008). Scatter correction for heart SPECT images using TEW method. *Journal of Applied Clinical Medical Physics*, 9, 136-140.

[26] Choe, Y. M., Choe, W., Lee, K. Y., Ahn, S. I., Kim, K., Cho, Y. U., Choi, S. K., Hur, Y. S., Kim, S. J., Hong, K. C., Shin, S. H., Kim, K. R., & Woo, Z. H. (2007). Tc-99m ciprofloxacin imaging in acute cholecystitis. *World Journal of Gastroenterol*, 13, 3249-3252.

[27] Cotti, E., & Campisi, G. (2004). Advanced radiographic techniques for the detection of lesions in bone. *Endodontic Topics*, 7, 52–72.

[28] Das, S. S., Hall, A. V., Wareham, D. W., & Britton, K. E. (2002). Infection imaging with radiopharmaceuticals in the 21th century. *Brazilian Archives of Biology and Technology*, 45, 25-37.

[29] Davies, J. (2006). Are antibiotics naturally antibiotics? *Journal of Industrial Microbiology and Biotechnology*, 33, 496–499.

[30] De Assis, D. N., Furtado Mosqueira, C. F., Carneiro Vilela, J. M., Andrade, M. S., & Cardoso, V. N. (2008). Release profiles and morphological characterization by atomic force microscopy and photon correlation spectroscopy of ^{99m}Technetium-fluconazole nanocapsules. *International Journal of Pharmaceutics*, 349, 152–160.

[31] De Backer, A. I., Mortele, K. J., De Keulenaer, B. L., & Parizel, P. M. (2006). Tuberculosis: Epidemiology, Manifestations, and the value of medical imaging in diagnosis. *JBR–BTR*, 89, 243-250.

[32] De Winter, F., Gemmel, F., Van Laere, K., De Winter, O., Poffijn, B., & Dierckx, R. A. (2004). 99mTc-ciprofloxacin planar and tomographic imaging for the diagnosis of infection in the postoperative spine: experience in 48 patients. *Europian Journal of Nuclear Medicin and Molecular Imaging*, 31, 233–239.

[33] Diamandis, E. P., & Christopoulos, T. K. (1991). The biotin-(strept)avidin system: principles and applications in biotechnology. *Clinical Chemistry*, 37, 625-638.

[34] Diniz, S. O. F., Siqueira, C. F., Nelson, D. L., Martin-comin, J., & Cardoso, V. N. (2005). Technetium-99m ceftizoxime kit preparation. *Brazulian archive of Biology and Technology*, 48, 89-96.

[35] El-Ghany, E. A., El-Kolaly, M. T., Amine, A. M., El-Sayed, A. S., & Abdel-Gelil, F. (2005). Synthesis of ^{99m}Tc-pefloxacin: A new targeting agent for infectious foci. *Journal of Radioanalytical and Nuclear Chemistry*, 266, 131-139.

[36] Fard-Esfahani, A., Beiki, D., Fallahi, B., Mohajeri-Tehrani, M. R., Gharaie, M. R., Rouhipour , N., Dehghanian, M., Saghari, M., Emami-Ardekani, A., & Eftekhari, M. (2010). Evaluation of ^{99m}Tc-ubiquicidin 29–41 scintigraphy in differentiation of bacte-

rial infection from sterile inflammation in diabetic foot. *Iranian Journal of Nuclear Medicine*, 18, 20-28.

[37] Finberg, R. W., Moellering, R. C., Tally, F. P., Craig, W. A., Pankey, G. A., Dellinger, E. P., West, M. A., Joshi, M., Linden, P. K., Rolston, K. V., Rotschafer, J. C., & Rybak, M. J. (2004). The importance of bactericidal drugs: Future directions in infectious disease. *Clinical Infectious Diseases*, 39, 1314–20.

[38] Fischman, A. J., Pike, M. C., Kroon, D., Fucello, A. J., Rexinger, D., Tenkate, C., Wilkinson, R., Rubin, R. H., & Strauss, H. W. (1991). Imaging focal site of bacterial infection in rats with indium-111-labeled chemotactic peptides analogs. *Journal of Nuclear Medicine*, 32, 483-491.

[39] Fortner, A., Taylor, A., Alazraki, N., & Datz, F. L. (1986). Advantage of indium-111 leukocytes over ultrasound in imaging an infected renal cyst. *Journal of Nuclear Medicine*, 27, 1147-1149.

[40] French, G. L. (2006). Bactericidal agents in the treatment of MRSA infections—the potential role of daptomycin. *Journal of Antimicrobial Chemotherapy*, 58, 1107–1117.

[41] Gal, O., Gmar, M., Ivanov, O. P., Laine, F., Lamadiec, F., Goaller, C. L., Mahe, C., Manach, E., & Stepanov, V. E. (2006). Development of a portable gamma camera with coded aperture. *Nuclear Instruments and Methods in Physics Research*, 563, 233–237.

[42] Gandomkar, M., Najafi, R., Shafiei, M., Mazidi, M., Goudarzi, M., Mirfallah, S. H., Ebrahimi, F., Heydarpor, H. R., & Abdie, N. (2009). Clinical evaluation of antimicrobial peptide [^{99m}Tc/Tricine/HYNIC] ubiquicidin 29–41 as a human-specific infection imaging agent. *Nuclear Medicine and Biology*, 36, 199–205.

[43] Gemmel, F., Dumarey, N., & Welling, M. (2009). Future diagnostic agents. *Seminars in Nucearl Medicine*, 39, 11-26.

[44] Giaffer, M. H. (1996). Labeled leucocyte scintigraphy in inflammatoty bowel disease: clinical applications. *Gut*, 38, 1-5.

[45] Gomes Barreto, V., Iglesias, F., Roca, M., Tubau, F., & Martin-Comin, J. (2000). Labeling of ceftizoxime with ^{99m}Tc. *Revista Espanola Medicine Nuclear*, 19, 479-83.

[46] Gomes Barreto, V., Rabiller, G., Iglesias, F., Soroa, V., Tubau, F., Roca, M., & Martin-comin, J. (2005). ^{99m}Tc-ceftizoxime scintigraphy in normal rats and abscess induced rats. *Revista Espanola Medicine Nuclear*, 24, 312-8.

[47] Gotthardt, M., Bleeker-Rovers, C. P., Boerman, O. C., & Oyen, W. J. G. (2010). Imaging of inflammation by PET, conventional scintigraphy, and other imaging techniques. *Journal of Nuclear Medicine*, 51, 1937–1949.

[48] Gyorke, T., Duffek, L., Bartfai, K., Mako, E., Karlinger, K., Mester, A., & Tarjan, Z. (2000). The role of nuclear medicine in inflammatory bowel disease. Review with experiences of aspecific bowel activity using immunescintigraphy with ^{99m}Tc anti-granulocyte antibodies. *European Journal of Radiology*, 35, 183–192.

[49] Hall, A. V., Solanki, K. K., Vinjamuri, S., Britton, K. E., & Das, S. S. (1998). Evaluation of the efficacy of ^{99m}Tc-Infecton, a novel agent for detecting sites of infection. *Journal of Clinical Pathology*, 51, 215–219.

[50] Hancock, R. E. W. (2005). Mechanisms of action of newer antibiotics for Gram-positive Pathogens. *Lancet Infectious Disease*, 5, 209–18.

[51] Hartwig, W., Carter, E. A., Jimenez, R. E., Werner, J., Fischman, A. J., Del Castillo, C. F., & Warshaw, A. L. (1999). Chemotactic peptide uptake in acute pancreatitis: correlation with tissue accumulation of leukocytes. *Journal of Applied Physiology*, 87, 743-749.

[52] Hernandez Serrano, P. (2005). Responsible use of antibiotics in aquaculture. Food and Agriculture Organization of the United Nation, Rome.

[53] Hricak, H. (2007). *Advancing nuclear medicine through innovation*. National Academy of Sciences, United States of America.

[54] IAEA, TECDOC-1414, (2004). *Development of kits for ^{99m}Tc radiopharmaceuticals for infection imaging*. International Atomic Energy Agency, Vienna, Austria.

[55] Ibrahim, I. T., Motaleb, M. A., & Attalah, K. M. (2010). Synthesis and biological distribution of ^{99m}Tc-norfloxacin complex, a novel agent for detecting sites of infection. *Journal of Radioanalytical and Nuclear Chemistry*, 285, 431–436.

[56] Jalilian, A. R., Novinrooz, A., Motamedi-Sedeh, F., Moradkhani, S., Rajamand, A. A., & Solati, J. (2009). Evaluation of [^{67}Ga] citrate in the detection of various microorganism infections in animal models. *Iran Journal of Nuclear Medicine*, 17, 34-41.

[57] Jordao, L. L., & Vieira, O. V. (2011). Tuberculosis: New aspects of an old disease. *International Journal of Cell Biology*, 1-13.

[58] Kamysz, W. (2005). Are antimicrobial peptides an alternative for conventional antibiotics? *Nuclear Medicine Review*, 8, 78–86.

[59] Kittigul, L., Suthchana, S., Kittigul, C., & Pengruangrojanachai, V. (1998). Immunoglobulin M-capture biotin-streptavidin enzyme linked immunosorbent assay for detection of antibodies to dengue viruses. *The American Society of Tropical Medicine and Hygiene*, 59, 352–356.

[60] Knight, L. C. (2003). Non-oncologic applications of radiolabeled peptides in nuclear medicine. *The Quarterly Journal of Nuclear Medicine*, 47, 279-91.

[61] Korkmaz, M., & Ozer, AY. (2006). DTPA liposomes in diagnostic imaging. *FABAD Journal of Pharmaceuticals Sciences*, 31, 210-219.

[62] Kumar, R., Basu, S., Torigian, D., Anand, V., Zhuang, H., & Alavi, A. (2008). Role of modern imaging techniques for diagnosis of infection in the era of ^{18}F-Fluorodeoxyglucose positron emission tomography. *Clinical Microbiology Reviews*, 21, 209–224.

[63] Kuo, C. L., Chuang, F. J., Hsu, C. H., Lee, Y. J., Lee, C. M., & Chang, N. C. (2002). Mycotic aneurysm in thoracic aorta detected by Gallium-67 scan: A case report. *Annals of Nuclear Medicine Sciences*, 15, 167-170.

[64] Kyprianidou, P., Tsoukalas, C., Chiotellis, A., Papagiannopoulou, D., Raptopoulou, CP., Terzis, A., Pelecanou, M., Papadopoulos, M,. & Pirmettis, I. (2011). First example of well-characterized Re and ^{99m}Tc tricarbonyl complexes of ciprofloxacin and norfloxacin in the development of infection-specific imaging agents. *Inorganica Chimica Acta*, 370, 236–242.

[65] Larikka, M. (2003). *Diagnosis of orthopaedic prosthesis infections with radionuclide techniques; clinical application of various imaging methods.* University of Oulu, Finland.

[66] Laverman, P., Boerman, O. C., Oyen, W. J. G., Dams, ETM., Storm, G., & Corstens, F. H. M. (1999). Liposomes for scintigraphic detection of infection and inflammation. *Advanced Drug Delivery Reviews*, 37, 225–235.

[67] Laverman, P., Bleeker-Rovers, C. P., Corstens, F. H. M., Boerman, O. C,. & Oyen, W. J. G. (2008). Development of Infection and Inflammation Targeting Compounds. *Current Radiopharmaceuticals*, 1, 42-48.

[68] Lazzeri, E., Manca, M., Molea, N., Marchetti, S., Consoli, V., Bodei, L., R.Bianchi, R., Chinol, M., Paganelli, G., & Mariani, G. (1999). Clinical validation of the avidin/indium-111 biotin approach for imaging infection/inflammation in orthopaedic patients. *Europian Journal of Nuclear Medicine*, 26, 606-614.

[69] Lazzeri, E., Erba, P., Perri, M., Tascini, C., Doria, R., Giorgetti, J., & Mariani, G. (2008). Scintigraphic imaging of vertebral osteomyelitis with ^{111}In-Biotin. *Spine*, 33, 198-204.

[70] Lin, Y., Zhang, X., Li, J., Yin, D., & Wang, Y. (2003). Preparation and radiolabeling of antimony sulfide nanocolloids with two different particle sizes. *Applied Radiation and Isotopes*, 58, 347–352.

[71] Livni, E., Berker, M., Hillier, S., Waller, S. C., Ogan, M. D., Discordia, R. P., Rienhart, J. K., Rubin, R. H., & Fischman, A. J. (2004). Preparation and pharmacokinetics of ^{11}C labeled stavudine (d4T). *Nuclear Medicine and Biology*, 31, 613–621.

[72] Lupetti, A., Welling, M. M., Mazzi, U., Nibbering, P. H., & Pauwels, E. K. (2002). Technetium-99m labeled fluconazole and antimicrobial peptides for imaging of Candida albicans and Aspergillus fumigates infections. *Europian Journal of Nuclear Medicine and Molecular Imaging*, 29, 674-9.

[73] Lupetti, A., Pauwels, E. K. J., Nibbering, P. H., & Welling, M. M. (2003a). 99mTc-Antimicrobial peptides: promising candidates for infection imaging. *The Quarterly Journal of Nuclear Medicine*, 47, 238-45.

[74] Lupetti, A., Nibbering, P. H., Welling, M. M., & Pauwels, E. K. J. (2003b). Radiopharmaceuticals: new antimicrobial agents. *Trends in Biotechnology*, 21, 70-73.

[75] Lupetti, A., Welling, M. M., Pauwels, E. K. J., & Nibbering, P. H. (2003c). Radiolabeled antimicrobial peptides for infection detection. *The Lancet Infectious Diseases*, 3, 223-229.

[76] Lupetti, A., De Boer, M. G. J., Erba, P., Campa, M., & Nibbering, P. H. (2011). Radiotracers for fungal infection imaging. *Medical Mycology*, 49, S62–S69.

[77] Lyra, M., Voliotopoulos, V., Skouroliakou, C., Stavraka, A., Vlahos, L., Frantzis, A., & Limouris, G. S. (1998). *Practical dosimetric condideration and imaging evaluation in infection scintigraphy*. Mediterra-Publishers, Athens, pp. 105-109.

[78] Malamitsi, J., Giamarellou, H., Kanellakopoulou, K., Dounis, E., Grecka, V., Christakopoulos, J., Koratzanis, C., Antoniadou, A., Panoutsopoulos, G., Batsakis, C., & Proukakis, C. (2003). Infecton: a ^{99m}Tc-ciprofloxacin radiopharmaceutical for the detection of bone infection. *Clinical Microbiology and Infection*, 9, 101-109.

[79] Malviya, G., De Vries, E. F. J., Dierckx, R. A., & Signore, A. (2007). Radiopharmaceuticals for imaging chronic lymphocytic inflammation. *The Brazilian Journal of Infectious Diseases*, 50, 1-13.

[80] Malviya, G., Anzola, K. L., Podestà, E., Laganà, B., Del Mastro, C., Dierckx, RA., Scopinaro, F., & Signore, A. (2011). 99mTc-labeled rituximab for imaging B lymphocyte infiltration in inflammatory autoimmune disease patients. *Molecular Imaging Biology*,

[81] Melendez-Alafort, L., Rodrıguez-Cortes, J., Ferro-Flores, G., De Murphy, C. A., Herrera-Rodrıguez, R., Mitsoura, E., & Martınez-Dunckerd, C. (2004). Biokinetics of ^{99m}Tc-UBI 29-41 in humans. *Nuclear Medicine and Biology*, 31, 373–379.

[82] Mirshojaei, S. F., Gandomkar, M., Najafi, R., Sadat Ebrahimi, S. E., Babaei, M. H., Shafiei, A., Talebi, M. H. (2011). Radiolabeling, quality control and biodistribution of ^{99m}Tc-cefotaxime as an infection imaging agent. *Journal of Radioanalytical Nuclear Chemistry*, 287, 21–25.

[83] Mora, F. R., Isunza, A. R., Lqpez, A. M., Palma, R. R., Guizar, S. C., Mora, I. M., Velazquez, V. P. (2010). Sensitivity and specificity of the Tc-99m ciprofloxacin scan in pediatric osteomyelitis. *Acta ortopedica Mexicana*, 24, 246-249.

[84] Mostafa, M., Motaleb, M. A., & Sakr, T. M. (2010). Labeling of ceftriaxone for infective inflammation imaging using ^{99m}Tc eluted from ^{99}Mo/^{99m}Tc generator based on zirconium molybdate. *Applied Radiation and Isotopes*, 68, 1959-1963.

[85] Motaleb, M. A. (2007a). Preparation of ^{99m}Tc-cefoperazone complex, a novel agent for detecting sites of infection. *Journal of Radioanalytical and Nuclear Chemistry*, 272, 167-171.

[86] Motaleb, M. A. (2007b). Preparation and biodistribution of ^{99m}Tc-lomefloxacin and ^{99m}Tc-ofloxacin complexes. *Journal of Radioanalytical and Nuclear Chemistry*, 272, 95–99.

[87] Motaleb, M. A. (2009). Preparation, quality control and stability of ^{99m}Tc-sparafloxacin complex, a novel agent for detecting sites of infection. *Journal of Labeled Compounds and Radiopharmaceuticals,* 52, 415-418.

[88] Motaleb, M. A., El-Kolaly, M. T., Ibrahim, A. B., & Abd El-Bary, A. (2011). Study on the preparation and biological evaluation of ^{99m}Tc–gatifloxacin and ^{99m}Tc–cefepime complexes. *Journal of Radioanalytical and Nuclear Chemistry,* 289, 57–65.

[89] Mufamadi, M. S., Pillay, V., Choonara, Y. E., Du Toit, L. C., Modi, G., Naidoo, D., & Ndesendo, V. M. K. (2011). A review on composite liposomal technologies for specialized drug delivery. *Journal of Drug Delivery,* 1-19.

[90] Naqvi, S. A. R., Ishfaq, M. M., Khan, Z. A., Nagra, S. A., Bukhari, I. H., Hussain, A. I., Mahmood, N., Shahzad, S. A., Haque, A. & Bokhari, T. H. (2012). ^{99m}Tc labeled levofloxacin as an infection imaging agent: a novel method for labeling levofloxacin using cysteine HCl as co-ligand and in vivo study. *Turkish Journal of Chemistry,* 36, 267 – 277.

[91] Niederman, M. S. (2009). Antibiotic therapy in critical illness. American College of Chest Physicians Critical Care Medicine Board Review, 20, 523-538.

[92] Okarvi, S. M. (2001). Recent progress in fluorine-18 labeled peptide radiopharmaceuticals. *Europian Journal of Nuclear Medicine,* 28, 929–938.

[93] Ono, M., Aranob, Y., Mukai, T., Fujioka, Y., Ogawa, K., Uehara, T., Saga, T., Konishi, J., Saji, H. (2001). ^{99m}Tc-HYNIC-derivatized ternary ligand complexes for ^{99m}Tc-labeled polypeptides with low in vivo protein binding. *Nuclear Medicine and Biology,* 28, 215–224.

[94] Oscariz, J. C., & Pisabarro, A. G. (2001). Classification and mode of action of membrane–active bacteriocins produced by gram-positive bacteria. *International Microbiology,* 4, 13-19.

[95] Oyen, W. J. G., Claessens, R. A. M. J., Van der Meer, J. W. M., Rubin, R. H., Strauss, H. W., & Corstens, F. H. M. (1992). Indium-111-labeled human nonspecific immunoglobulin G: A New Radiopharmaceutical for Imaging Infectious and Inflammatory Foci. *Clinical Infectious Diseases,* 14, 1110-8.

[96] Oyen, W. J. G., Boerman, O. C., & Corstens, F. H. M. (2001). Animal models of infection and inflammation and their role in experimental nuclear medicine. *Journal of Microbiological Methods,* 47, 151–157.

[97] Oyen, W. J. G., Corstens, F. H. M., & Boerman, O. C. (2005). Discriminating infection from sterile inflammation: can radiolabeled antibiotics solve the problem. European *Journal of Nuclear Medicine and Molecular Imaging,* 32, 151–152.

[98] Palestro, C. J., Love, C., & Miller, T. T. (2006). Imaging of musculoskeletal infections. *Best Practice & Research Clinical Rheumatology,* 20, 1197-1218.

[99] Palestro, C. J., & Love, C. (2009). Nuclear medicine and diabetic foot infections. Seminars in Nuclear Medicine, 39, 52-65.

[100] Patei Riddhi, D., Patel, P. M., & Patel, N. M. (2011). A review on radiopharmaceuticals and radiochemical method in analysis. *International Journal of Pharmaceutical & Biological Archives*, 2, 1062-1067.

[101] Peterson, J. J. (2006). Postoperative infection. *Radiologic Clinics of North America*, 44, 439-450.

[102] Petruzzi, N., Shanthly, N., & Thakur, M. (2009). Recent trends in Soft-tissue infection imaging. *Seminars in Nuclear Medicine*, 39, 115-123.

[103] Phillips, W. T., Goins, B. A., & Bao, A. (2009). Radioactive liiposomes. *WIREs Nanomedicine and Nanobiotechnology*, 1, 69–83.

[104] Price, R. W., Satio, Y., & Fox, J. J. (1983). Prospects for the use of radiolabeled antiviral drugs in the diagnosis of herpes simplex encephalitis. *Biochemical Pharmacology*, 32, 2455-2461.

[105] Reddy, K. V. R., Yedery, R. D., & Aranha, C. (2004). Antimicrobial peptides: premises and promises. *International Journal of Antimicrobial Agents*, 24, 536–547.

[106] Rennen, H. J. J. M., Boerman, O. C., Oyen, W. J. G., & Corstens, F. H. M. (2001). Imaging infection/inflammation in the new millennium. *Europian Journal of Nuclear Medicine*, 28, 241-252.

[107] Rennen, H. J. J. M., Boerman, O. C., Oyen, W. J. G., & Corstens, F. H. M. (2002). Scintigraphic Imaging of Inflammatory Processes. *Current Medical Chemistry – Anti-Inflammatory & Anti-Allergy Agents*, 1, 63-75.

[108] Riaz, S. S., Faisal, M., & Hasnain, S. (2011). Antibiotic susceptibility pattern and multiple antibiotic resistances (MAR) calculation of extended spectrum β-lactamase (ESBL) producing Escherichia coli and Klebsiella species in Pakistan. *African Journal of Biotechnology*, 10, 6325-6331.

[109] Richter, W. S., Ivancevic , V., Meller, J., Otto Lang, O., Le Guludec , D., Szilvazi, I., Amthauer, H., Chossat, F., Dahmane, A., Schwenke, C., & Signore, A. (2011). 99mTc-besilesomab (Scintimun®) in peripheral osteomyelitis: comparison with 99mTc-labeled white blood cells. *European Journal of Nuclear Medicine and Molecular Imaging*, 38, 899–910.

[110] Robinson, R. J., & Scarsbrook, A. F. (2009). Radionuclide imaging of joint prostheses: established & emerging applications. *Orthopaedics and Trauma*, 23, 77-87.

[111] Roohi, S., Mushtaq, A., & Malik, S. A. (2005). Synthesis and biodistribution of ^{99m}Tc-vancomycin in model of bacterial infection. *Radiochemistry*, 93, 415-418.

[112] Roohi, S. (2006). *Preparation and quality control of Technethium-99m labeled compounds for diagnostic purpose*. Quaid-I-Azam University, Islamabad, Pakistan, pp. 33-34.

[113] Roohi, S., Mushtaq, A., Jehangir, M., & Malik, A. (2006). Synthesis, quality control and biodistribution of ^{99m}Tc-kanamycin. *Journal of Radioanalytical and Nuclear Chemistry*, 267, 561-566.

[114] Roper, J. R., Bowsher, J. E., Wilson, J. M., Turkington, T. G., Yin, F. F. (2012). Target localization using scanner-acquired SPECT data. *Journal of Applied Clinical Medical Physics*, 13, 108-123.

[115] Rotem, S., & Mor, A. (2009). Antimicrobial peptide mimics for improved therapeutic properties. *Biochimica et Biophysica Acta*, 1788, 1582–1592.

[116] Saito, Y., Rubenstein, R., Price, R. W., Fox, J. J., & Watanabe, K. A. (1984). Diagnostic imaging of herpes simplex virus encephalitis using a radiolabeled antiviral drug: autoradiographic assessment in an animal model. *Annual Neurology*, 15, 548-58.

[117] Sanchez, F., Benlloch, J. M., Escat, B., Pavon, N., Porras, E., Kadi-Hanifi, D., & Ruiz, JA. (2004). Design and tests of a portable mini gamma camera. (2004). *American Association of Physicists in Medicine*, 31, 1384-1397.

[118] Sarda, L., Cremieux, A. C., Lebellec, Y., Meulemans, A., Lebtahi, R., Hayem, G., Genin, R., Delahaye, N., Huten, D., Le Guludec, D. (2003). Inability of ^{99m}Tc-ciprofloxacin scintigraphy to discriminate between septic and sterile osteoarticular diseases. *Journal of Nuclear Medicine*, 44, 920-926.

[119] Sarda-Mantel, L., Saleh-Mghir, A., Welling, M. M., Meulemans, A., & Vrigneaud, J. M. (2007). Evaluation of ^{99m}Tc-UBI 29-41 scintigraphy for specific detection of experimental Staphylococcus aureus prosthetic joint infections. *European Journal of Nuclear Medicine and Molecular Imaging*, 34, 1302-1309

[120] Sascha A. Kristian, S. A., Timmer, A. M., Liu, G. Y., Lauth, X., Sal-Man, N., Rosenfeld, Y., Shai, Y., Gallo, R. L., & Nizet, V. (2007). Impairment of innate immune killing mechanisms by bacteriostatic antibiotics. *The FASEB Journal*, 21, 1107-1117.

[121] Saxena, S. K., Mirsha, N., & Saxena, R. (2009). Advances in antiviral drug discovery and development. *Future Virology*, 4(2), 101-107.

[122] Schillaci, O., Filippi, L., Danieli, R., & Simonetti, G. (2007). Single-photon emission computed tomography/computed tomography in abdominal diseases. Seminars in Nuclear Medicine, Vol. 37, pp. 48-61.

[123] Shah, S. Q., Khan, A. V., & Khan, M. R. (2010). Radiosynthesis and biodistribution of ^{99m}Tc-rifampicin a novel radiotracer for in-vivo infection imaging. *Applied Radiation and Isotopes*, 68, 2255-2260.

[124] Shah, S. Q., Khan, M. R. (2011a). Radiolabeling of gemifloxacin with technetium-99m and biological evaluation in artificially Streptococcus pneumoniae infected rats. *Journal of Radioanalytical and Nuclear Chemistry*, 288, 307–312.

[125] Shah, S. Q., & Khan, M. R. (2011b). Radiocharacterization of the ^{99m}Tc–rufloxacin complex and biological evaluation in Staphylococcus aureus infected rat model. *Journal of Radioanalytical and Nuclear Chemistry*, 288, 373–378.

[126] Shah, S. Q., & Khan, M. R. (2011c). Synthesis of techentium-99m labeled clinafloxacin (^{99m}Tc–CNN) complex and biological evaluation as a potential Staphylococcus aureus infection imaging agent. *Journal of Radioanalytical and Nuclear Chemistry*, 288, 423–428.

[127] Shah, S. Q., Khan, A. U., & Khan, M. R. (2011a). Radiosynthesis of ^{99m}Tc-nitrofurantoin a novel radiotracer for in vivo imaging of Escherichia coli infection. *Journal of Radioanalytical and Nuclear Chemistry*, 287, 417–422.

[128] Shah, S. Q., Khan, A. U., & Khan, M. R. (2011b). Synthesis, biological evaluation and biodistribution of the ^{99m}Tc–Garenoxacin complex in artificially infected rats. *Journal of Radioanalytical and Nuclear Chemistry*, 288, 207–213.

[129] Shoham, S., & Levitz, S. M. (2005). The immune response to fungal infections. *British Journal of Haematology*, 129, 569–582.

[130] Siaens, R. H., Rennen, H. J., Boerman, O. C., Dierckx, R., & Slegers, G. (2004). Synthesis and comparison of ^{99m}Tc-enrofloxacin and ^{99m}Tc-ciprofloxacin. *Journal of Nuclear Medicine*, 45, 2088-2094.

[131] Signore, A., Procaccini, E., Annovazzi, A., Chianelli1, M., Van der Laken, C., & Mire-Sluis, A. (2000). The developing role of cytokines for imaging inflammation and infection. *Cytokine-Academic Press*, 12, 1445–1454.

[132] Signore, A., D'Alessandria, C., Lazzeri, E., & Dierckx, R. (2008). Can we produce an image of bacteria with radiopharmaceuticals? *Europian Journal of Nuclear Medicine and Molecular Imaging*, 35, 1051–1055.

[133] Signore, A., Soroa, V. E., De Vries, E. F. J. (2009). Radiolabeled white blood cells or FDG for imaging of inflammation and infection? The *Quarterly Journal of Nuclear Medicine and Molecular Imaging*, 53, 1-3.

[134] Silindir, M., Ozer, Y. A. (2008). Recently developed radiopharmaceuticals for positron emission tomography (PET). *FABAD Journal of Pharmaceuticals Sciences*, 33, 153-162.

[135] Singh, A. K., Verma, J., Bhatnagar, A., Sen, S., Bose, M. (2003). Tc-99m isoniazid: A specific agent for diagnosis of tuberculosis. *World Journal of Nuclear Medicine*, 2, 292-305.

[136] Singh, B., Mittal, B. R., Bhattagharya, A., Aggarwal, A., Nagi, O. N., & Singh, A. K. (2005). Technetium- 99m ciprofloxacin imaging in the diagnosis of postsurgical bony infection and evaluation of the response to antibiotic theraoy: A case report. *Journal of Orthopaedic Surgery*, 13, 190-194.

[137] Singh, N., & Bhatnagar, A. (2010). Clinical evaluation of efficacy of ^{99m}Tc ethambutol in tubercular lesion imaging. *Tuberculosis Research and Treatment*, Hindawi Publishing Corporation, 1-9.

[138] Solanki, K. K., Bomanji, J., Siraj, Q., Small, M., & Breitton K. E. (1993). ^{99m}Tc-infecton. A new class of radiopharmaceutical for imaging infection. *Journal of Nuclear Medicine*, 34, 119p.

[139] Sonmezoglu, K., Sonmezoglu, M., Halac, M., Akgun, I., Turkman, C., Onsel, C., Kanmaz, B., Solanki, K., Britton, K. E., & Uslu, I. (2001). Usefulness of ^{99m}Tc-ciprofloxacin (Infecton) scan in diagnosis of chronic orthopedic infections: Comparative study with ^{99m}Tc-HMPAO leukocyte scintigraphy. *Journal of Nuclear Medicine*, 42, 567-574.

[140] Truluck, C. A. (2007). Nuclear Medicine Technology: Inflammation and Infection Imaging. *Journal of Radiology Nursing*, 26, 77-85.

[141] Turpin, S., & Lambert, R. (2001). Role of scintigraphy in muscloskeletal and spinal infections. *Radiologic Clins of North America*, 39, 168-189.

[142] Vallejo, E., Martinez, I., Tejero, A., Hernandez, Jimenez, L., Bialostozky, Sanchez, G., Ilarraza H., & Ferro-Flores, G. (2008). Clinical utility of ^{99m}Tc-labeled ubiquicidin 29-41 antimicrobial peptide for the scintigraphic detection of mediastinitis after cardiac surgery. *Archives of Medical Research*, 39, 768-774.

[143] Verma, J., Singh, A. K., Bhatnagar, A., Sen, S., & Bose, M. (2005) Radiolabeling of ethambutol with technetium-99m and its evaluation for detection of tuberculosis. *World Journal of Nuclear Medicine*, 4, 35-46.

[144] Vinjamuri, S. H., Hall, A. V., Solanki, K. K., Bomanji, J., Siraj, Q., O'Shaughnessy, E., Das, S. S., & Britton, K. E. (1996). Comparison of ^{99m}Tc Infecton imaging with radiolabeled white-cell imaging in the evaluation of bacterial infection. *Lancet*, 347, 233-235.

[145] Wareham, D., Michael, J., & Das, S. S. (2005). Advances in bacterial specific imaging. *Brazilian Archives of Biology and Technology*, 48, 145-152.

[146] Welling, M. M., Nibbering, P. H., Paulusma-Annema, A., Hiemstra, P. S., Pauwels, E. K. J., & Calame, W. (1999). Imaging of bacterial infections with ^{99m}Tc-labeled human neutrophil peptide-1. *Journal of Nuclear Medicine*, 40, 2073–2080.

[147] Welling, M. M., Lupetti, A., Balter, H. S., Lanzzeri, S., Souto, B., Rey, A. M., Savio, E. O., Paulusma-Annema, A., Pauwels, E. K. J., & Nibbering, P. H. (2001). ^{99m}Tc-labeled antimicrobial peptides for detection of bacterial and candida albicans infections. *The Journal of Nuclear Medicine*, 42, 788–794.

[148] Welling, M. M., Visentin, R., Feitsma, H. I. J., Lupetti, A., Pauwelsa, E. K. J., & Nibbering, P. H. (2004). Infection detection in mice using ^{99m}Tc-labeled HYNIC and N2S2 chelate conjugated to the antimicrobial peptide UBI 29-41. *Nuclear Medicine and Biology*, 31, 503-509.

[149] Wu, Y. C., Wu, P. S., Chiu, N. T., Lee, B. F., Yao, W. J., & Chiou, Y. Y. (2003). Comparison of ^{99m}Tc-DMSA renal SPECT and ultrasonography for diagnosis of acute pyelonephritis in children. *Annals Nuclear Medicine Scienses*, 16, 111-116.

[150] Wyss, M. T., Honer, M., Spath, N., Gottschalk, J., Ametamey, S. M., Weber, B., Von Schulthess, G. K., Buck,A. & Kaim, A. H. (2004). Influence of ceftriaxone treatment on FDG uptake—an in vivo [^{18}F]-fluorodeoxyglucose imaging study in soft tissue infections in rats. *Nuclear Medicine and Biology*, 31, 875–882.

[151] Yap, M. H., Edirisinghe, E. A., & Bez, H. E. (2008). A novel algorithm for initial lesion detection in ultrasound breast images. *Journal of Applied Clinical Medical Physics*, 9.

[152] Yapar, Z., Kibar, M., Yapar, A. F., Togrul, E., Kayaselcuk, U., & Sarpel, Y. (2001). The efficacy of technetium-99m ciprofloxacin (Infecton) imaging in suspected orthopaedic infection: a comparison with sequential bone/gallium imaging. *Europian Journal of Nuclear Medicin*, 28, 822–830.

[153] Yurt Lambresht, F., Yilmaz, O., Unak, P., Seyitoglo, B., Durkan, K., & Baskan, H. (2008a). Evaluation of ^{99m}Tc-cefuroxime axetil for imaging of inflammation. *Journal of Radioanalytical and Nuclear Chemistry*. 277, 491-494.

[154] Yurt Lambresht, F., Durkan, K., & Unak, P. (2008b). Preparation, quality control and stability of ^{99m}Tc-cefuroxime axetil. *Journal of radioanalytical and nuclear chemistry*, 275, 161-164.

[155] Yurt Lambrecht, F., Yilmaz, O., Durkan, K., Unak, P., & Bayrak, E. (2009). Preparation and biodistribution of [^{131}I] linezolid in animal model infection and inflammation. *Journal of Radioanalytical and Nuclear Chemistry*, 281, 415–419.

[156] Zhuang, H., Yu, JQ., & Alavi, A. (2005).Applications of fluorodeoxyglucose-PET imaging in the detection of infection and inflammation and other benign disorders. *Radiological Clinics of North America*, 43, 121–134.

Section 3

Specific Clinical Applications

Chapter 10

Quantitative Assessment of Peripheral Arteries in Ultrasound Images

Marco Antonio Gutierrez, Maurício Higa,
Paulo Eduardo Pilon, Marina de Sá Rebelo and
Silvia Gelás Lage

Additional information is available at the end of the chapter

http://dx.doi.org/10.5772/53310

1. Introduction

Ultrasound imaging is widely used to assess carotid, brachial, femoral, as well as other arteries. There are major advantages of using ultrasound in comparison to other imaging techniques, such as its non invasiveness and its capability to produce real-time visualization of the arterial lumen and vessel wall that is not possible with any other imaging modality [1]. Recent clinical studies have benefited from continuous improvements in ultrasound image quality, new imaging techniques and signal processing algorithms with the aim of identifying the vulnerable carotid plaque based on the mechanical wall motion behavior [2,3].

The vulnerable arterial plaque may cause atherothrombotic events, myocardial infarction and stroke, which are responsible for approximately 35% of the total mortality in the western world, and are the leading causes of morbidity world-wide [4]. The first indication of cardiovascular disease is a thickening of the intimal and medial layers of the arterial wall. It involves lipid accumulation and the migration and proliferation of many cells in the sub-intimal and medial layers, which results in the formation of plaques. It is the rupture of such plaques that causes myocardial infarcts, cerebrovascular events, peripheral vascular disease and kidney infarcts. The impact of the intima-media thickness (IMT) on the incidence of cardiovascular events in the Rotterdam study by B-mode ultrasound indicates that the risk of myocardial infarction increases 43% per standard deviation increase (0.163 mm) in common carotid IMT [4]. The main conclusions resulting from this study were supported by other independent investigations which reveal that an IMT higher than 0.9-1.0 mm indicates a potential atherosclerotic disease, which translates into an increased risk of a cardiovascular event. Hence, the robust segmentation and measurement of IMT by B-mode ultrasound has a considerable impact in the early diagnosis of atherosclerosis, prognosis prediction, and in the monitoring of responses to lifestyle and prescribed pharmacological treatments.

Ultrasound signals have also been extensively used in clinical sites, by exploiting Doppler effect to measure vascular blood velocity and flow, among other applications [5,6]. Typically, a spectrum of frequencies related to the different velocities of the blood cells is presented as a curve of velocity versus time. The analysis of this curve can reveal important relationships between the frequency spectral pattern along the cardiac cycle and the presence of cardiovascular diseases [7,8], among other examples [9,10].

2. Arterial vessels image analysis

2.1. Problem statement

The current clinical practice in the assessment of the early cardiovascular diseases involves acquisition of B-mode ultrasound data from large superficial arterial vessels such as the common carotid artery (CCA). The image acquisition process generates sequences of two dimensional ultrasound images along the time (2D+time) that are currently interpreted using either manual annotation procedures or commercially available semi-automatic image processing environments. While the manual annotation generally results in accurate IMT measurements, it is subject to intra and inter-observer variability. Moreover, this procedure requires annotating multi-frame ultrasound data, which is not only labor intensive but also highly dependent on the experience of the observer. All these factors stimulated the investigation of automatic segmentation techniques, which can greatly support the clinical practitioners in their evaluation and may have substantial benefits in the quality of the medical act. As a consequence of this clinical interest, a large number of studies were focused on the development of automatic IMT segmentation algorithms in order to provide an accurate analysis of IMT measurements [11-31].

The IMT complex is best visualized in longitudinal sections of the CCA. Fig. 1 shows a representative B-mode ultrasound image of the CCA and a schematic illustration of the relevant leading edges of echo responses. Previous studies [10-12] have shown that the leading edges can be mapped to the following interfaces: near-wall media-adventitia, far-wall lumen-intima and far-wall media-adventitia. The lumen diameter (LD) is defined as the distance between the intima-lumen interface of the near-wall and the lumen-intima interface of the far-wall. The far-wall IMT is defined as the distance between the far-wall lumen-intima (FWLI) and the far-wall media-adventitia interfaces (FWMA).

The determination of ultrasonic measurement of the artery becomes equivalent to accurately detecting the echo boundaries presented in Fig. 1. However, the existence of ultrasonic imaging artifacts such as speckle, reverberations and dropouts make the accurate definition of a boundary very difficult.

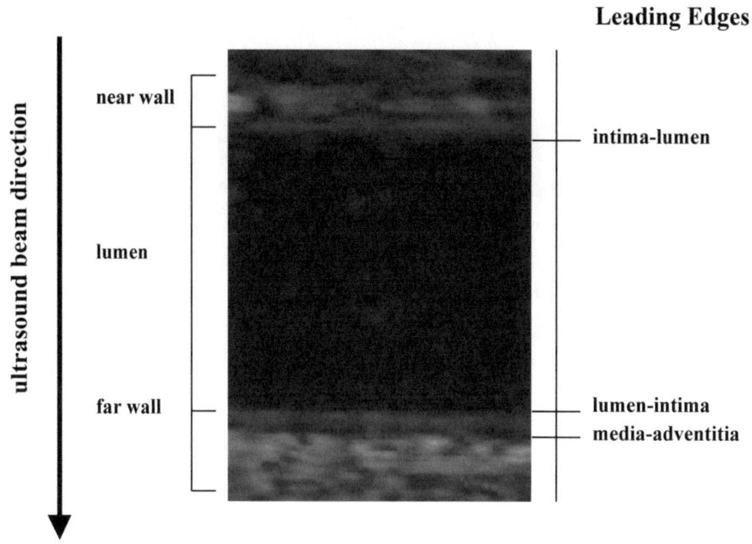

Figure 1. Interfaces between carotid tissue layers obtained from B-mode ultrasound.

2.2. IMT segmentation algorithms

Since the IMT complex is defined by two distinguishable interfaces in the ultrasound image data, the majority of studies that addressed the IMT segmentation were built on several assumptions regarding the intensity profiles associated with each interface. The automatic detection of such interfaces requires a priori knowledge that implies a certain amount of user intervention. In recent studies, substantial efforts have been dedicated to reduce the level of user intervention during the IMT segmentation process. A review of the methods in this area is presented by Molinari et al. [13], which address the main directions of research in the field of IMT segmentation. The published methods in this area can be classified in three classes: edge-based, dynamic programming and probabilistic IMT segmentation methods. The edge based segmentation schemes aim to reconstruct the IMT complex from gradient data and in this process prior knowledge relating to the intensity profiles is enforced in the process of selecting the FWLI and FWMA interfaces. The early segmentation schemes that addressed the identification and measurement of the IMT were based on semi-automatic methods where the user intervention was critical to obtain accurate results. De Groot et al. [14] analyzed the contribution of the patient and observer variability in the process of the IMT measurement in serial carotid and femoral B-mode ultrasound scans. Through the use of variance components analysis they found that 75% of the variance in the measurement of the far-wall thickness could be attributed to the differences among patients and a 7% variability recorded in the analysis of the mean IMT thickness was caused by the ultrasound equipment. In a study presented by Selzer et al. [15], the initial IMT boundary position was manually selected and this information was used to guide an IMT edge-based segmentation process. Dwyer et al. [16] developed a semi-automatic IMT segmentation algorithm that was applied in B-mode ultrasound images. In the algorithm the average distance between the FWLI and FWMA interfaces was used to approximate the IMT. A selection of the frames used in this study was carried out by the user to ensure that there would be a clear identification of the interfaces.

Liguori et al. [17] proposed a multi-step semi-automatic IMT segmentation algorithm that has been developed for the analysis of single frames B-mode ultrasound data. The first step of their method involves the manual selection of the region of interest (ROI) followed by a threshold procedure that is applied to set all pixels with intensity values lower than a predefined threshold. The IMT detection entails an analysis of the intensity profiles associated with the gradient data under the assumption that all pixels corresponding to the lumen are anechoic and the image areas that define the tunica intima and tunica adventitia are the most reflective arterial layers.

The two IMT interfaces are selected by analyzing the strength of the gradient in the direction of the ultrasound beam, the FWLI interface corresponds to the first relative maximum, while the FWMA is given by the second one. A similar approach was employed in [18,19], where the authors also analyzed the pixel intensity profiles to detect the salient intensity transitions that are characteristic for the two IMT interfaces. Ilea et al. [20] adopted a multiscale approach that embeds a statistical shape model with the aim of identifying the two interfaces that form the IMT without any user intervention. The developed algorithm was validated on 49 single frame B-mode ultrasound images and results were compared against manually annotated data. Delsanto et al. [21] implemented a hybrid algorithm where active contours were applied to refine the initial FWLI and FWMA estimates. The reported results indicate the efficiency of this approach in reducing the level of outliers, but several problems that are caused by the gaps in the IMT structure started to surface. The assumption that in longitudinal images of the carotid artery the IMT is defined by a pair of active contours was used in subsequent contributions [22-26]. However, all contributions require a user interaction in the process of initializing the active contours.

Gutierrez et al. [27] proposed a different semi-automatic active contour-based IMT segmentation algorithm where the edge information is extracted using a multiresolution approach. The major objective of this paper was to measure the lumen diameter and the IMT and in their experiments the authors assessed the performance of their semi-automatic algorithm against the manually segmented ultrasound data using metrics such as the coefficient of variability and correlation.

Dynamic programming algorithms were proposed [28,29] as a computationally efficient alternative to the standard heuristic search methods when applied in the context of boundary tracing, and due to their intrinsic properties they positioned as an attractive approach for IMT segmentation. An example is represented by the work of Liang et al. [29] where the authors addressed the IMT segmentation problem by adopting a multiscale approach. Rocha et al. [30] applied a related segmentation scheme to more challenging ultrasound images that exhibit arterial plaques. Their approach starts with the detection of the media adventitia layer by searching for the best fit of a cubic spline to the edge data by taking into account the anatomical

http://dx.doi.org/10.5772/53310

characteristics of the adventitia. This is followed by the segmentation of the lumen boundary by applying a hybrid dynamic programming-based active contour technique.

A distinct category of algorithms relied on probabilistic schemes to identify the IMT interfaces such as the work of Destrempes et al. [31]. Their algorithm was developed based on the assumption that the echogenicity of the region of interest where the IMT is located can be modeled using a mixture of three Nakagami distributions and the parameters of the distributions are estimated using an expectation maximization (EM) algorithm. The proposed method proved accurate but it requires user interaction for the ROI initialization.

The discussion will be continued with a technical presentation of an artery boundary segmentation method to measure lumen diameter and IMT.

2.3. Artery boundary enhancement

One of the first steps in to segment artery leading edges is to enhance such interfaces from B-mode ultrasound images. To enhance border detection accuracy, a multiscale border identification can be implemented using filters in the form of scaled convolution operators [32,33]. The scale space of an image is constructed through convolution of the image with a two-dimensional (2D) Gaussian density kernel with zero mean and standard deviation:

$$G(\vec{x},\sigma)=\frac{1}{\sqrt{2\pi\sigma^2}^{D}}e^{-\frac{\|\vec{x}\|^2}{2\sigma^2}} \tag{1}$$

where D denotes the dimension of the input domain. A blurred replica of the original image is obtained by convolution with $G(\vec{x};\sigma)$ for a specific σ. The stack of images as a function of increasing scale parameter σ is coined a linear scale space. Hence, as σ increases the detailed object structures vanish while gross structures persist. Fig.2 shows the 2D gradient magnitude calculated for a carotid vessel image (B-mode ultrasound) in three different scales.

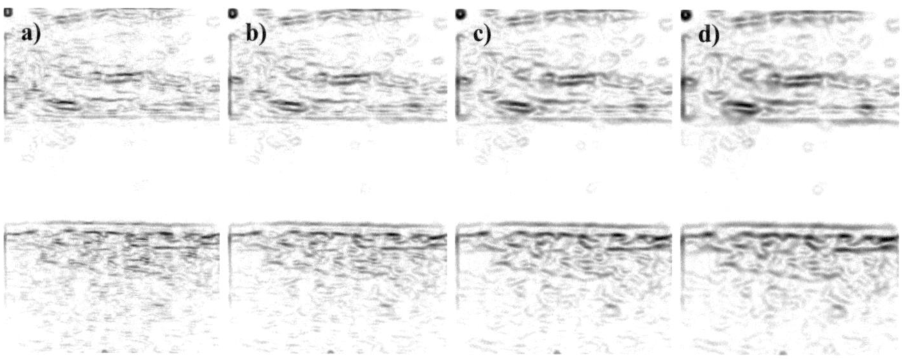

Figure 2. gradient magnitude calculated for a carotid vessel image (B-mode ultrasound) in three different scales: a); b); c); d).

Based on these features a scaled artery image is used to identify the approximated position of the near and far walls. Two complementary images are obtained based on the gradient value in y-direction: one that enhances pixel values transitions from high to low echoes, such as edges encountered in near wall tissue interfaces, and other that enhances pixel values transitions from low to high echoes (such as edges encountered in far wall tissue interfaces). Fig. 3 shows the boundary enhancement of the near and far wall.

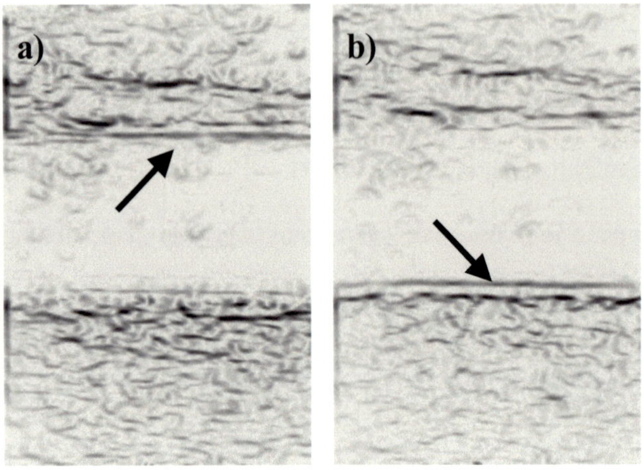

Figure 3. Boundary enhancement of the near wall a) and far wall b)

2.4. Contour modeling

The contour of each wall can be modeled following the Geometrically Deformed Model proposed by Lobregt and Viergever [34]. In this model, a set of vertices connected by straight line segments or edges forms the basic contour structure (Fig. 4).

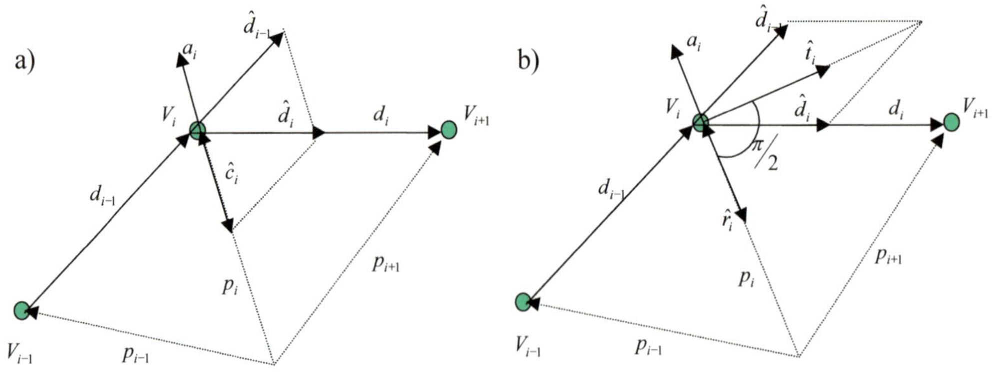

Figure 4. Contour model consisting of a set of vertices V_i which are connected by segments or edges.

In Fig. 4, the position of a vertex V_i is represented by a vector p_i, and the edge between V_i and V_{i+1} by a vector d_i. The contour deformation is caused by a combination of forces which act on the vertices. The resulting acceleration in vertex V_i is denoted by a vector a_i.

The contour local curvature at a vertex V_i is defined as the difference between the directions of the two edge segments that join at that location:

$$\hat{c}_i = \hat{d}_i - \hat{d}_{i-1} \tag{2}$$

The local tangential unit vector is defined as the normalized sum of the unit vectors of two joining edge segments:

$$\hat{t}_i = \frac{\hat{d}_i + \hat{d}_{i-1}}{\left\| \hat{d}_i + \hat{d}_{i-1} \right\|} \tag{3}$$

The local radial direction at a vertex V_i is obtained from $\hat{t}_i$ by a rotation over $\pi/2$ radians:

$$\hat{r}_i = \begin{bmatrix} 0 & 1 \\ -1 & 0 \end{bmatrix} \hat{t}_i \tag{4}$$

2.5. Dynamic force formulation

In the model definition, the dynamic in each vertex V_i must satisfy the Newton´s second law,

$$\begin{aligned} F_i &= F_{\text{int},i} + F_{ext,i} + F_{damp,i} \\ F_i &= \mu_i a_i \end{aligned} \tag{5}$$

Where μ_i is a coefficient that has a mass unit, $F_{damp,i}$, $F_{\text{int},i}$ and $F_{ext,i}$ and are the damping (or viscous), the internal and the external forces, respectively.

The internal force can be estimated from the local contour curvature along the local r-axis :

$$F_{\text{int},i} = \left(c_i \cdot \hat{r}_i \right) \tag{6}$$

The external force acting in each vertex can be approximated by some image feature. In this paper we used the information obtained from the local image gradient as the external force.

The damping force is proportional to the velocity of the vertex and points in opposite direction:

$$F_{damp,i} \approx -k.v_i \tag{7}$$

The total force F_i acting on a vertex is a weighted combination of damping, internal and external forces :

$$F_i = w_{\text{int}} F_{\text{int},i} + w_{ext} F_{ext,i} + w_{damp} F_{damp,i} \qquad (8)$$

where w_{int}, w_{ext} and w_{damp} are the weighting factors.

The deformation process over the contour is implemented as a numerical time integration process in which the complete state of the contour is calculated at a sequence of discrete positions in time [34]. A set of state equations controls the deformation process in terms of position, velocity and acceleration of each vertex on the contour:

$$\begin{cases} p_i(t+\Delta t) = p_i(t) + v_i(t) \\ v_i(t+\Delta t) = v_i(t) + a_i(t).\Delta t \\ a_i(t+\Delta t) = \dfrac{1}{m_i} F_i(t+\Delta t) \end{cases} \qquad (9)$$

Where $p_i(t+\Delta t)$, $v_i(t+\Delta t)$ and $a_i(t+\Delta t)$ define the position, velocity and acceleration, respectively, of the vertex in a incremental time Δt. The vertex mass, m_i, is setting constant for all vertices and the resulting force, F_i, is calculated using equation (8).

Fig. 5 shows the result of the deformation of the active contours during the process of detection the FWLI and FWMA in two patients in systole and diastole. The vessel's lumen diameter and IMT can be obtained by automatic measurement of the distance between segments estimated from the linear regression of the contours in each interface.

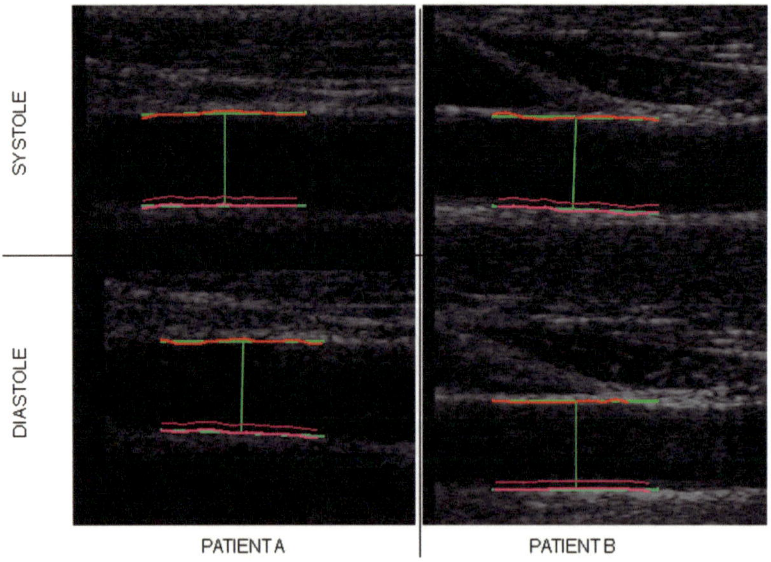

Figure 5. The detection of FWLI and FWMA using active contours in two patients during systole and diastole (in red) and the automatic measurement of the distance between segments obtained from the linear regression (in green) of the contours in each interface.

http://dx.doi.org/10.5772/53310

2.6. Vascular blood velocity and flow

As presented in the previous sections, B-mode ultrasound is capable of reliably and accurately imaging peripheral arteries and can be used for vessel diameter measurement. Ultrasound signals have also been extensively used in clinical sites by exploiting Doppler effect to measure vascular blood velocity and flow.

The Doppler effect refers to an increase or decrease in the frequency of a wave that is traveling toward or away from the observer, respectively. This principle is applied in Doppler ultrasound to measure the direction and velocity of blood flow in the vessels. The relationship between the Doppler shift and blood flow velocity is:

$$v = \frac{c\left(f - f_0\right)}{2 f_0 \cos\theta} \tag{10}$$

where c is the speed of sound in blood (1540 m/s), θ is the angle between the ultrasound beam and the direction of blood flow, and f and f_0 are the frequencies of the transmitted and returned signals, respectively. Due to the angle dependency, alignment of the ultrasound beam parallel with the direction of blood flow is essential to obtain accurate flow estimates.

In vascular studies using commercial ultrasound equipment, a spectrum of frequencies related to the different velocities of the blood cells is presented as a curve of velocity versus time (Fig. 6). This information can reveal important relationships between the frequency spectral pattern along the cardiac cycle and the presence of cardiovascular diseases [7-10].

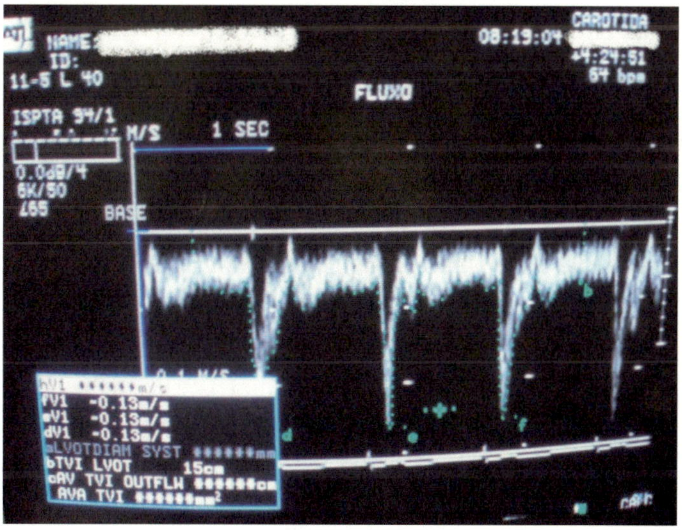

Figure 6. Typical screen of an ultrasound system showing a curve of vessel's blood velocity versus time.

However, commercial ultrasound systems are primarily dedicated to get instantaneous data for individual patients, and they have, in general, low flexibility to perform large-scale researches. Thus, to make this kind of study easier in clinical protocols involving hundreds of patients, computational tools have to be developed to extract quantitative data from spectral display of Doppler ultrasound images.

Higa et al. [35] proposed a methodology used to extract blood velocity and flow automatically from images of the type shown in Fig. 6. A brief description of the method proposed is presented below.

After two steps defined by the user: calibration and selection of the region of interest (ROI), a Gaussian filter (σ=1 pixel, precision ≥ 90%) can be applied to the grayscale input image to attenuate high frequency noise.

The detection process of the time axis ('X') considers the smallest variation of the pixels intensities occurs in the horizontal direction. Thus, equations (11), (12) and (13) calculates the ordinate 'y' expected for the axis 'X', which will be the reference (0 m/s) to the velocity calculation.

$$g(i,j) = \begin{cases} \dfrac{1}{\left|I(i,j) - I(i+1,j)\right| + 1}, & I(i,j) > z \\ 0, & I(i,j) \le z \end{cases} \tag{11}$$

$$f(j) = \sum_{i=0}^{m-2} g(i,j), \quad j \in \left[y_{\min}, y_{\max}\right] \tag{12}$$

$$y = \left\{ j \in \left[y_{\min}, y_{\max}\right] \mid f(y) = \max f(j) \right\} \tag{13}$$

where I(i, j) is the image intensity (grayscale level) at i and j coordinates; m is the image width (in pixels); y_{min} and y_{max} are, respectively, the ordinates of the superior and inferior lines that delimit the rectangular ROI defined by the user; z is an empirical pre-defined threshold to reject the graphic background;

The image can be transformed to a binary image depending on a threshold level that can be defined by the user. After image binarization, a median filter (size: 3 x 3 pixels) can be applied to edge smoothing and spurious suppression.

An envelope detection step can be initialized with horizontal lines at the top and at the bottom of the ROI. Each point of these lines is moved down or up to the border of the binary curve. Then, the algorithm holds either the superior or the inferior contour (Fig. 7), assuming that, in general, the desired one has higher amplitude variation.

Finally, after automatic detection of the peaks (Fig. 7), the algorithm can compute the mean peak velocity ($\overline{V}_P$), the mean envelope velocity ($\overline{V}_N$) and the velocity time integral (VTI), according to the equations (14), (15) and (16), respectively.

http://dx.doi.org/10.5772/53310

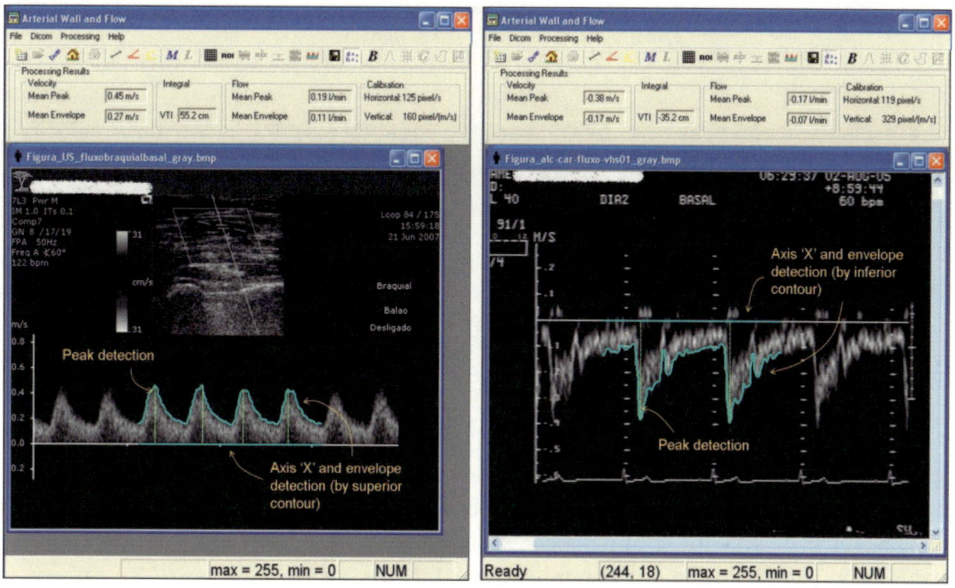

Figure 7. Detection of the axis 'X', envelope (by superior or inferior contour) and peaks in the vessel's blood velocity vs. time curve.

$$\bar{V}_P = \frac{1}{P \cdot YCal} \sum_{p=1}^{P} A_p \,(\mathrm{m/s}) \tag{14}$$

$$\bar{V}_N = \frac{1}{N \cdot YCal} \sum_{n=1}^{N} A_n \,(\mathrm{m/s}) \tag{15}$$

$$VTI = \frac{100}{XCal \cdot YCal} \sum_{n=1}^{N} A_n (\mathrm{cm}) \tag{16}$$

where P is the total number of peaks detected in the curve; N is the total number of pixels in the curve; $XCal$ and $YCal$ are the calibrations in pixels for the time and the velocity axes, respectively; A is the amplitude in pixels for each point in the curve.

In addition, if B-Mode images are available, an arterial wall interface detection module can determine the vessel diameter and the mean peak blood flow ($\bar{\phi}_P$) and the mean blood flow ($\bar{\phi}_N$) can be estimated using (16) and (17).

$$\bar{\phi}_P = 0{,}06 \cdot \bar{V}_P \cdot \frac{\pi D_{\max}^2}{4} (\mathrm{l/min}) \tag{17}$$

$$\bar{\phi}_N = 0,06 \cdot \bar{V}_N \cdot \frac{\pi\left(D_{\max} + D_{\min}\right)^2}{16} (\text{l/min}) \tag{18}$$

where $\overline{V}_P$ is the mean peak velocity obtained by equation (14); $\overline{V}_N$ is the mean velocity obtained by equation (15); $D_{\max}$ and $D_{\min}$ are de vessel's maximum and minimum diameters;

3. Clinical applications

3.1. Automatic IMT measurement

The method presented in the previous section can be used in clinical applications to assess large sequences of 2D+time B-mode ultrasound images of the CCA. We performed an experiment that comprised the analysis of 180 images from 30 patients (3 images in diastole and 3 images in systole for each patient), all of which included manually defined interfaces for reference. The minimum and maximum artery diameters were measured for each patient using the manual and the automatic procedure.

In order to study the variability between the automatic and manual definition of artery boundaries, the pooled mean, $\bar{\mu}$, and the standard deviation, σ, for the difference between automated and manual measurements of lumen diameter were computed. The coefficient of variation (CV) was calculated according equation (19).

$$CV = \left(\frac{\sigma}{\bar{\mu}\sqrt{2}} \times 100\right)\% \tag{19}$$

The strength of the relationship between automated and manual methods is indicated by the correlation, $R_{a,m}$, between the two measurements:

$$R_{a,m} = \frac{Cov_{a,m}}{\sigma_a . \sigma_m} \tag{20}$$

where $Cov_{a,m}$ is the covariance between the automated and manual measurements. σ_a and σ_m are the standard deviation of automated and manual measurements, respectively.

Means ($\mu_{a,m}$) and standard deviations ($\sigma_{a,m}$) for the differences between the automatic and manual methods were calculated for the population (n=30). The coefficients of variability ($CV_{a,m}$) and the correlation ($Corr_{a,m}$) between both methods were also obtained.

The results obtained for the parameters $\mu_{a,m}$, $\sigma_{a,m}$, $CV_{a,m}$ and $Corr_{a,m}$ are summarized in Table 1.

	Automatic $\mu_a \pm \sigma_a$ (mm)	Manual $\mu_m \pm \sigma_m$ (mm)	Difference Δ $\mu_{a,m} \pm \sigma_{a,m}$ (mm)	Variability CV (%)	Correlation $Corr_{a,m}$
Lumen Diameter diastole)	7,85 ± 1,01	7,78 ± 1,01	0,13 ± 0,09	0,83	0,99
Lumen Diameter (systole)	6,81 ± 1,06	6,77 ± 1,05	0,12 ± 0,10	1,00	0,99
Intima Media Thicknes	0,72 ± 0,14	0,63 ± 0,12	0.09 ± 0,06	6,16	0,90

Table 1. Lumen diameter (LD) and Intima-Media thickness measured using automatic and manual methods (n=30). The difference (Δ), the coefficient of variability (*CV*) and the correlation ($Corr_{a,m}$) between both measurements are also presented.

A comparative analysis between commercial ultrasound systems operated by specialists and the method presented in the previous section to measure blood velocity and flow automatically can be performed. A new experiment was performed using systolic mean peak velocities (102 samples) and velocity time integrals (75 samples) of common carotid and brachial arteries under basal condition, brachial arteries in the reactive hyperemic response and echocardiographic exams. Table 2 shows the number of images and samples used in this analysis.

Artery	Number of images	Number of samples	
		Peak velocity	Velocity time integral
Common carotid arteries	30	39	31
Brachial arteries under basal condition	23	35	24
Brachial arteries in the reactive hyperemic response	10	15	15
Echocardiographic exams	11	13	5
Total	74	102	75

Table 2. Composition of samples used to validate the methodology.

According to the procedure described in the previous section, the peak velocities measured from the carotid arteries were negative (average: -0.59 m/s), while from the brachial arteries under basal condition, as well as in the reactive hyperemic response, the peak velocities were positive (averages: 0.63 m/s and 1.18 m/s, respectively). In the echocardiographic images the measurements were either positive or negative and the average of the absolute values was 1.48 m/s.

Similarly, positive or negative velocity time integrals were dependent on the exam type. However, the number of cardiac cycles used to get these measurements was not standardized, leading to a range of the samples, from -150 to 91 cm.

Fig. 8 shows Bland-Altman's [36] and Linear Regression graphics for the systolic peak velocity analysis, where 'A' refers to the measurements done with a commercial ultrasound system and 'B' refers to the methodology described in section 2.6. Bias, standard-deviation, correlation coefficient, and linear equation results are presented in Table 3. Like peak velocity, Figure 9 and Table 4 were obtained for velocity time integral analysis.

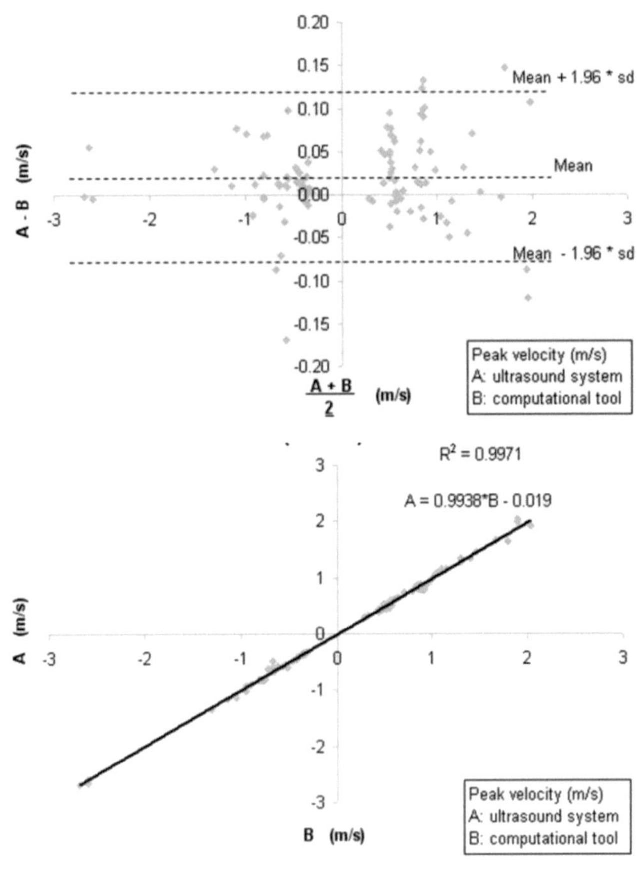

Figure 8. Bland-Altman's (up) and Linear Regression (down) analysis of the systolic peak velocity (102 samples) measured by the ultrasound system and by the proposed methodology.

Systolic Peak Velocity (N=102)			
Bias (m/s)	sd (m/s)	rAB (p<0.001)	Linear Regression Equation
0.02	0.05	0.9985	A = 0.9938*B – 0.0190

Table 3. Summary of systolic peak velocity statistics.

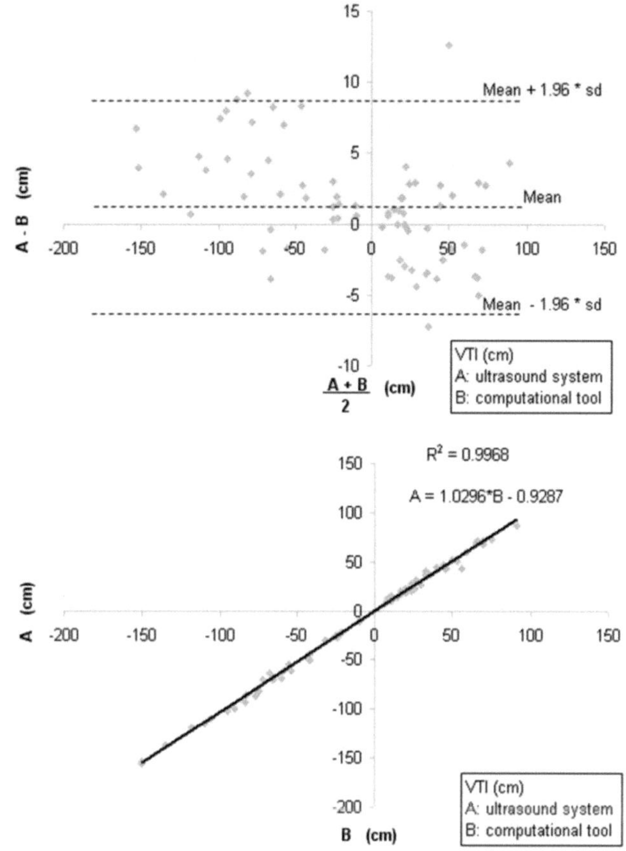

Figure 9. Bland-Altman's (left) and Linear Regression (right) analysis of the VTI (75 samples) measured by the ultrasound system and by the proposed methodology.

VTI (N=75)			
Bias (cm)	sd (cm)	rAB (p<0.001)	Linear Regression Equation
1.25	3.86	0.9984	A = 1.030*B – 0.9287

Table 4. Summary of VTI statistics.

4. Conclusion

Measurements of lumen diameter (LD) and intima-media thickness (IMT) of carotid, brachial and femoral arteries from B-mode ultrasound are defined as the average distance of interfaces between vessel tissue layers. In order to determine the interfaces location, manual tracing is commonly used. However, this approach is a time consuming procedure and based on subjective operator assessment. Besides, it inevitably results in inter and intra-observer variability due to the complex nature of the echogenic zones, especially at the lumen-intima interface, which frequently present weak echoes, echo dropouts and irregularities caused by scattering.

In this chapter, we have reviewed some methods for automatic or semi-automatic interface detection and presented in detail an approach that uses the active contour technique. In this technique, external forces are proportional to the local image gradient obtained from a multiscale analysis. The automated measurements, when compared to those obtained by manual tracing, are equally accurate and the coefficients of variability between both methods are below 1,0% for Lumen Diameter and 6,5% for IMT thickness measurements.

Vascular blood velocity can be measured by using Doppler effect, and if lumen diameter is available the blood flow can also be estimated. However, commercial ultrasound systems are primarily dedicated to get instantaneous data for individual patients, and they have, in general, low flexibility to perform large-scale researches. Thus, to make this kind of study easier in clinical protocols involving hundreds of patients, computational tools have to be developed to extract quantitative data from spectral display of Doppler ultrasound images.

We briefly presented a methodology to extract automatically blood velocity and flow from Doppler ultrasound images that permits extensive clinical studies. The small bias and high correlation for both, peak velocity and VTI, indicate the reliability of this methodology and these findings are better than those presented by Tschirren et al. [37] (bias: 0.40 m/s for peak velocity and 7 cm for VTI), though their results refers to a dilatation study of the brachial artery, where data values were about ten times higher than the present study.

It is important to note that for VTI statistics shown in Table 4, the threshold used to get the binary image was 60, instead of the default 40 used to extract the systolic peak velocity. This change was motivated by the higher bias (1.70 cm) and standard deviation (6.78 cm) obtained with the default value for VTI. Despite these numerical results, it is not possible to conclude that the threshold of 60 is more appropriate than 40, since the human operation to get measurements using the ultrasound equipment may also be subject to systematic errors and deviations. For instance, visual results showing the envelopes drawn on the blood velocity graphics point that, by using the proposed methodology (Fig. 7), the envelope line is more refined than that obtained by manual operation of an ultrasound system (Fig. 6). In the latter case the user does not notice or simply disregards small image brightness variations, which means that this procedure is highly dependent on the user's subjective evaluation and it is hardly reproducible.

By processing a diversity of common carotid, brachial and echocardiographic Doppler image samples, collected from four different commercial ultrasound systems, the proposed methodology to measure peak velocity and VTI was validated by the Bland-Altman's analysis and by the correlation coefficient. Visual analysis also confirmed that the spectrum envelope detection is very satisfactory.

http://dx.doi.org/10.5772/53310

The methodology was implemented in a user friendly graphical interface that has a semi-automatic characteristic. The delivery of this tool was intended to help clinicians in their studies based on Doppler ultrasound images with the following advantages: to save operational time, to lower subjective results, and to support measurement reproducibility.

However, ultrasound is still an observer-dependent modality in which the image quality depends on an experienced observer, appropriated technique and equipment. Automated systems and algorithms which can improve measurement accuracy and reproducibility, without the observers input, still remains an open area of study and research.

Acknowledgements

This work was supported in part by the National Institute of Science and Technology—Medicine Assisted by Scientific Computing INCT MACC, and the Zerbini Foundation.

Author details

Marco Antonio Gutierrez[1,2], Maurício Higa[2], Paulo Eduardo Pilon[2],
Marina de Sá Rebelo[1] and Silvia Gelás Lage[1]

1 Heart Institute (InCor) - University of Sao Paulo Medical School, Brazil

2 Polytechnic School - University of Sao Paulo, Brazil

References

[1] Sonka, M., Stolpen, A., Liang, W., Stefancik, R. M. Vascular imaging and analysis. In: Sonka, M., Fitzpatrick, J. M. (ed.) Handbook of medical imaging. Bellingham: SPIE Press; 2000. p809-906.

[2] Richardson P. D. Biomechanics of plaque rupture: progress, problems, and new frontiers. Annals Biomedical Engineering 2002;30(4) 524-536.

[3] Ramnarine K. V., Hartshorne T., Sensier Y., Naylor M., Walker J., Naylor A. R., Panerai R. B., Evans D. H. Tissue Doppler imaging of carotid plaque wall motion: a pilot study. Cardiovascular Ultrasound 2003;1(1) 17.

[4] van der Meer I. M., Bots M. L., Hofman A., del Sol A. I., van der Kuip D. A., Witteman J. C.Predictive value of noninvasive measures of atherosclerosis for incident myocardial infarction: The Rotterdam Study. Circulation 2004;109(9) 1089-1094.

[5] Gerhard-Herman, M.; Gardin, J. M.; Jaff, M.; Mohler, E.; Roman, M.; Naqvi, T. Z. Guidelines for noninvasive vascular laboratory testing: a report from the American

Society of Echocardiography and the Society for Vascular Medicine and Biology. Vascular Medicine 2006;11(3) 183-200.

[6] Nichols, W.; O'Rourke, M. Doppler ultrasound for arterial blood flow measurement. In:. McDonald's blood flow in arteries: theoretic, experimental and clinical principles. 3rd ed. Malvern, Philadelphia, USA: Lea & Febiger; 1990.

[7] Hoskins, P. R. Measurement of arterial blood-flow by Doppler ultrasound. Clinical Physics and Physiological Measurement 1990;11(1) 1-26.

[8] Yao, J. S. T. Noninvasive studies of peripheral vascular disease. In: Hobson, R. W.; Wilson, S. E.; Veith, F. J. (Eds.). Vascular surgery: principles and practice. 3rd ed. Marcel Dekker, Inc.; 2004.

[9] Corretti, M. C.; Aanderson, T. J.; Benjamin, E. J.; Celermajer, D.; Charbonneau, F.; Creager, M. A.; Deanfield, J.; Drexler, H.; Gerhard-Herman, M.; Hierrington, D.; Vallance, P.; Vita, J.; Vogel, R. Guidelines for the ultrasound assessment of endothelial-dependent flow-mediated vasodilation of the brachial artery: A report of the International Brachial Artery Reactivity Task Force. Journal of the American College of Cardiology 2002; 39(2) 257-265.

[10] Lage, S. G.; Kopel, L.; Medeiros, C. C.; Carvalho, R. T.; Creager, M. A. Angiotensin II contributes to arterial compliance in congestive heart failure. American Journal of Physiology – Heart and Circulatory Physiology 2002;283(4) H1424-H1429.

[11] Liang Q., Wendelahg I., Wikstrand J., Gustavsson T. A multiscale dynamic programming procedure for boundary detection in ultrasonic artery images. IEEE Transactions on Medical Imaging 2000;19:127-142.

[12] Gustavsson T., Liang Q., Wendelhag I., Wikstrand J. A dynamic programming procedure for automated ultrasonic measurement of the carotid artery. IEEE Computers in Cardiology 1994;297-300.

[13] Molinari F., Zeng G., Suri J.S. A State of the art review on intima-media thickness (IMT) measurement and wall segmentation techniques for carotid ultrasound. Computer Methods and Programs in Biomedicine 2010;100(3) 201-221.

[14] De Groot E., Zwinderman A.H., Van Der Steen A.F.W., Ackerstaff R.G.A., Van Swijndregt A.D.M., Bom N., Lie K.I., Bruschke A.V.G., Variance components analysis of carotid and femoral intima-media thickness measurements. Ultrasound in Medicine and Biology 1998;24(6) 825-832.

[15] Selzer R.H., Hodis H.N., Kwong Fu H., Mack W.J., Lee W.J., Liu W.J., Liu C.H., Evaluation of computerized edge tracking for quantifying intima-media thickness of the common carotid artery from b-mode ultrasound images. Atherosclerosis 1994;111 1–11.

[16] Dwyer J.H., Sun P., Kwong-Fu H., Dwyer K.M., Selzer R.H., Automated intima-media thickness: The Los Angeles atherosclerosis study. Ultrasound in Medicine and Biology 1998;24(7) 981-987.

[17] Liguori P., Paolillo A., Pietrosanto A. An automatic measurement system for the evaluation of carotid intima-media thickness. IEEE Transactions on Instrumentation and Measurement 2001;50(6) 1684-1691.

[18] Hangiandreou N.J., James E.M., McBane R.D., Tradup D.J., Persons K.R. The effects of irreversible JPEG compression on an automated algorithm for measuring carotid artery intima-media thickness from ultrasound images. Journal of Digital Imaging 2002;15(1) 258-60.

[19] Faita F., Gemignani V., Bianchini E., Giannarelli C., Demi M. Real-time measurement system for the evaluation of the intima media thickness with a new edge detector. Proceedings of the 28th Annual International Conference of the IEEE Engineering in Medicine and Biology Society 2006; 715-718.

[20] Ilea D.E., Whelan P.F., Brown C., Stanton A. An automatic 2D CAD algorithm for the segmentation of the IMT in ultrasound carotid artery images. Proceedings of the 31st Annual International Conference of the IEEE Engineering in Medicine and Biology Society: Engineering the Future of Biomedicine 2009; 515-519.

[21] Delsanto S., Molinari F., Giustetto P., Liboni W., Badalamenti S., Suri J.S. Characterization of a completely user-independent algorithm for carotid artery segmentation in 2D ultrasound images. IEEE Transactions on Instrumentation and Measurement 2007;56(4) 1265-1274.

[22] Loizou C.P., Pattichis C.S., Pantziaris M., Tyllis T., Nicolaides A. Snakes based segmentation of the common carotid artery intima media. Medical and Biological Engineering and Computing 2007; 45(1) 35-49.

[23] Cheng D.C., Schmidt-Trucksäss A., Cheng K.S., Burkhardt H. Using snakes to detect the intimal and adventitial layers of the common carotid artery wall in sonographic images. Computer Methods and Programs in Biomedicine 2002;67(1) 27-37.

[24] Chan R.C., Kaufhold J., Hemphill L.C., Lees R.S., Karl W.C. Anisotropic edge-preserving smoothing in carotid B-mode ultrasound for improved segmentation and intima-media thickness (IMT) Measurement. Computers in Cardiology 2000;27 37-40.

[25] Shah J. A common framework for curve evolution, segmentation and anisotropic diffusion. Proceedings of the IEEE Computer Society Conference on Computer Vision and Pattern Recognition 1996;136-142.

[26] Bastida-Jumilla M.C., Morales-Sánchez J., Verdú-Monedero R., Larrey-Ruiz J., Sancho-Gómez J.L. Detection of the intima and media walls of the carotid artery with geodesic active contours. Proceedings of the 17th International Conference on Image Processing 2010; 2213-2216.

[27] Gutierrez M.A., Pilon P.E., Lage S.G., Kopel L., Carvalho R.T., Furuie S.S. Automatic measurement of carotid diameter and wall thickness in ultrasound images. Computers in Cardiology 2002; 359-362.

[28] Cheng D.C., Jiang X. Detections of arterial wall in sonographic artery images using dual dynamic programming. IEEE Transactions on Information Technology in Biomedicine 2008; 12(6) 792-799.

[29] Molinari F., Zeng G., Suri J.S. An Integrated Approach to Computer-Based Automated Tracing and Its Validation for 200 Common Carotid Arterial Wall Ultrasound Images. Journal of Ultrasound in Medicine JUM 2010; 29(3) 399-418.

[30] Rocha R., Campilho A., Silva J., Azevedo E., Santos R. Segmentation of the carotid intima-media region in B-mode ultrasound images. Image and Vision Computing 2010;28(4) 614-625.

[31] Destrempes F., Meunier J., Giroux M.F., Soulez G., Cloutier G. Segmentation in ultrasonic B-mode images of healthy carotid arteries using mixtures of Nakagami distributions and stochastic optimization. IEEE Transactions on Medical Imaging 2009; 28(2) 215-229.

[32] Koenderink J. J. The structure of images. Biological Cybernetics 1984;50 363-370.

[33] Lindeberg T. Discrete derivation approximations with scale-space properties: a basis for low-level feature extractions. Journal of Mathematical Imaging and Vision 1993;3 349-376.

[34] Lobregt S, Viergever M. A discrete dynamic contour model. IEEE Transactions on Medical Imaging 1995;14:12-24.

[35] Higa M., Pilon, E., Lage, S.G., Gutierrez, M.A. A Computational tool for quantitative assessment of peripheral arteries in ultrasound Images. Computers in Cardiology 2009: 41-44.

[36] Bland J.M., Altman D.G. Statistical methods for assessing agreement between two methods of clinical measurement. The Lancet 1986; 327(8476) 307-310.

[37] Tschirren J, Lauer R.M., Sonka M. Automated analysis of Doppler ultrasound velocity flow diagrams. IEEE Transactions on Medical Imaging 2001; 20(12) 1422-1425.

Chapter 11

The Top Ten Cases in Cardiac MRI and the Most Important Differential Diagnoses

Patricia Carreño-Morán, Julian Breeze and
Michael R. Rees

Additional information is available at the end of the chapter

http://dx.doi.org/10.5772/53444

1. Introduction

Noninvasive imaging plays a central role in the diagnosis of heart failure, assessment of prognosis, and monitoring of therapy. Cardiovascular magnetic resonance (CMR) offers a comprehensive assessment of heart failure patients and is now the gold standard imaging technique to assess myocardial anatomy, regional and global function, and viability. Furthermore, it allows assessment of perfusion and acute tissue injury (edema and necrosis), whereas in nonischemic heart failure, fibrosis, infiltration, and iron overload can be detected [1]. The American College of Cardiology/American Heart Association have recently updated their guidelines for imaging techniques used to assess patients with HF [2]. According to it, two-dimensional echocardiography is currently the imaging modality most commonly used in clinical practice to meet the ACCF/AHA requirements. It provides a good general assessment of LV function but is limited in patients with poor acoustic windows, it requires geometric assumptions in quantifying global LV systolic function, and its ability to provide specific tissue characterization is modest. CMR is the gold standard to LV and RV global and regional dysfunction, dilation, viability and what is the underlying etiology of HF. CMR makes it particularly well suited to studying the RV, which is difficult to assess with echocardiography.

The CE-MARC study [3,4] defines the role of Cardiac MR: 752 patients with suspected heart disease were recruited and scheduled for MR and SPECT as well as for an X-ray coronary angiogram used as the reference standard. Angiography identified 39% of the patients with CAD. Cardiac MR had a sensitivity and specificity of 86.5% and 83.4%, respectively. In comparison, SPECT delivered a sensitivity and specificity of 66.5% and 82.6 %, respectively. Viability/post-myocardial infarction scarring can be described with unprecedented resolution, and highly specific patterns of fibrosis and scarring have been described for many nonischemic cardiomyopathic processes. DE-CMR appears to offer advantages in detecting small or subendocardial infarcts with high accuracy and is well validated. Late studies showed that the sensitivity of DE-CMR increased with increasing gadolinium dose, reaching 99% and 94% in acute and chronic MI, respectively. These surveys have shown that unrecognized MIs are common, comprising as many as 40% to 60% of all MIs.

Nearly one-half of HF patients have abnormalities in diastolic function with preserved ejection fraction CMR can assess diastolic function in several ways. In an analogous manner to echocardiography, MR tagging is a sophisticated method for quantitative analysis of regional systolic and diastolic function.

2. Background

Cardiac MR is increasingly becoming the modality of choice in the diagnosis of coronary and cardiac disease. The aim of this guide is to cover the most frequent conditions encountered, highlight technical issues, differential diagnoses, and the most common pitfalls found when diagnosing patients.

Cardiovascular disease is the most frequent cause of mortality in the developed world. Although diverse, many techniques exist for diagnosing cardiac diseases, and it is frequently necessary to request several tests to reach a conclusive diagnosis. Magnetic resonance (MR) is a well tolerated and safe technique, which is currently available in a majority of hospitals. This technique makes it possible in a single exploration to study the anatomy of the heart, allowing qualitative, semi-quantitative, and quantitative assessments to be made of the parameters of cardiac anatomy and function. It provides information of cardiac and vascular anatomy and function in complex congenital and acquired cardiopathies. With the administration of intravenous contrast, it also enables us to visualize the extent of ischemic cardiopathies and assess myocardial viability. As such, cardiac magnetic resonance is emerging as one of the most promising techniques for the study of congenital and acquired cardiac pathology.

According to the American College of Cardiology [1], the proposed indications for CMR Imaging in patients with Heart Failure are:

- Serial assessment of biventricular structure, size, and function (anatomy, LV/RV volumes, global and regional systolic function, mass)
- Evaluation of native and prosthetic cardiac valves (planimetry of stenotic disease, estimation of peak stenotic velocities and gradients, quantification of regurgitant disease)
- Evaluation of cardiac masses, differentiation between tumour and thrombus
- Evaluation of great vessels and pulmonary veins

http://dx.doi.org/10.5772/53444

- Determination of the location and extent of acute (including no-reflow regions) and chronic myocardial necrosis
- Viability assessment before revascularization (LGE or low-dose dobutamine)
- Determination of the area at risk in patients with acute myocardial infarction and the salvageable area post-revascularization with percutaneous coronary intervention
- Identification of the presence and quantification of the extent of inducible ischemia (vasodilator perfusion or high-dose dobutamine stress CMR)
- Evaluation of suspected anomalous coronary origins (MR coronary angiography)
- Differentiation of ischemic versus non-ischemic cardiomyopathy
- Evaluation of myocarditis
- Evaluation of specific cardiomyopathies (in vivo tissue characterization)
- Dilated cardiomyopathy
- Hypertrophic cardiomyopathy
- Arrhythmogenic right ventricular cardiomyopathy
- Cardiac amyloidosis
- Cardiac sarcoidosis
- Anderson-Fabry disease
- Iron overload cardiomyopathy
- Left ventricular noncompaction
- Other less common diseases (e.g., Chagas disease, endomyocardial fibrosis, Churg-Strauss syndrome, and so on)
- Assessment of mechanical dyssynchrony before resynchronization therapy
- Patients with technically limited images from echocardiogram
- Discordant information that is clinically significant from prior tests

3. A survival guide to cardiac MRI

3.1. Protocol

a. Sequences: SE (black blood), gradient ECHO: CineMRI, perfusion, viability, flow quantification, motion tagging, and others.

b. Planes: SA, 2CH, 3CH, 4CH, inflow and outflow.

c. How to review:

- Structure (size, thickness)
- Function (motility, volumes, EF, cardiac output)
- Valves (morphology, flow)
- Ischemia: T2 STIR, perfusion first pass and stress, viability (DHE)

3.2. Sequences

BLACK BLOOD: SE (Spin echo) is the most suitable sequence to analyze the morphology of the heart and great vessels. The blood is black and fat is white. Variations are fast (or turbo). Spin echo (FSE or TSE) allows the acquisition of an entire image in a single heartbeat.

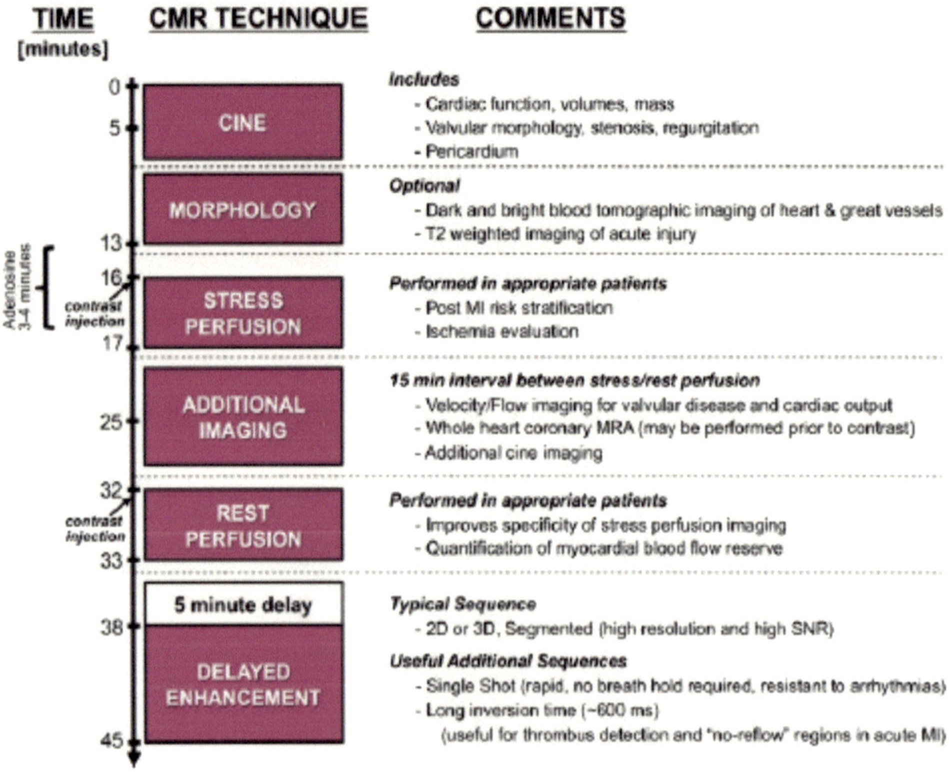

Figure 1. Protocol cardiac MR. Timeline and potential components of a multitechnique CMR examination for Cardiac imaging. 2D=2-dimensional; 3D= 3-dimensional; CMR= cardiovascular magnetic resonance; MI= myocardial infarction; MRA= magnetic resonance anglography; SNR= signal-to-nolse ratio.

http://dx.doi.org/10.5772/53444

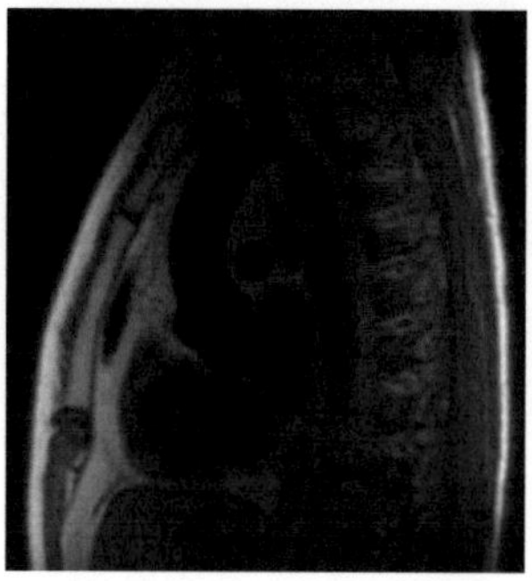

Figure 2. T1 Black Blood image using SENSE aortic outflow plane: coarctation of the aorta.

WHITE BLOOD: GE (Gradient echo). Blood and fat appear white. Variations: b-SSFP (balanced Steady-State Free Precession Imaging), FLASH and velocity mapping. b-SSFP cine sequence can also be applied 2D (single shot), as a real time technique (does not require breath holding or ECG triggering) and 3D volume scan.

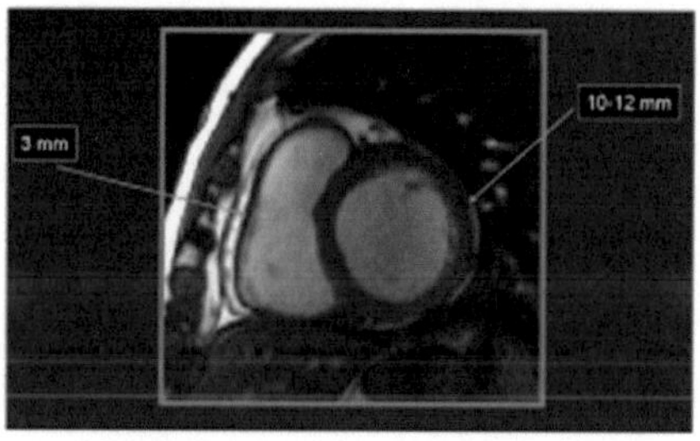

Figure 3. b-SSFP: 2 CH short axis: measure thickness RV and LV. Normal thickness RV 3mm LV 10-12mm.

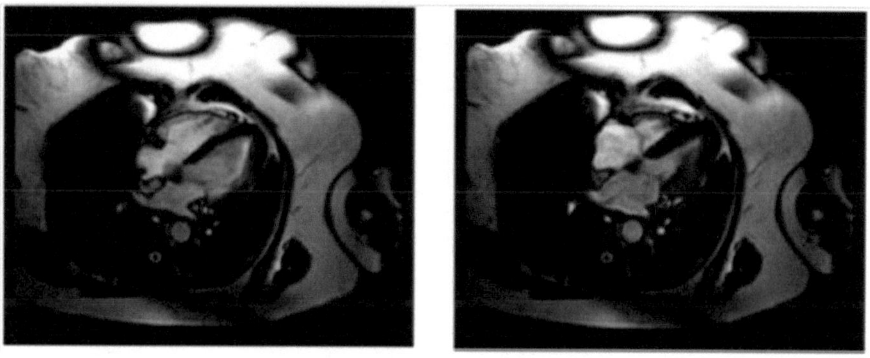

Figure 4. b-SSFP cine (diastole and systole): Global and segment analysis of movement and thickness.

It is used to analyze global and regional cardiac function, detecting abnormal flow, such as jets from stenoses of the valves or insufficiency, to study flows and quantify the degree of stenosis and regurgitation, to quantify Qp:Qs between pulmonary and systemic flow, and is also useful in detecting congenital malformations. CineMR: To analyze the contractility of the heart wall. Analysis is performed for each segment (hypokinesia, akinesia, dyskinesia): There must also be evidence of wall thickening.

We can see jets (turbulent flow) in the valves or from the outflow of left or right ventricles.

- AV valves:

- Insufficiency or regurgitation, if the flow of the jet is directed into the ventricles.
- Stenosis: the flow of the jet originates from inside the ventricles.

- Aortic and pulmonary valves:

- Insufficiency, the flow of the jet is directed into the ventricles
- Stenosis: the origin of the jet comes from outside the ventricles from the vessels.

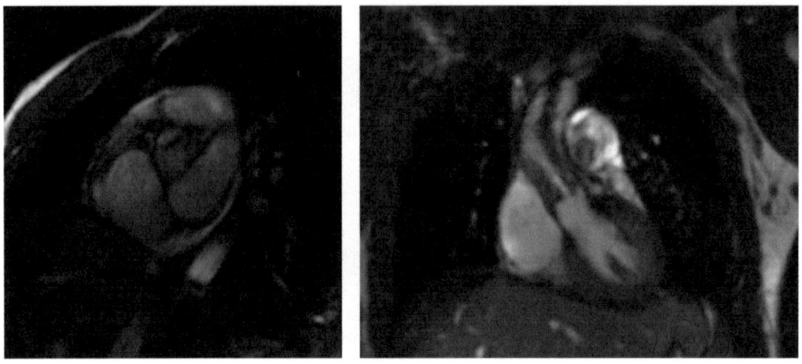

Figure 5. Plane aortic valve (bicuspide aortic valve) and plane outflow LV with yet of aortic insufficiency

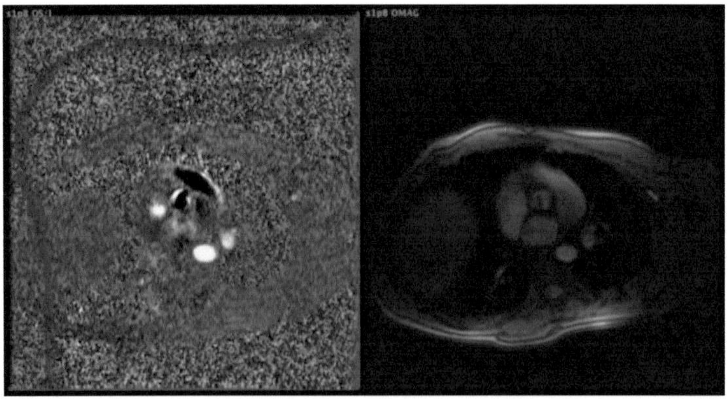

Figure 6. Q-Flow magnitude and phase encoding (velocity mapping): bicuspid aortic valve with regurgitation

http://dx.doi.org/10.5772/53444

VELOCITY MAPPING (Flow velocity mapping):

- Detect and quantify peak velocity in valvular stenosis.
- Calculate overflow in a mayor vessel through the cardiac cycle
- Quantification in regurgitation or valvular incompetence.
- Confirm abnormal chamber communication and the ratio of pulmonary to systemic flow in shunts, such as septal defects.
- Determine the average velocity: The operator selects the plane and sets a maximal encoding velocity (VENC), the initial VENC used is an approximation upper of the velocity expected.

INVERSION RECOVERY TECHNIQUE AND CONTRAST ENHANCEMENT MR (CE-MR): Uses a pre-pulse to create high T1 tissue contrast to visualize infarct imaging (black myocardium), compound of gadolinium (Gd-DTPA) to detect insufficient perfusion in first pass, followed by a delayed DHE to detect scar or inflammatory changes (white myocardium in infarct, myocarditis and infiltrative diseases.) Stress MR can be obtained using adenosine or dobutamine as chemical stressors.

Furthermore, this can be used to evaluate cardiovascular physiology and anatomy, characterize tissues, and vascular angiography.

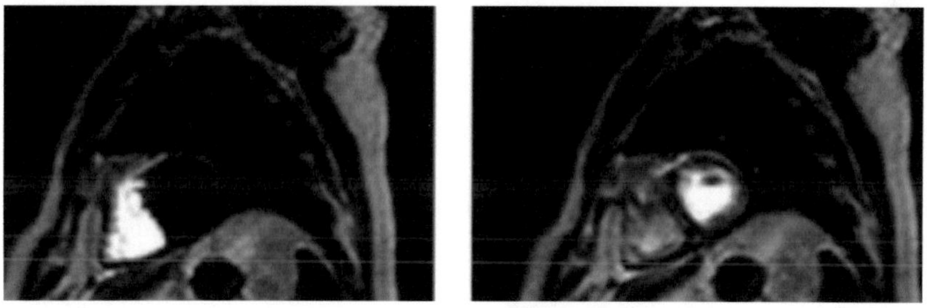

Figure 7. Early Enhancement Perfusion Short Axis SENSE (TR: 2, TE: 1)

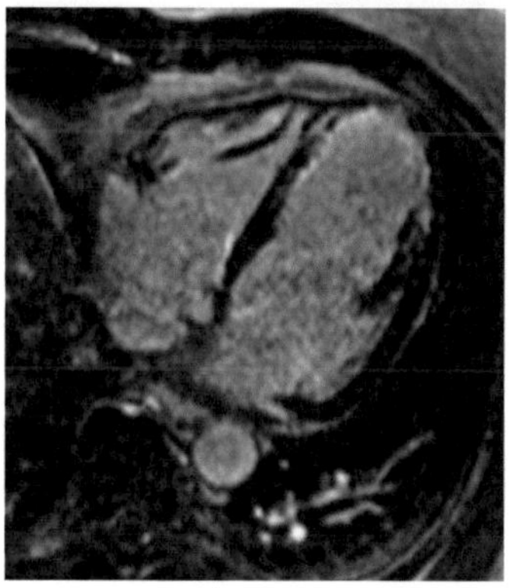

Figure 8. DHE Late contrast enhancement 8 minutes after injection of Gadolinium. Apical enhancement: scar of inferior infarction.

OTHERS:

- Contrast-enhanced MR angiography: study of aortic aneurism and dissection, congenital anomalies of great vessels, vasculitis evaluation, central thoracic veins, pulmonary artery anatomy, postsurgical follow-up and contraindications to computed tomography
- TAGGING IMAGING: Measurement the contractility of myocardium; T2 STIR: In edema, and T2* for quantification of haemochromatosis; Sequences fat suppression (SPIR), etc

3.3. Planes in cardiac imaging

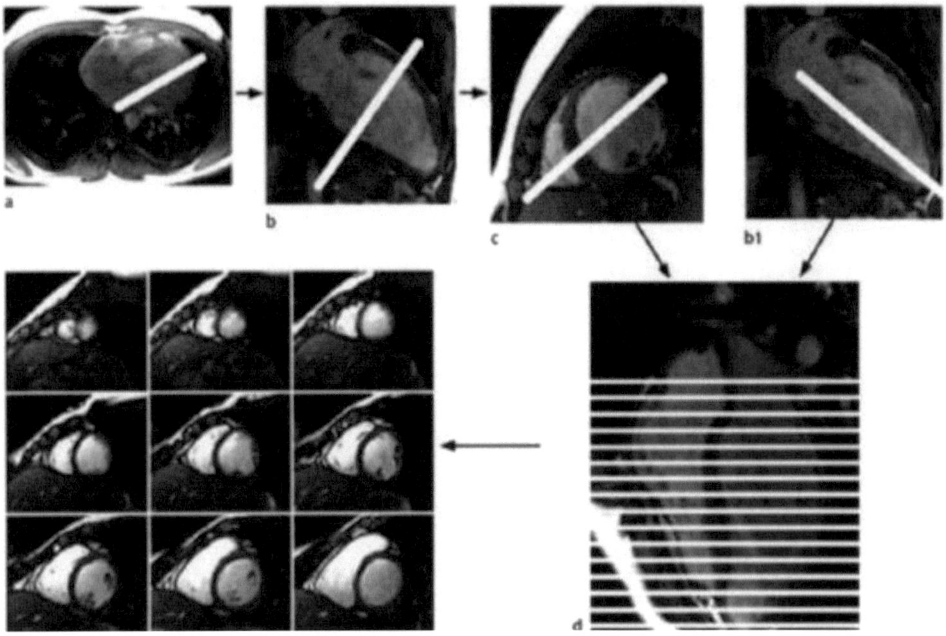

Figure 9. Protocols for cardiac imaging: a,b,c. Rapid pilot scans in the 3 orthogonal planes (axial, coronal and sagittal) in a breath-hold, FSE 1 imaging per cardiac cycle; d. Anatomical coverage from the diaphragm up to the thoracic inlet into the 3 orthogonal planes.

3.3.1. Specific standard cardiac planes (intrinsic) with GE cines and SE sequences

From the axial plane:

- 2CH (2 chamber) and LA (ventricular long axis) to acquire HA (horizontal long axis), inflow (mitral plane) and outflow (aortic plane)
- SA (Short Axis): inflow HA and 4CH (4 chambers).
- Real 4CH: from SA (short axis) between papillary muscles and inflow LA (mitral valve)
- 3CH (3 chambers): from LA and perpendicular aortic valve.

http://dx.doi.org/10.5772/53444

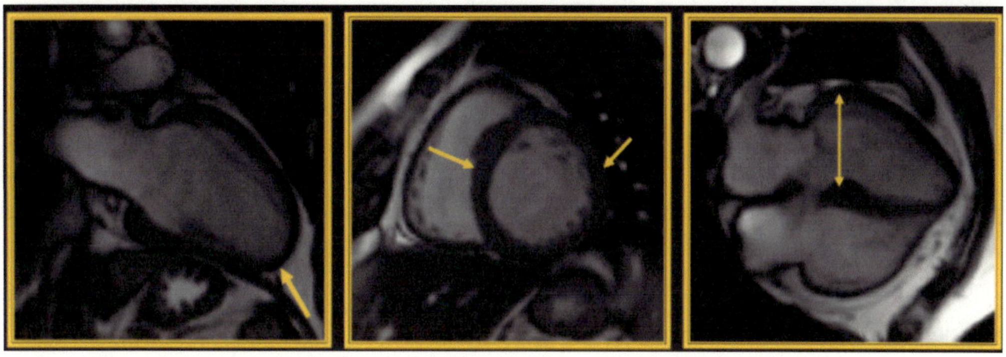

Figure 10. Ventricles size and wall thickness measurement procedure. First and second images: 2CH LA apex 3mm, SA lateral wall and septum 10-12 mm; Third image: 4CH LV size 50mm

3.3.2. Target CMR with additional planes and sequences, such inversion recovery

Sagittal, coronal or oblique planes, LV and RV outflow, valves plane, etc.

3.4. Topics to review

3.4.1. Structure

Size is measured in 4CH in systole and in diastole. Size of chambers in systole and diastole (ant-post): LV 50mm, RV 32mm and LA (left atrium) inferior a 40mm.

The thickness of the wall is measured (end of diastole) in SA (basal and middle) and LA (apical). Left ventricle 10-12mm (< 15mm hypertrophy) and right ventricle > 6mm.

3.4.2. Function

CINE SA and LA:

REGIONAL FUNCION:

Visual assessment of wall motion patterns using cardiac short axis b-SSFP cine: End- diastolic, mid- diastolic and end-systolic.

- Normokinesia: normal wall motion.
- Hypokinesia: Decreased wall motion.
- Akinesia: absent wall motion.
- Dyskinesia: wall motion in the opposite direction.
- Hyperkinesia: increased wall motion.

GLOBAL FUNCION:

CINE MRI SA and LA using b-SSFP is probably the best technique to quantify ventricular volumes, function, and mass. The most commonplace is the Simpson method: drawing epicardial and endocardial borders of LV in systole and diastole, this can also be used for the RV.

The following items are to be analyzed:

- LV undergoes a circumferential and longitudinal ventricular shortening and an extensive wall thickening during systole. The sequence allows the obtention of the ejection fraction (EDV – ESV = SV (mL); SV/EDV = EF (%).
- Ventricular mass to be measured in diastole.

	Male		Female	
	LV	**RV**	**LV**	**RV**
EDV (end diastolic volume)	77-195	88-227	52-141	
ESV (end systolic volume)	19-72	23-103	12-51	
SV (systolic volume)	51-133	52-138	33-97	
EF (%)(ejection fraction)	56-78	47-74	56-87	
Mass index (g/m^2)	< 113	< 36	< 95	< 33

Table 1. Parameters of ventricular function in the population.

3.4.3. Study valves

CINE: jet and direction. Stenosis: through chamber and regurgitation through proximal chamber.

VELOCITY MAPPING: Imaging plane perpendicular to the vessel.

- Quantification volume in both ventricles in SA. N 1:1
- Quantitative velocity mapping: Flow measurement, LV and RV outputs quantification and comparison with ascending aorta and pulmonary trucks.
- Ventricular function EF ejection fraction.

3.4.4. Study ischemia

- T2 STIR: Hyperintensity in edema. It could appear in acute infarct or myocarditis.

- PERFUSION:

- FIRST PASS or EGE (early Ga enhancement): ischemic areas no enhancement. Stress perfusion with adenosine or dobutamine: Induced ischemia (revascularizable)
- VIABILITY or DHE (delayed enhancement) or LGE (late Ga enhancements) after 10-20 min Ga in interstitial space. This is present in an acute infarct because of edema and rup-

http://dx.doi.org/10.5772/53444

ture of the membrane, and in chronic infarcts due to scarring of the tissue. Necrosis ("The White is dead") is typically ischemic, and occurs within the endocardium or can be transmural, and extend across the entire wall.

- INVERSION RECOVERY TECHNIQUE AND CONTRAST ENHANCEMENT MR (CE-MR). This uses a pre-pulse to create high T1 tissue contrast to visualize infarct imaging (black myocardium) and chelats of gadolinium (Gd-DTPA) to detect damage in PERFUSION in first pass and delayed at 10 mins DHE to detect scarring or inflammatory changes (white myocardium in infarct, myocarditis, infiltrative diseases...). Also be can be used with Stress MR using adenosine or dobutamine.

CMR imaging technique	Morphological correlates	Clinical application
▪ Cine imaging ▪ Rest/stress (LDD)	contractile function	▪ LV function ▪ ischemia / viability
T2/weighted	myocardial oedema	▪ tissue at risk ▪ inflammation
First pass perfusion rest/stress	regional myocardial blood flow	▪ myocardial ischemia ▪ microvascular obstruction
Early Gadolinum enhancement	microvascular integrity	▪ No reflow ▪ MVO
Late Gadolinium Enhancement	Myocardial necrosis / fibrosis	▪ Infarct size ▪ Viability

Table 2. Evaluation of CAD (Coronary artery disease) with cardiac MRI

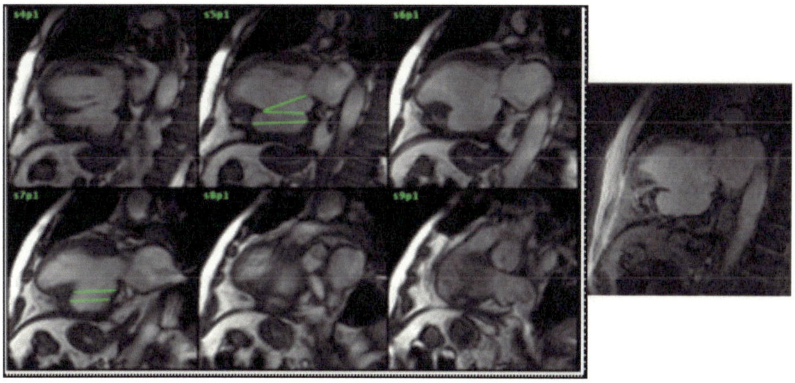

Figure 11. SSFP Cine: enormous aneurism with thrombus in the wall. Huge dilatated LV 163ml/m^2. Systolic dysfunction FE 20%. On the right: GDHE apical and inferior aneurism (no enhancement) with apical thrombus. Transmural inferior myocardium.enhancement suggest microvascular obstruction

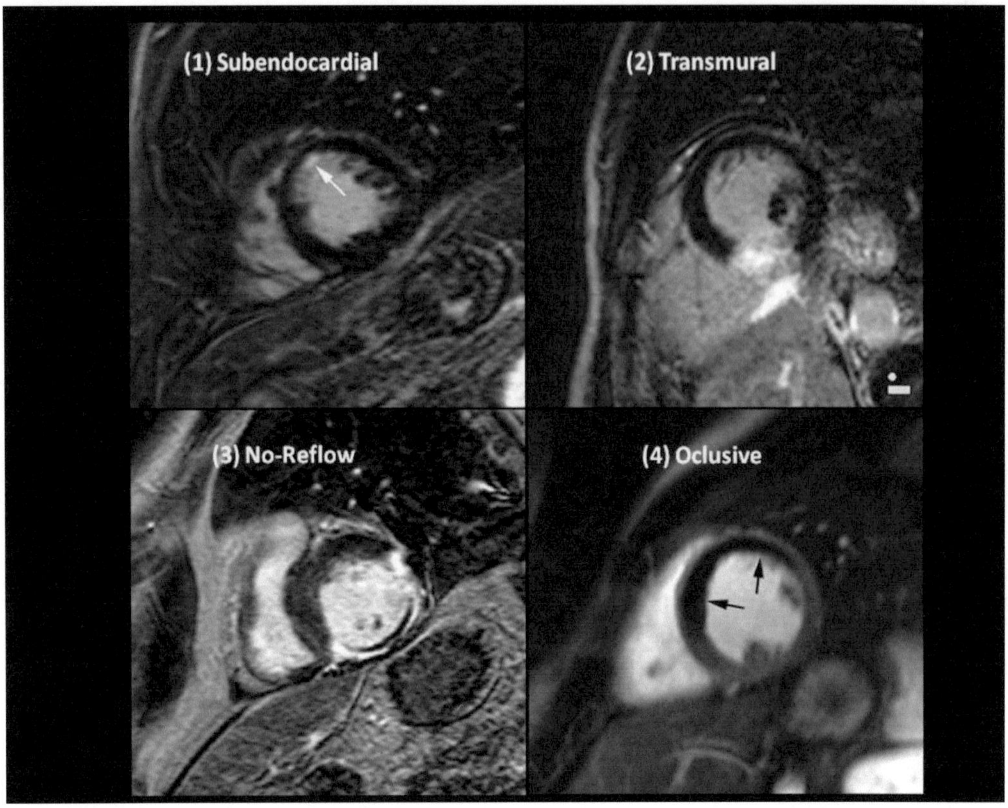

Figure 12. Types of DHE in ischemic cardiopathy: (1) Subendocardial infarction: enhancement only in endocardium and thinness of wall; (2) Transmural infarction: enhancement all the thickness of the inferior wall; (3) No-reflow; (4) Occlusive infarction.

"The no reflow phenomenon": Early DHE 5-7mins could be transient: This pattern represents a transmural infarction, in which the reperfusion was only partially successful, with a residual lack of reperfusion at the tissue level. This can show evidence of important edema or necrosis with microvascular damage, and predicts against a functional recovery.

Non-reperfused occlusive infarcts: DHE Peripheral enhancement surrounding a dark core of non-perfused myocardium.

4. The top 10 cases

4.1. Ischemic cardiopathy

In patients with known or suspected myocardial infarction (MI), cardiovascular magnetic resonance (CMR) provides a comprehensive, multifaceted view of the heart.

http://dx.doi.org/10.5772/53444

Recent multicenter clinical trial indicates that delayed-enhancement cardiac magnetic resonance imaging (DE-CMR) is a well-validated, robust technique that can be easily implemented on scanners that are commonly available worldwide with an effectiveness that clearly rivals the best available imaging techniques for the detection and assessment of acute and chronic MI. When patients present with symptoms outside the usual diagnostic window of cardiac troponins, DE-CMR may be especially useful. Moreover, because DE-CMR can uniquely differentiate between ischemic and various nonischemic forms of myocardial injury, it may be helpful in cases of diagnostic uncertainty, such as in patients with classical features of MI, in whom coronary angiography does not show a culprit lesion. Even once a diagnosis of MI has been made, CMR can also provide clinically relevant information such as identifying residual viability, microvascular damage, stunning, and right ventricular infarction. In addition, post-MI complications, including left ventricular thrombus and pericarditis, are easily identified. Given that quantification of infarct size by DE-CMR is highly reproducible, this technique may provide a useful surrogate end point for clinical trials with appreciable reductions in sample size compared with alternative methods. [5]

Study of ischemia sequences

- *T2 weighted STIR:* edema-weighted imaging. Hyper intensity could appear in acute infarct or myocarditis.
- CINE b-SSFP: motility: Hypokinesia dyskinesia of ischemic areas
- Perfusion: first pass of EGE (early Ga enhancement): ischemic areas no enhancement. Stress perfusion with adenosine and dobutamine: Induced ischemia.
- Viability DHE (delayed enhancement) or LGE (late Ga enhancement) after 10-20 mins. Gadolinium in interstitial space in acute infarct because of edema and rupture of membrane and in chronic infarct due to scarring, showing the extension of the scar.

Scarring less than 25% of the thickness of the wall (subendocardial), 25-50%, greater than 50% (transmural). This usually associates with thinning of the wall and is a prognosis factor that predicts functional recovery after revascularization.

Patterns of ischemic enhancement

The distribution of DHE from ischemia is typically subendocardial to transmural. Differential diagnosis with myocarditis: diffuse multifocal enhancement, often epicardial The morphology of an area of DHE is also relative to the longitudinal distribution of the blood supply of the coronary artery.

- Inferior infarctions: area of enhancement basal and mid-ventricular myocardium. May extend towards the infero-lateral RV right ventricular wall
- Lateral wall infarctions: mid ventricular and apical portions
- Anterior infarctions: antero-basal wall and may include the apex

Imaging Technique cardio RM	Morphologic correlation	Clinical applications	Normal	Acute IAM	Chronic IAM	Induced Ischemia
Cine Rest/stress (LDD)	Contractile Function	LV Function Ischemia/ viability	Normal	Normal/ decrease contractile function	Normal/ decrease contractile function	Normal decrease with stress
Weighted T2	Myocardial edema	Tissue in risk Inflammation (swelling)	●	○	●	●
Perfusion first pass: Rest and stress	Regional myocardial flow	Myocardial ischemia Microvascular obstruction	○	N. I.	○	○
Early enhancement EHG	Normal microvascular	No reflow. Microvascular obstruction	○	●	○	○
Late enhancement DHE	Myocardial necrosis/ fibrosis	Infarct size Viability	●	○	○	●

Table 3. Ischemic cardiomyopathy differential diagnosis between normal, acute or chronic infarct and induced ischemia (black circle: hypointensive; White circle: hyperintensive; N. I.: not indicated)

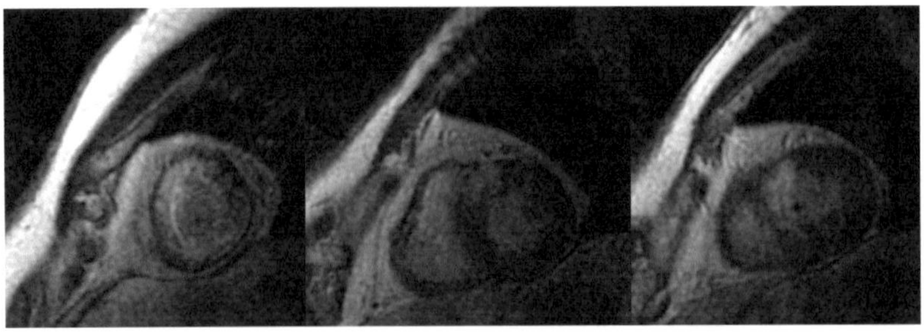

Figure 13. Ischemic cardiomyopathy. DHE. Enhancement inferior infarction: area of enhancement basal and mid-ventricular myocardium.

http://dx.doi.org/10.5772/53444

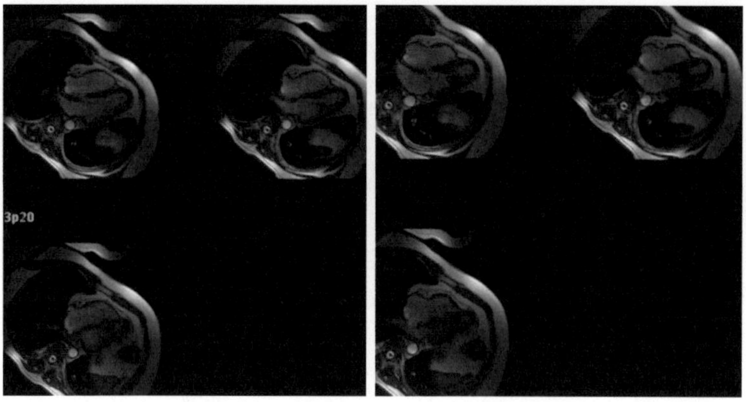

Figure 14. Cine b-SSFP Diastole and systole: apical aneurism (diskinetic area)

4.2. Dilated cardiopathy

The main differential diagnosis is between ischemic and non-ischemic dilated cardiopathies.

Non-ischemic: idiopathic, amyloidosis, haemochromatosis end stage, metabolic toxic alcohol

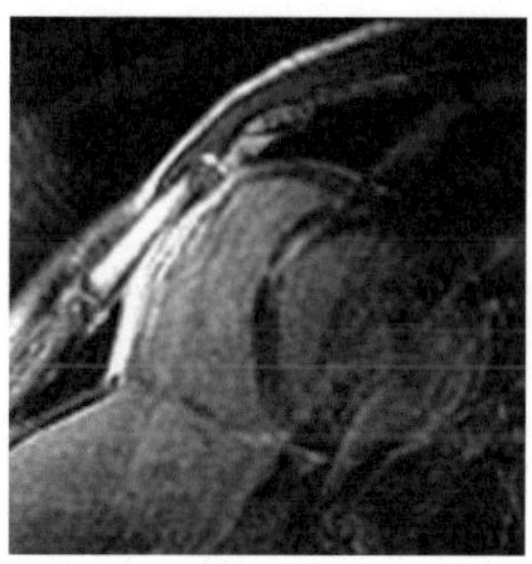

Figure 15. DHE: Chagas Disease. American trypanosomiasis. Severe LV dysfunction, heart failure and tachycardia MR Ga: high signal of inflammation in infero-lateral wall of the LV.

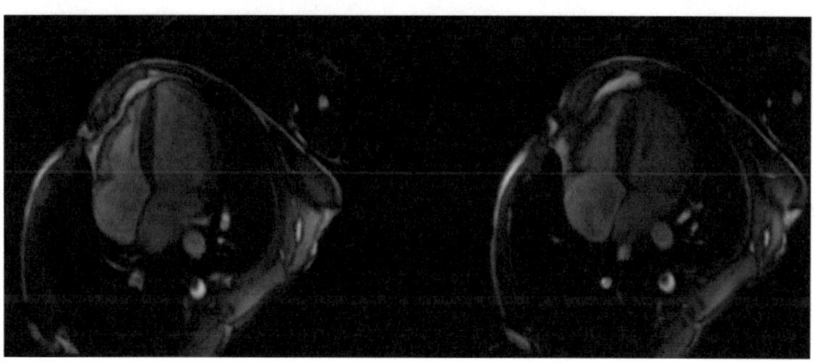

Figure 16. SSFP systole: dilated four chamber hypokinesia

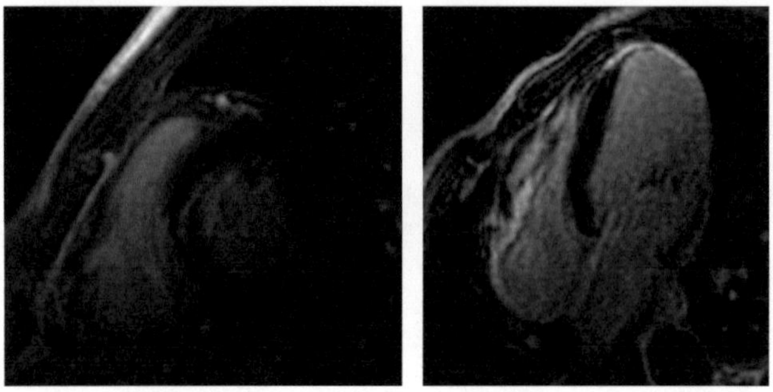

Figure 17. Ischemic dilated myocardiopathy: 2CH SA and 4CH Dilated chambers and DHE inf basal because of an infarct.

4.3. Hypertrophic MC

Criteria:

Morphological: measure diastolic myocardial thickness LV > 15mm, RV > 5mm in absence of Hypertension, aortic stenosis, amyloidosis or pulmonary hypertension. Measure left chambers.

MR is used when a cardio echogram cannot determinate the severity and risk.

Functional: mitral valvulopathy, obstruction left ventricle outflow and motility dysfunction.

DHE: detect fibrosis and perfusion disorders as a prognosis factor. Non-enhanced is good prognosis.

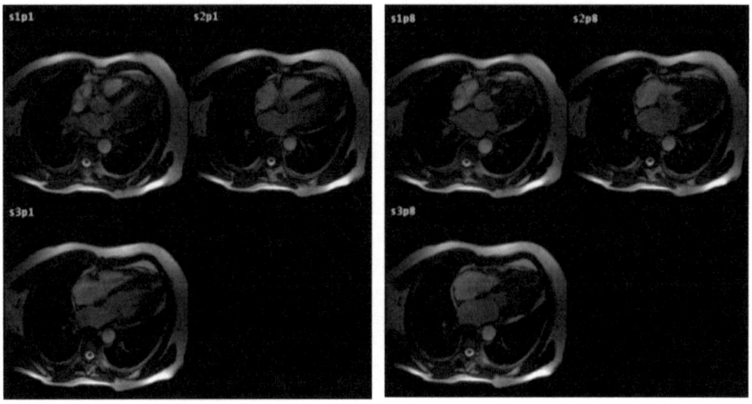

Figure 18. Cine b-SSFP Diastole and systole: Hypertrophic myocardiopathy. Measure diastolic myocardial thickness LV > 15mm

4.4. RVAD (Right ventricle arrythmogenic dysplasia)

Etiology: inherence diseases (1:5000). A. D. Transmission variability. The diagnosis criteria proposed by RVAD Task Force in 1994 are based on the presence of major and minor criteria

http://dx.doi.org/10.5772/53444

encompassing structural, histologic, electrocardiographic, arrhythmic and genetic factors: 2 major criteria, 1 major plus 2 minor, or 4 minor. MR allows multiplanar evaluation of the right ventricle (RV), enabling accurate morphologic and functional assessment.

- RV and outflow dilated
- Aneurisms
- Global systolic dysfunction
- Regional dysfunction contraction
- Fibro fatty transformation

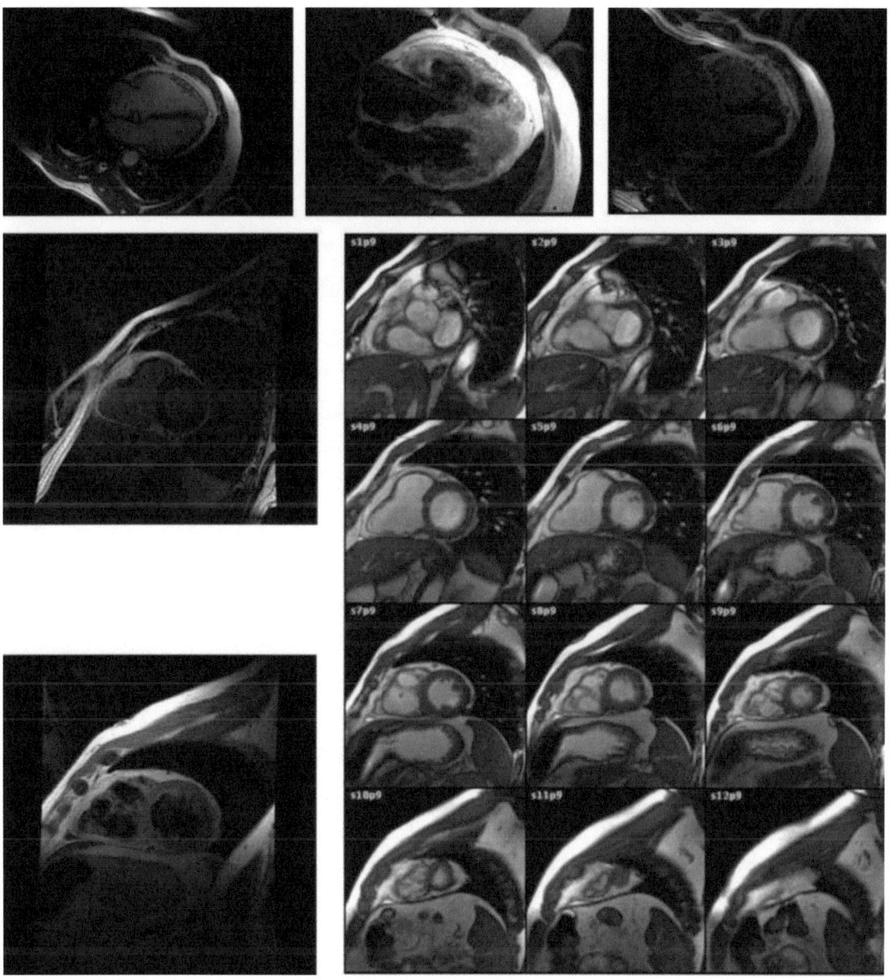

Figure 19. b-SSFP sequences fat suppression, cine and DHE of a ADRV. Criteria: RV 129 ml/m^2 global dysfunction of RV (FE RV 29%), dyskinesia, saccular granulations, fibro fatty transformation and late enhancement of gadolinium (DHE).

4.5. Restricted cardiopathy

Restrictive cardiomyopathies constitute a heterogeneous group of heart muscle conditions that all present with the symptoms of heart failure, showing diastolic dysfunction with preserved systolic function.

The majority of restrictive cardiomyopathies are secondary to a systemic disorder such as amyloidosis, sarcoidosis, scleroderma, haemochromatosis, eosinophilic heart disease, or as a result of radiation treatment. The more rare diagnosis of idiopathic restrictive cardiomyopathy is supported only by the absence of specific pathology or endomyocardial biopsies.

The classic anatomical features of a restrictive cardiomyopathy are: small left ventricle (not dilated) with marked atrial dilatation and normal systolic function in the absence of pericardial disease.

MRI can demonstrate the underlying anatomical lesion:

- Pericardial thickening, though the presence of a pericardium or normal thickning does not entirely exclude the possibility of constriction. The main differential diagnosis is with constrictive pericarditis.
- Additional imaging features such as abnormal right ventricular shape, vena cava dilatation, and paradoxical movement of the intraventricular septum, during operator guided deep respiration.
- Characteristic tissues, especially the demonstration of interstitial or nodular fibrosis based on the underlying etiology. In the presence of constrictive pericarditis from pericardial inflammation, fibrosis or calcifications, diastolic expansion is impaired resulting in poor diastolic ventricular filling, resulting in a characteristic type of diastolic impairment.
- Amyloidosis: Homogenous increased thickness of ventricular and atrial walls. The ventricular cavities are normal or reduced in size. Severe concentric hypertrophy of both normal sized ventricles in absence of hypertension or valvular heart disease is suggestive of amyloidosis. The atria are usually enlarged owing to the diastolic dysfunction and /or valvular dysfunction due to amyloid deposition. Atrial septum usually > 6mm. Pleural and epicardial effusions are frequent. Inhomogeneous enhancement, patchy, subepicardial or subendocardial, and irrespective of coronary territories.

The differential diagnosis from constrictive pericarditis may be necessary.

MR imaging can serve as a noninvasive examination for the definitive diagnosis of constrictive pericarditis and can help distinguish between constrictive pericarditis and restrictive cardiomyopathy on the basis of pericardial thickness. Mean thickness 1mm.

- The most frequent site of pericardial thickening is over the right ventricle. In Constrictive pericarditis, the signal intensity of the thickened pericardium is similar or decreased compared with that of the myocardium.

http://dx.doi.org/10.5772/53444

• Indirect findings of impaired right ventricular diastolic filling (e.g., dilatation of the inferior vena cava and right atrium) identified in constrictive pericarditis and restrictive cardiomyopathy.

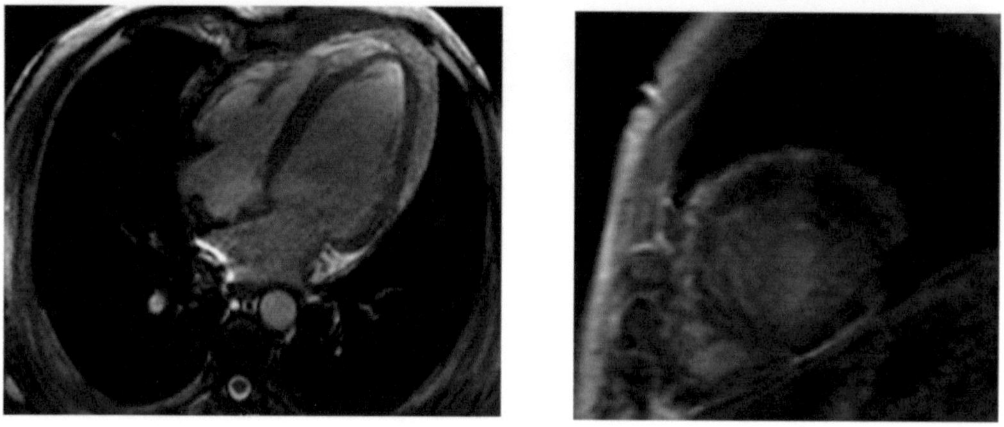

Figure 20. b-SSFP and DHE in Amyloidosis: patchy, subepicardial or subendocardial enhancement irrespective of coronary territories.

Miocardiopathies

Etiology: Primary or secondary to systemic diseases. [6]

Cardiac MR is very useful in myocardiopathies (MC):

• Genetics: hypertrophic MC (MCI I), RVDA arrhythmogenic dysplasia of the RV, non-compacted MC.

• Mixed: dilated MC (MCD), restrictive MC.

• Acquired: inflammatory MC (myocardytis), stress MC (apical ballooning: Tako-Tsubo): transient apical dilatation and dysfunction.

4.6. Pericarditis and myopericarditis

Pericardial inflammation can be caused by infectious diseases viral/bacterial/tuberculosis/fungal); can be manifestation of various systemic diseases (e.g. Rheumatoid arthritis, lupus scleroderma, in patients with uremia, following an acute myocardial infarction, as a result of radiation exposure, or idiopathic.

• Acute may result in diastolic heart failure

• Chronic: fibrosing pericardium ending in stiffening of the pericardium constricting the heart.

Constrictive pericarditis is a thickening (greater than 4 mm), fibrotic and/or calcified pericardium constricting heart.

Normal pericardial thickness is 2mm or less.

Myopericarditis is frequently associated with pericarditis. With a third of cases developing into dilated myocardiopathy. Global dysfunction of myocardium with non coronary distribution.

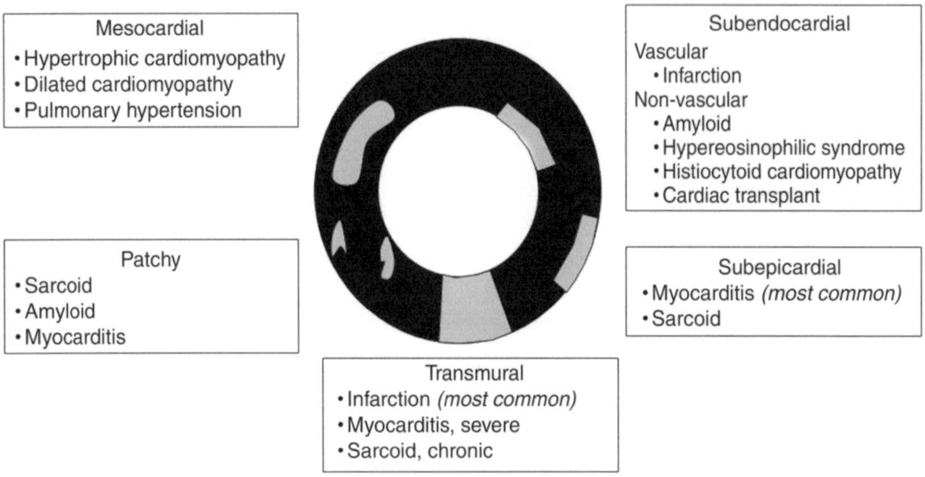

Figure 21. A pattern-based approach to assessment of delayed enhancement in nonischemic cardiomyopathy using MR imaging. [7]

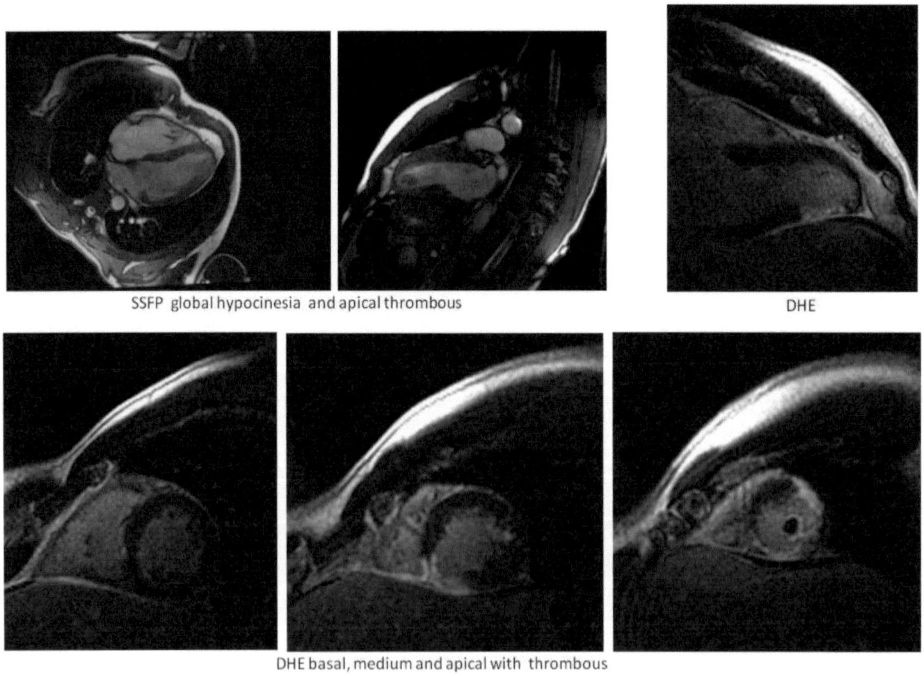

Figure 22. Miocarditis: SSFP apical hypokinesia and thrombus. DHE basal, medium and apical

http://dx.doi.org/10.5772/53444

4.7. Valvular diseases

- Cardiac MR provides good functional information about both valvular stenosis and regurgitation, and allows accurate assessment of ventricular function and relevant cardiac and vascular anatomy. Cardiovascular MR is the gold standard for non invasive imaging of regurgitation: can image the regurgitant volume in any plane, and thus 3D appreciation of the jets can be acquired. Furthermore, it can quantify the regurgitant volume and regurgitant fraction, as well as ventricular function. Transthoracic echocardiography remains the most important and accessible, and easily performed, quantification of valvular heart disease, measuring valvular stenosis and valve area. However this technique is less accurate in quantifying valvular regurgitation with a semi quantitative assessment and only provides an estimate of ventricular function. In addition, imaging planes may be restricted with this technique. X-ray–Angiography (AGF) has been regarded the gold standard but the assessment of valvular regurgitation is both imprecise, inaccurate, and invasive.

- Qualitative assessment of signal loss on cine MR images

- GE technique: For regurgitant lesions signal loss can be grades in a similar way to X-ray AGF: grade 1 = signal loss close to the valve; grade 2 = signal loss extending into the proximal chamber; grade 3 = signal loss filling the whole of the proximal chamber; grade 4 = signal loss in the receiving chamber throughout the relevant half of the cardiac cycle.

Quantitative assessment by measurement of ventricular volumes. MR is the gold standard technique. Using a set of SA cuts covering the length of the ventricles, in combination with Simpson`s rule, the stroke volumes of both right and left ventricle can be measured. There is a 1:1 relationship between these stroke volumes; any discrepancy between the ventricular volumes in a patient with regurgitation will identify the regurgitant volume.

- Quantitative assessment by phase-contrast velocity mapping can be applied in any direction for flow quantification of RV and LV outputs can be compared from the proximal ascending aorta and pulmonary trunk. The severity of the regurgitation fraction: 15-20% mild, 20-40% moderate and >40% severe regurgitation.

- Valvular stenosis can be identified by signal loss in cine-MR. Velocity mapping is used to establish an accurate peak velocity across the valve and to quantify the severity of the stenosis. The mean velocity across caval veins and the mitral valve can be used to describe the inflow curves for the A-V valves.

4.8. Cardiac masses

Cardiac mass may be a neoplasm or non-neoplasmic swelling, such as a thrombus

Cardiac tumors may be secondary with direct extension, venous, with lymphatic extension, malignant primary tumors, or benign, such as mixoma. The most frequent mass found in clinical practice is due to a thrombus, while the second most frequent is due to mixoma.

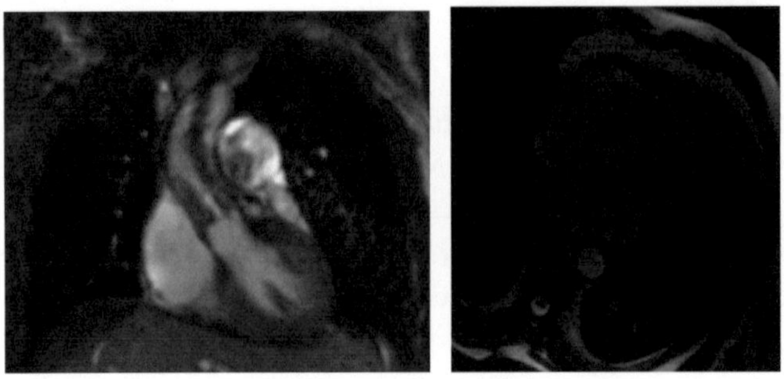

Figure 23. Aortic stenosis and tricuspid regurgitation.

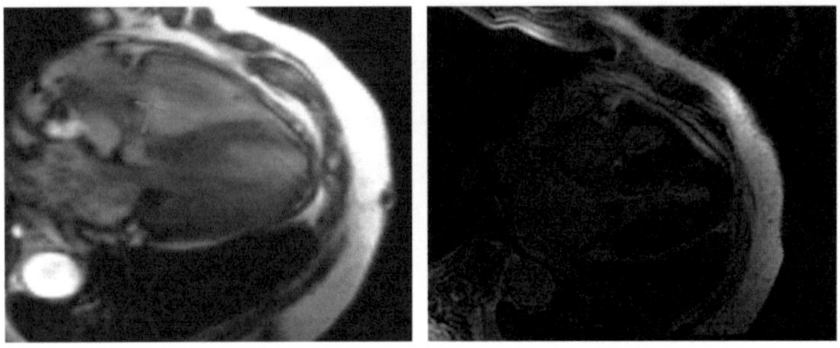

Figure 24. Mixoma: b-SSFP pedunculated mass in LA with heterogeneous DHEg

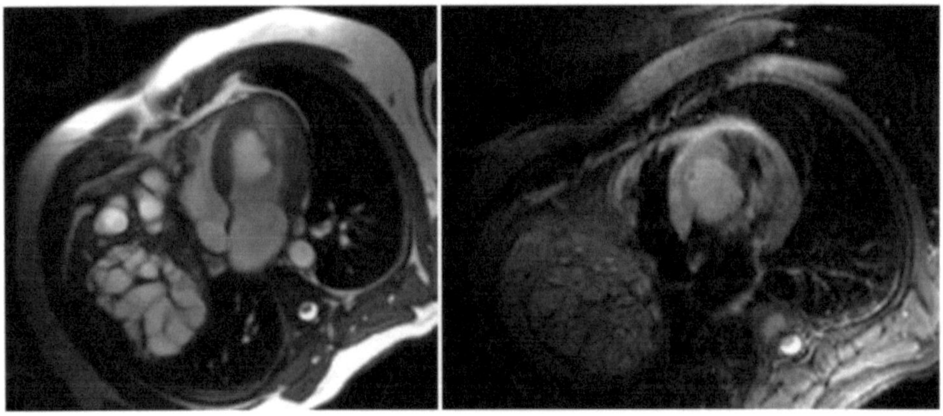

Figure 25. b-SSFP and DHE hidatidic cyst in myocardium and liver.

http://dx.doi.org/10.5772/53444

LOCATION	TUMOR	MR FINDINGS	CHARACTERISTICS
INTRACAVITARY	Myxoma	Oval, mobile, LA (left atrium) heterogeneous enhancement	Fosa ovalis
	Thrombus	LA, orejuela, ventricles in IAM	Low signal in DHE
	Valvular vegetations	Irregular masses valvular or perivalvular	Signal similar to thrombus.
	Metastases	Transvenous spread	Continued spread Primary tumor
INTRAMURAL CHILDREN	Rabdomioma	Several masses similar signal to muscles	Children with E.T
	Fibroma	Solitary mass disturbing anatomy. Ventricles. Intramural	Low signal T2
INTRAMURAL ADULTS	Metastases	Pericardial effusion mass with enhancement	Melanoma hight signal T1
	Lipomatous hypertrophy of the interatrial septum	Septum >2cm, high signal in T1	Loose signal in fat suppression sequences
	Lipoma	Epicardial or intramural high signal in T1	Loose signal in fat suppression sequences
	Paraganglioma	Well defined in atrial walls or septum	Light-bulb in T2
Epi or PERICARDIAL	Metastases	Pericardial effusion	Direct spread of tumour
	Pericardial cyst	Well defined cyst no enhancement	Signal liquid in all sequences
	Hemangioma	Multiple cysts with enhancement	High signal in T1 y T2

Table 4. Differential diagnosis of cardiac masses by location [8]

4.9. Aortic diseases and great vessels

- MR is the non invasive method of choice for the assessing the great vessels of the thorax.
- MR angiography provides exquisite 3D imaging.
- Assessment of ventricular function and intracardiac anatomy may be important.
- Aortic aneurism: sinus of valsalva > 3.3cm; ascending aorta: mid > 3cm and distal > 2.4cm.

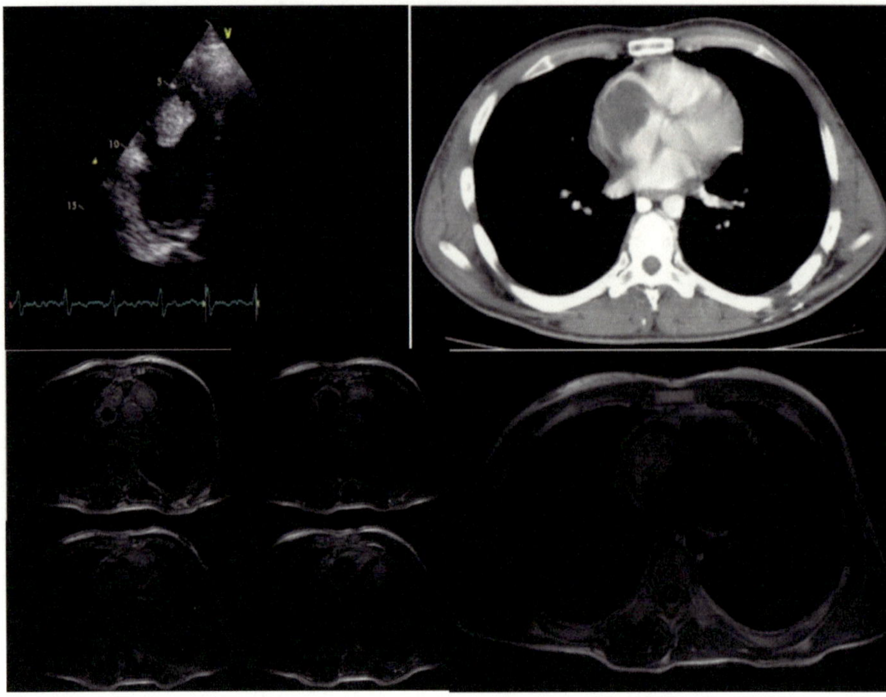

Figure 26. Metastases of germinal tumor: eco and TC peduculated mass in RA. MR: SE and DHE with enhancement of a large mass.

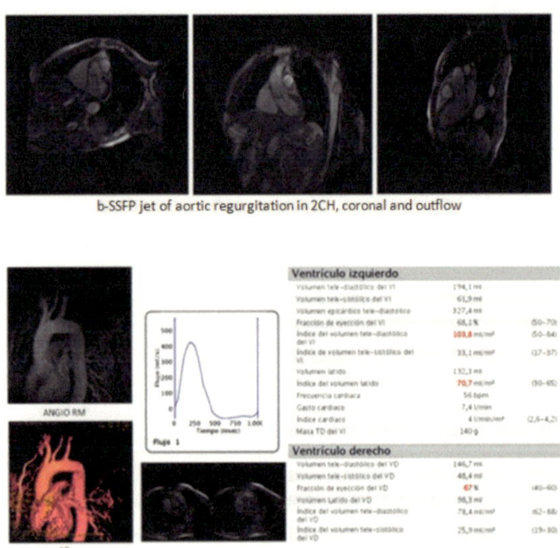

Figure 27. b-SSFP, cine SSFP, RM angiography and QFlow: Dilated ascending aortic with moderate aortic regurgitation. EF and % regurgitation

http://dx.doi.org/10.5772/53444

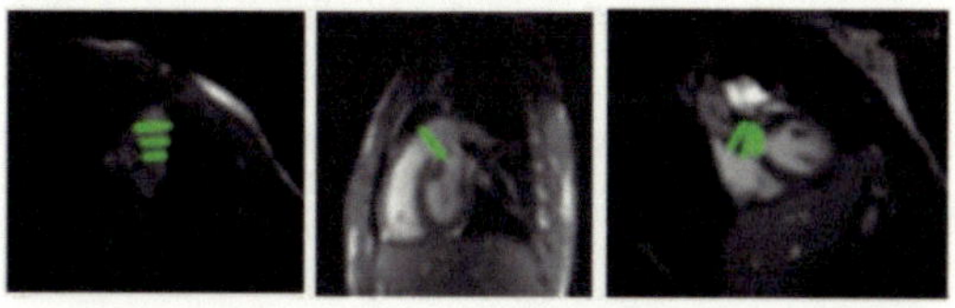

Figure 28. Aortic aneurism: sinus of valsalva > 3.3cm, mid ascending aorta > 3cm and distal ascending aorta > 2.4cm

- Aortic coarctation: area of narrowing of the thoracic aorta in the region of inserction of the arterial duct with or without additional abnormalities.

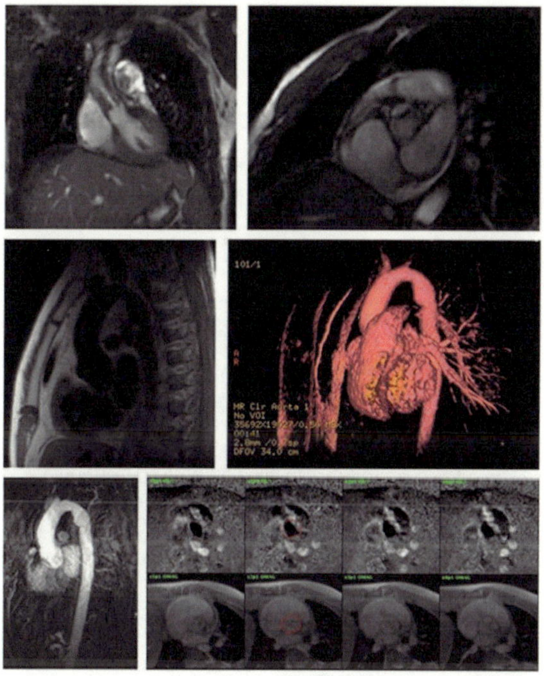

Figure 29. SE blackblood coartation.Volume-rendered 3D. AGF-MR:colateral vessel. Magnitude and velocity map: Bicuspid aortic valve (jet of aortic stenisis) and aortic coarctation after sugery

- Others:Aortic arch anomalies, interrupted aortic arch, vascular rings, aortic disection, ulceration and intramural hematoma, Marfan.
- Anomalous pulmonary veins (PV): anomalous pulmonary venous return or systemic venous abnormalities.

4.10. Congenital diseases

Cardiac MR is increasingly becoming an important tool for the diagnosis and follow-up of children and adult patients with congenital heart disease. Its main role is as an adjunct to echocardiography. MR can provide an accurate, non-invasive method of imaging for assessment of form (3D assessment of anatomy) and function, and is the best method for quantification of ventricular function and vascular flow. The use of (VENC) velocity-encoded-phase-contrast MR allows accurate non invasive quantification of blood flow and pressure gradients, Qp:Qs, and assessment of myocardial perfusion and coronary artery anatomy. Best method for ventricular volumetry (in particular of the RV).

SEQUENTIAL SEGMENTAL ANALYSIS: the nomenclature of complex congenital diseases is based in segmental analysis. Require description of atrial situs, atrio-ventricular connections, and other associated lesions. Increasing ability to assess myocardial perfusion and coronary artery anatomy.

- ASD (Atrial septal defect) are the most common congenital heart defects detected in adults. Cause left-to-right shunting at the atrial level. There are three types: Ostium secundum (80% of ASD), Ostium primum and sinus venous defect.
- AVSD atrio-ventricular septal defect. Partial with a defect of the atrial septum or complete with defect of atrial and ventricular septum there are also abnormalities of the AV valves.

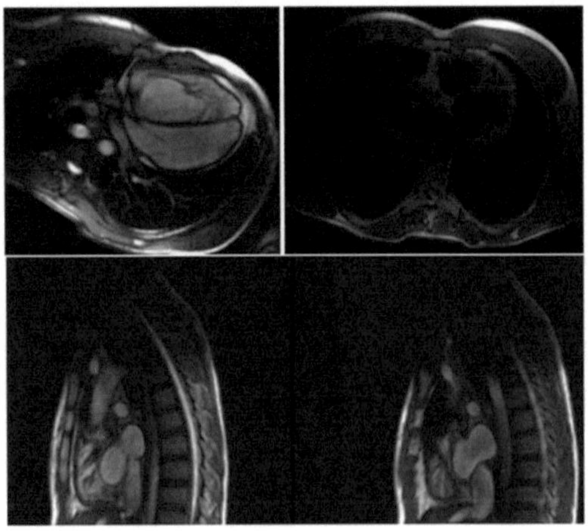

Figure 30. TGV: transposition great vessels after the Mustard procedure. SE black blood LA left atrium connection after surgery. SSFP: RV anatomic (left functionally) dilated 145ml/m^2, hypertrophic FE 60%. Anatomic LV dilated FE 50%

- TGV is the second-commonest cyanotic congenital heart diseases in the first year of life.It is defined as ventriculoarterial discordance with an anterior aorta arising from de RV, and the pulmoray artery arising from the LV.40% have a VSD and 30% subpulmonary stenosis
- VSD ventricular septal defect depends of the shunt volume the left sided heart failure and pulmonary vascular disease. Quantification of left-to-right shunts using VENC MR as a non invasive method. Perimembranous lesions make up 80% of VSD.20% muscular septum.

http://dx.doi.org/10.5772/53444

- Congenital aortic supravalvular stenosis: area of narrowing of the thoracic aorta in the region of inserction of the arterial duct. There are three types; hourglass, membranous and diffuse coarctation.

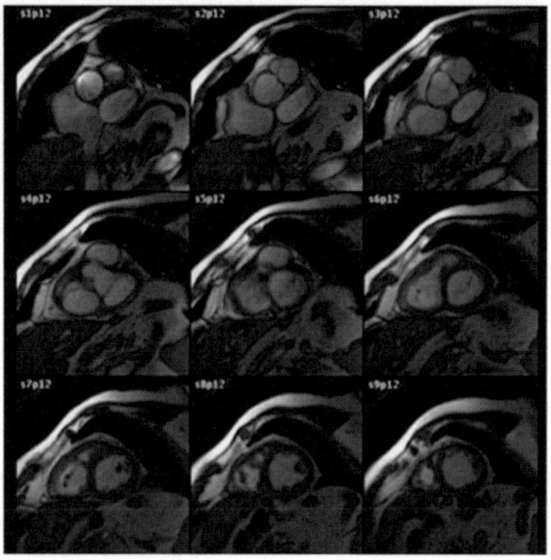

Figure 31. b-SSFP SA outflow. Jet of tricuspid regurgitation Ventricular septal defect and hypertrophy of RV. Tetralogy of Fallot: is the most common cyanotic congenital heart defect, caused by malalignment of the infundibular septum, which leads to right ventricular outflow (RVOT) obstruction, a subaortic VSD (ventricular septal defect) with aortic override, and right ventricular hypertrophy. The role of MR is assesment of postoperative complications besides accurate diagnosis.

Others: pulmonary atresia, double outlet RV, common arterial trunk, anomalous coronary artery, etc.

5. Conclusion

Cardiovascular MR has become a revolutionary technique for the management of cardiac disease. With new sequences the development of this technique has become very important in the diagnosis and management of multiples cardiac diseases and conditions, complementing echocardiography and cardiac angiography.

It has become one of the most accurate techniques (the gold standard) in quantification volumes, mass, study of the right ventricle, and the most complete in the diagnosis of ischemic diseases and congenital diseases. The development of the science in this area has widened the indications and reduced exploration times. Cardiologists and Radiologists must work closely together, and have a widespread knowledge of the most frequent cases and possible differential diagnoses, with a clear understanding of MR sequences and their uses and limitations of this technique.

Acknowledgements

The authors acknowledge Dr J. M. Fernández García-Hierro (University Hospital of Salamanca, Spain) for kindly providing many of the images discussed in this chapter. P. Carreño-Morán also acknowledges the European Society of Radiology for the award of a Fellowship in Cardioimaging in Bangor (UK) in 2010.

Author details

Patricia Carreño-Morán[1], Julian Breeze[2] and Michael R. Rees[2,3]

1 University Hospital of Salamanca, Spain

2 School of Medical Sciences, Bangor University, Gwynedd, UK

3 Ysbyty Gwynedd, Betsi Cadwaladr University Health Board, Gwynedd, UK

References

[1] Karamitsos TD, Francis JM, Myerson S, Selvanayagam JB, Phil D, Neubauer S. The Role of Cardiovascular Magnetic Resonance Imaging in Heart Failure. J. Am. Coll. Cardiol. 2009; 54(15): 1407-1424

[2] Jessup M, Abraham WT, Casey DE. Focused update: ACCF/AHA guidelines for the diagnosis and management of heart failure in adults. A report of the American College of Cardiology Foundation/ American Heart Association Task Force on Practice Guidelines. J. Am. Coll. Cardiol. 2009; 53: 1343-82

[3] Greenwood JP, Maredia N, Younger JF, Brown JM, Nixon J, Everett CC, Bijsterveld P, Ridgway JP, Radienovic A, Dickinson CJ, Ball SG, Plein S. Cardiovascular magnetic resonance and single-photon emission computed tomography for diagnosis of coronary heart disease (CE-MARC): a prospective trial. The Lancet. 4 February 2012; 379: 453-60

[4] Kwong RY et all. Defining Roles: Where Does Cardiac MR Fit in? Health Imaging. http://www.healthimaging.com/index.php?option=com_magazines&task=showmag&id=240 (accessed August 2012)

[5] Kim HW et al. Cardiovascular Magnetic Resonance in Patients With Myocardial Infarction. Current and Emerging Applications. J Am Coll. Cardiol. 2010; 55: 1–16

[6] Bogaert J, Taylor AM. Nonischemic Myocardial Disease in Cardiovascular Magnetic Resonance Imaging. Springer: 2005

http://dx.doi.org/10.5772/53444

[7] Cummings KW et al. A Pattern-based Approach to Assessment of Delayed Enhancement in Nonischemic Cardiomyopathy at MR Imaging. Radiographics; january-february 2009; 29: 189

[8] Grizzard JD, Ang GB. Magn Reson Imaging Clin N Am. 2007; 15: 579–607

Chapter 12

Determination for the Comprehensive Arterial Inflows in the Lower Abdomen Assessed by Doppler Ultrasound: Methodology, Physiological Validity and Perspective

Takuya Osada

Additional information is available at the end of the chapter

http://dx.doi.org/10.5772/53239

1. Introduction

The splanchnic circulation has been described as the "blood-giver of circulation" and is believed to play a major role in overall cardiovascular regulation. The splanchnic cicrculatory system contains a fifth of the total blood volume [1]. The splanchnic system receives nearly 30% of the cardiac output through three large arteries: the coeliac and the superior and inferior mesenteric arteries at rest [2]. The splanchnic blood flow is controlled intrinsically by metabolic and myogenic regulation and extrinsically by neural factors [3]. Hemodynamics in the splanchnic organs are altered under various stressful conditions, such as during physical activity [4] and in the postprandial state [5], due to balancing of tone between sympathetic and vagus activity [6]; consequently, clinical assessment of the splanchnic circulation could potentially provide valuable information regarding hepato-gastrointestinal disease [7-9] and cardiac dysfunction [10].

Doppler ultrasonographic techniques represent a major advance, enabling the measurement of blood flow noninvasively in subjects and the monitoring of flow changes in response to physiological and pathological stresses. Previous Doppler ultrasound studies that measured splanchnic blood flow in a "single vessel with small size volume", such as the superior mesenteric, coeliac artery, or portal vein, were concerned solely with the target organ in the gastrointestinal area or liver; therefore, evaluation of alterations in these single arterial blood flows under the various states were sometimes limited to small blood volumes, even though there was a relatively large change in hemodynamics. Evaluation of the comprehensive arterial blood flow in the lower abdomen, including the liver, spleen, gastro-intestine, kidney, and pelvic organs as a multiple arterial function (Figure 1), may potentially be a feasible method of determining the distribution of abdominal blood-flow volume or disorder in cases of splanchnic or cardiovascular dysfunction, as well as the distribution following nutritious meal intake or physical exercise.

Our previous studies used ultrasonography to assess whole arterial blood flow in the lower abdominal hemodynamics: the comprehensive arterial blood flow in the lower abdomen was obtained by subtracting blood flow in the bilateral proximal femoral arteries [left femoral artery and right femoral artery] from blood flow in the upper abdominal aorta above the coeliac artery bifurcation [11-16].

This method of quantitative assessment is a challenging but unique and non-invasive procedure for determining the comprehensive inflows of all abdominal organs, and is a potentially useful indicator of blood flow redistribution in cardiovascular and hepato-gastrointestinal disease in the clinical state, in the postprandial period, and in relation to physical exercise.

The focus in this chapter will be the variability in the hemodynamics (blood velocity, vessel diameter and blood flow) of the three target arteries which is valuable information for determining the comprehensive arterial blood flow in the lower abdomen as assessed by Doppler ultrasound. Furthermore, in this chapter we will summarize a methodology for determining comprehensive arterial blood flow in the lower abdomen using validated data of three target arteries, discuss methodological considerations regarding physiological aspects and limitations in view of previously reported findings, and consider the potential clinical usefulness and application of measurements for the comprehensive lower abdominal flows.

2. Participants

The expressed data from participants were : total number of participants, 154 healthy males; mean age, 24.5 (range: 19-41) years; mean height, 172.7 (range: 158.3-185.4) cm; and mean body weight, 68.0 (range: 51.4-92.4) kg. Participants had no previous history of cardiovascular disease, gastrointestinal disease, hypertension, or anaemia, and no abnormality of the peripheral vasculature. The studies were conducted according to the principles of the Declaration of Helsinki (1976) and with the approval of the Institutional Ethics Committee of the author's institution. All participants gave their written consent and were informed of the nature and purpose of the study, as well as potential risks and discomfort. The participants also understood that they could withdraw from the study at any time without consequence. The study populations represented in this chapter do not include the elderly.

3. Measurement for comprehensive arterial blood flow in the lower abdomen

3.1. Approach for Doppler ultrasound assessment of three target arteries

The target vessels were the following three conduit arteries: 1) the abdominal aorta (Ao) at ~3 cm above the coeliac artery trunk, 2) the proximal left femoral artery (LFA), and 3) the proximal right femoral artery (RFA) (Figure 1). The Ao region was most commonly measured just below the diaphragm in longitudinal section view (from the sub-sternal area) to enable Ao sample volume to be maintained at the end of the expiratory phase during spontaneous breathing (Figure 2) [14]. Detection of the Ao was relatively constant and free from interference from intestinal gas. For both femoral arteries, measurement location was chosen to minimize turbulence and the influence of the inguinal region on blood flow above the bifurcation, thereby enabling easy and reliable measurement (Figure 2) [11-15,17-21]. Blood velocity (pulsed wave) and vessel diameter (2-dimensional) measurements were obtained using a curvilinear array probe (3.5 MHz) for Ao and a linear array probe (7.5 MHz) for the LFA and RFA. The insonation angle was maintained below 60º for each participant and remained constant throughout the experiments [11-15,22]. The sample volume was placed in the precise centre of the vessel before being adjusted to cover the width of the vessel diameter and blood velocity distribution.

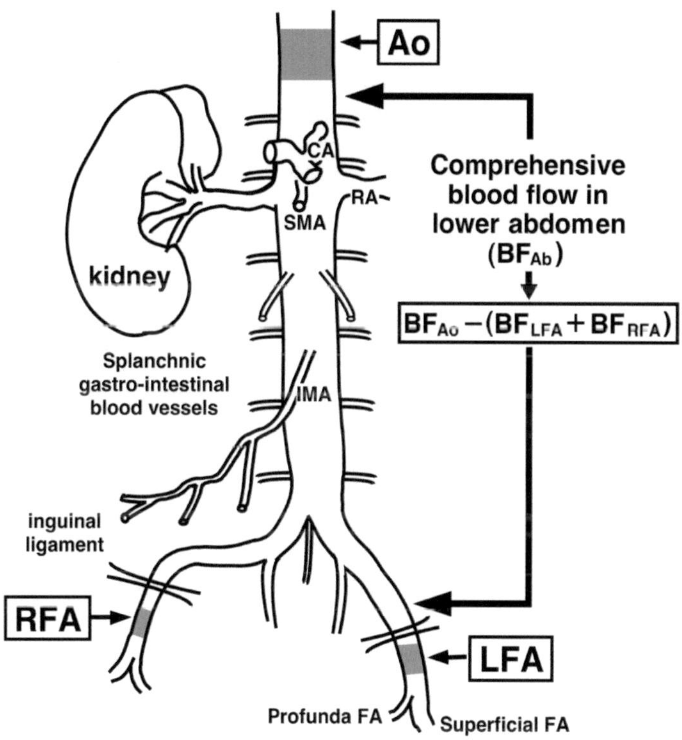

Figure 1. Schematic illustration of the anatomical region for the three target arteries. Blood flow (BF) measurements were obtained for the upper abdominal aorta (Ao) above the coeliac artery trunk (CA) and for the bilateral femoral arteries (right and left femoral arteries; RFA and LFA, respectively) above the bifurcation. Comprehensive BF in the lower abdomen (BF_{Ab}) was calculated by subtracting bilateral femoral arterial flow (BF_{LFA} + BF_{RFA}) from BF_{Ao}. The splanchnic gastrointestinal blood vessels include the renal (RA), CA and the superior and inferior mesenteric arteries (SMA and IMA, respectively). Figure modified from Osada T. et al. [12], reproduced with permission from IOP Publishing Ltd.

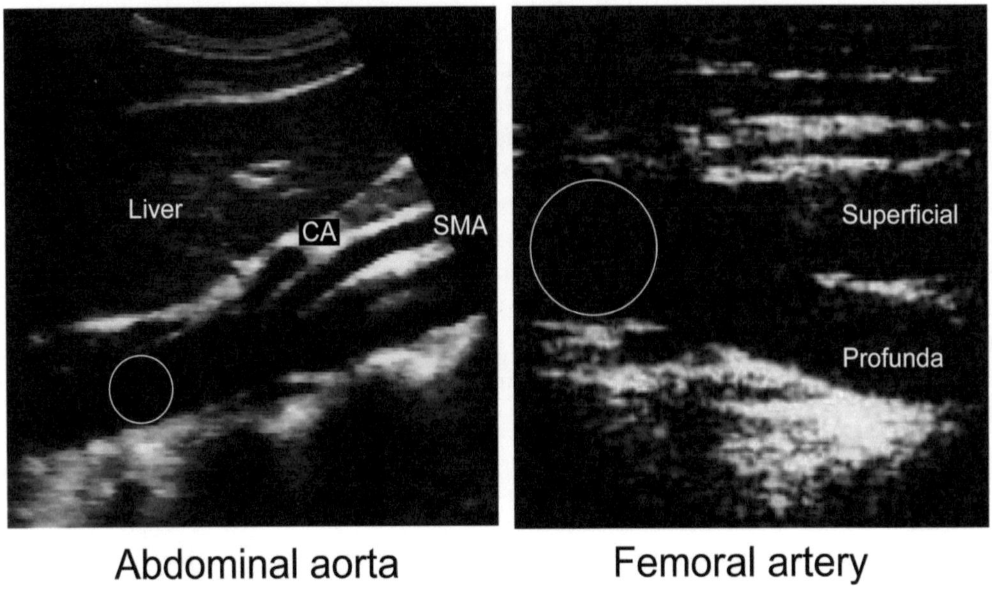

Figure 2. Two-dimensional vascular images in longitudinal view. The target areas (circled) in the blood flow measurements were above the coeliac artery trunk for the upper abdominal aorta (left panel) and above the bifurcation to superficial and profunda femoral arteries for the femoral arteries (right panel). CA, coeliac artery; SMA, superior mesenteric artery.

The presented data were obtained using an ultrasound unit (SONOS 1500, HP77035A; Hewlett-Packard, Tokyo, Japan) with a real-time two-dimensional ultrasonic imager and a pulsed-Doppler flowmeter for calculating maximum envelope in the blood velocity profile. The principle of blood flow measurement using Doppler ultrasound is the calculation of instantaneous mean blood velocity over the cardiac cycle using analysis of the waveform of Doppler-shifted ultrasound reflected from cellular elements of the moving blood within the blood vessel.

The Doppler instrument used in this chapter, however, could not determine time- and spatial-averaged and amplitude (signal intensity)-weighted mean blood velocities; thus, the measured blood velocity determined by integration of the outer envelope (maximum velocities) would have reflected the higher (maximum) velocity component at the centre of the vessel through the cardiac cycle. Because this procedure takes no account of the lower velocity component of the flow profile, the blood velocity values in this chapter have potentially been overestimated. On the basis of this physiological phenomenon, the above-mentioned measure of mean blood velocity, which expresses the averaged speed for all red blood cells within the vessel, is more precise; however, the present procedure used to determine blood velocity also provides acceptable data.

Recent developments in ultrasound instrumentation include an auto-tracing programme for determining mean and maximum blood velocity (outer envelope). Maximum (envelope) blood velocity in the femoral artery is previously reported as being ~1.53 [23] and 1.3–1.8

http://dx.doi.org/10.5772/53239

[24,25] times higher than mean blood velocity. An in vitro study that used a silicon tube to model the conduit artery found that maximum (envelope) blood velocity was approximately 1.75 times higher than mean blood velocity [26].

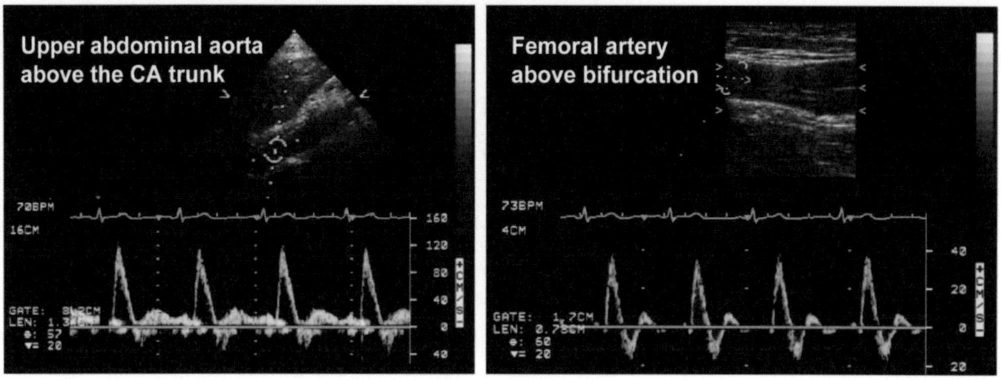

Figure 3. The blood velocity profile in the upper abdominal aorta and femoral artery. The beat-by-beat flow profile was detected at the target area in the arteries. Sampling point as target area was as shown in the vascular image above within in the view. CA, coeliac artery.

3.2. Measurement procedure of blood velocity, vessel diameter, and blood flow in the arteries at resting condition

For the measurement in the base state of hemodynamics with minimal influence (for instance, gastrointestinal hyperemia) from meal digestive and absorptive response, the measurement for the base state was conducted in the morning following a 12-h fast. Prior to measurement, colour Doppler was used to check for unsuspected pathology in each conduit artery. For each of the three conduit arteries, blood velocity was measured for 2–3 minutes and vessel diameter for 1–2 minutes via image observation using a wide expanded view in longitudinal section, by a single operator (the author). Blood velocity was analysed by integrating the outer envelope of the maximum velocity values from the flow profile for each beat, for approximately 20–40 beats [11,27-29]. Blood velocity and vessel diameter analyses were performed using the phase that demonstrated similar heart rate and blood pressure values among measurements from the three conduit arteries. The systolic and diastolic vessel diameter of each conduit artery was measured in relation to the electrocardiograph displayed on the monitor of the ultrasound unit.

Vessel diameter was also measured under perpendicular insonation and calculated in relation to the temporal duration of the electrocardiography recording curve, as follows: [(systolic vessel diameter × 1/3) + (diastolic vessel diameter × 2/3)] [17-19]. The mean vessel diameter for each beat was calculated over approximately 20–40 beats. Blood flow was determined by multiplying the cross-sectional area [area = $\pi \times$ (vessel diameter/2)^2] by the amplitude (signal intensity)-weighted blood velocity (time- and spatial-averaged outer envelope of the maximum velocity). To determine BF_{Ab} precisely, blood pressure and heart rate should remain in a steady state during measurement of the three target arteries.

3.3. Determination of comprehensive blood flow in lower abdomen

Blood flow in the Ao, LFA, and RFA is defined as BF_{Ao}, BF_{LFA}, and BF_{RFA}, respectively. The comprehensive blood flow in lower abdomen (BF_{Ab}) was calculated by subtracting the sum of BF_{RFA} and BF_{LFA} from BF_{Ao}, as follows: $BF_{Ab} = [BF_{Ao} - (BF_{LFA} + BF_{RFA})]$ [11-15].

4. Day-to-day reliability and variability in hemodynamics of the three arteries and BF_{Ab} via repeated measurements

The variability in the hemodynamics (blood velocity, vessel diameter and blood flow) of the three target arteries is valuable information for determining the comprehensive arterial blood flow in the lower abdomen assessed by Doppler ultrasound. In addition, the reliability and reproducibility in the hemodynamics measurement is also required for its measurement.

Hemodynamic measurements (blood velocity, vessel diameter, and blood flow) in the three arteries were performed on three consecutive days. BF_{Ab} can then be determined for each day by the formula $BF_{Ao} - (BF_{LFA} + BF_{RFA})$, with blood flow calculated by multiplying blood velocity by the cross-sectional area.

Hemodynamic s variable	Target artery	1st		2nd		3rd		Mean CV (%)	Relative reliability, SM-ICC	*F (2, 118, 0.05)*	*p<0.05*
		Mean	SD	Mean	SD	Mean	SD				
Blood velocity (cm/sec)	Ao	26.0	6.6	26.2	6.3	26.0	7.0	4.9	0.94	0.18	ns
	LFA	8.4	2.5	8.3	2.3	8.2	2.5	7.8	0.90	0.48	ns
	RFA	8.4	2.5	8.2	2.2	8.3	2.6	8.7	0.85	1.15	ns
Vessel diameter (mm)	Ao	15.5	1.3	15.6	1.2	15.5	1.2	1.3	0.95	3.63	ns
	LFA	9.0	0.7	9.1	0.7	9.0	0.7	1.4	0.94	3.09	ns
	RFA	9.1	0.8	9.1	0.7	9.0	0.8	1.2	0.97	1.35	ns
Blood flow (ml/min)	Ao	2946	774	2989	740	2931	818	4.9	0.95	1.65	ns
	LFA	322	104	324	105	317	113	8.6	0.90	0.66	ns
	RFA	323	103	317	94	319	106	8.6	0.90	0.57	ns
	Ab	2301	699	2348	666	2295	721	6.2	0.94	1.87	ns

Table 1. Reliability and coefficients of variation in hemodynamics for repeated measurements. Mean coefficients of variation (CV) in hemodynamics were obtained from the average CV values of 60 participants among three repeated measurements over three different days. Single-measure intra-class correlation coefficient (SM-ICC) was evaluated by three repeated measurements over three different days. All measurements were performed by a single operator. SD, standard deviation; ns, not significant; Ao, abdominal aorta; LFA, left femoral artery; RFA, right femoral artery; Ab, lower abdomen. This material is reproduced from Osada T. et al. [12,16], with permission from IOP Publishing Ltd. and BioMed Central.

First, relative reliability was estimated by analysing the three hemodynamic measurements repeated on three different days [12], for 60 healthy male participants [16]. As shown in Table 1, F-test revealed no significant difference in blood velocity, vessel diameter, or blood flow values among the three measurements. Consequently, the single-measure intra-class correlation coefficient was significantly high for relative reliability estimated by repeated hemodynamics measurements [30]. This indicates that Doppler assessment of hemodynamic parameters in the three target arteries has potential as a stable and acceptable procedure for determining BF_{Ab}.

Second, Bland–Altman analysis [31] was used for statistical analysis of mean values (x-axis) and difference values (y-axis) in hemodynamics (blood velocity, vessel diameter, and blood flow) between two measurements over three different days (Figure 4). Figure 4 shows that no systematic bias (fixed bias and proportional bias) was found between any two measurements over three different days. The limits of agreement (mean ± 1.96 SD) in terms of the difference between two hemodynamics measurements and the 95% confidence interval also indicate validity in the present study population within an acceptable and permissible range and true mean values (Table 2). Bland–Altman analysis revealed that the acceptable range in difference (bias) between two measurements may be less than 8.9 cm/s for Ao and less than 5.3 cm/s for blood velocity in the femoral arteries; less than 1.5 mm for Ao and less than 0.95 mm for vessel diameter in the femoral arteries; and less than 1.0 l/min and less than 0.18 l/min for blood flow in the Ao and femoral arteries, respectively. It is considered that this range takes into account day-to-day physiological variation as well as measurement error. The results for repeated measurements on three different days reveals that the range in blood flow values in the three arteries remained similar for individual participants under similar testing conditions; thus, mean BF_{Ab} is considered a reliable value with the acceptable range in difference (bias) between two measurements may be less than 0.9 l/min for blood flow in the lower abdomen. (Table 1, 2; Figure 5).

Hemodynamics variable		Ao	LFA	RFA	Ab
Blood velocity (cm/sec)	Limit of agreement	0.00 ± 8.93	0.00 ± 4.37	0.00 ± 5.24	—
	95%CI	0.00 ± 0.67	0.00 ± 0.33	0.00 ± 0.39	—
Vessel diameter (mm)	Limit of agreement	0.00 ± 1.49	0.00 ± 0.95	0.00 ± 0.77	—
	95%CI	0.00 ± 0.11	0.00 ± 0.07	0.00 ± 0.06	—
Blood flow (ml/min)	Limit of agreement	0.00 ± 1008.42	0.00 ± 186.78	0.00 ± 180.71	0.00 ± 922.08
	95%CI	0.00 ± 75.16	0.00 ± 13.92	0.00 ± 13.47	0.00 ± 68.73

Table 2. Acceptable range in difference (bias) in hemodynamics via three repeated measurements from Bland-Altman analysis. Results are based on 180 samplings (comparison between 1st and 2nd, 2nd and 3rd, and 3rd and 1st measurements) in 60 participants. All measurements were performed by a single operator. The mean difference (bias) in each hemodynamic parameter (blood velocity, vessel diameter, and blood flow) between two measurements almost corresponds to zero. Therefore, the limit of agreement is expressed as 0.00 ± 1.96 SD. The 95% of confidence interval (95%CI) is expressed as 0.00 ± 1.96 SE. Ao, abdominal aorta; LFA, left femoral artery; RFA, right femoral artery; Ab, lower abdomen; SD, standard deviation; SE, standard error. This material is reproduced from Osada T. et al. [12,16], with permission from IOP Publishing Ltd. and BioMed Central.

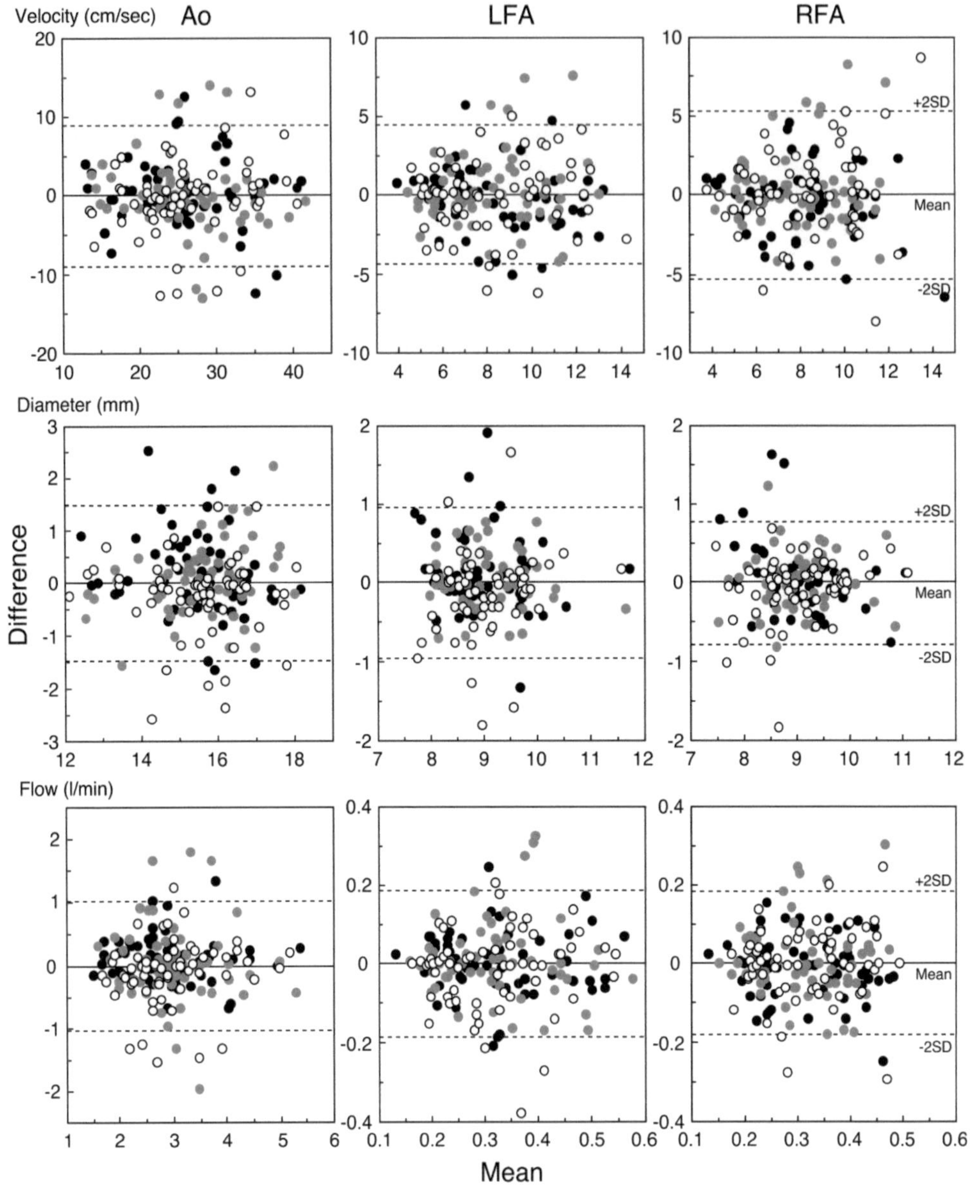

Figure 4. Bland–Altman analysis of three arterial hemodynamics for repeated measurement. The difference (y-axis) and mean (x-axis) are shown for hemodynamics (blood velocity, vessel diameter, and blood flow, respectively) in the three arteries between two measurements obtained over three different days. Results are based on 180 samplings (comparison between 1st and 2nd, 2nd and 3rd, and 3rd and 1st measurements) in 60 participants. The solid line indicates bias (close to zero) and the dashed lines are the limits of agreement of ± 1.96 SD (± 2 SD on the figure). The open circles correspond to 1st *vs.* 2nd measurement. The grey circles correspond to 2nd *vs.* 3rd measurement. The closed circles correspond to 3rd *vs.* 1st measurement. All measurements were obtained by a single operator, using the same ultrasound instrument. Thus, no systematic bias (fixed bias or proportional bias) exists between two measurements. Ao, abdominal aorta; LFA, left femoral artery; RFA, right femoral artery. Reprinted figure and material from Osada T. et al. [12,16], with permission from IOP Publishing Ltd. and BioMed Central.

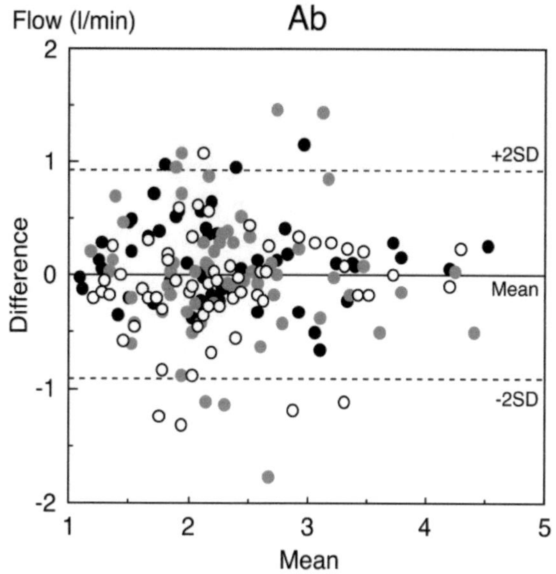

Figure 5. Bland–Altman analysis of blood flow in the lower abdomen for repeated measurements Bland–Altman analysis revealed no systematic bias (fixed bias or proportional bias) between two measurements. The difference (y-axis) and mean (x-axis) in blood flow in lower abdomen (Ab) between two measurements over three different days. Results are based on 180 samplings (comparison between 1st and 2nd, 2nd and 3rd, and 3rd and 1st measurements) in 60 participants. The solid line indicates bias and the dashed lines are the limits of agreement of ± 1.96 SD (± 2 SD on the figure). The open circles correspond to 1st *vs.* 2nd measurement. The grey circles correspond to 2nd *vs.* 3rd measurement. The closed circles correspond to 3rd *vs.* 1st measurement. SD, standard deviation. Reprinted figure and material from Osada T. et al. [12,16], with permission from IOP Publishing Ltd. and BioMed Central.

5. Validity of target arterial blood flows and blood flow in the lower abdomen compared with previous findings

5.1. Abdominal aorta

Values for vessel diameter, estimated cross-sectional area, and blood flow of the upper abdominal aorta obtained in the present method were 15.6 ± 1.2 mm, 1.91 ± 0.29 cm^2, and 2951 ± 767 ml/min, respectively (Table 3).

The present values for diameter and cross-sectional area are similar to those of 15.5–17.6 mm and 1.88–2.43 cm^2, respectively, measured by Gabriel and Kindermann [32]. Nimura et al. [33] reported blood flow values obtained by Doppler ultrasound of the upper abdominal aorta and the sum total blood flow of the coeliac, superior mesenteric and both renal arteries as 2470–3246 ml/min and 2450–3549 ml/min, respectively. These values are similar to those for BF_{Ao} expressed in the present review.

5.2. Femoral artery

The present values for the diameter of the femoral arteries were 9.0 ± 0.7 mm in the LFA and 9.1 ± 0.7 mm in the RFA (Table 3), which is in the same range as the previously reported values of 7.5 ± 0.3 mm measured using angiography [34] and 8.1 ± 0.11 mm measured by Duplex Doppler [35]. In the present review, cross-sectional area of the femoral arteries was 0.65 ± 0.1 cm^2 in the LFA and 0.65 ± 0.11 cm^2 in the RFA. Mean blood velocity in the femoral arteries was 8.3 ± 2.4 cm/s in the LFA and 8.1 ± 2.1 cm/s in the RFA; these values are in the same range as that of 10.2 ± 0.39 cm/s previously measured by pulsed Doppler [35]. Blood flow in the femoral arteries was 316 ± 97 ml/min in the LFA and 313 ± 83 ml/min in the RFA. These values are in the same range as those of 450–886 ml/min [36], 301 ± 81 ml/min [37], and 390 ± 20 ml/min [38] measured using indicator dilution; and 376 ± 154 ml/min [39], 226.5 ± 28.6 ml/min [35], 344 ml/min [40], and 350–367 ml/min [41] measured by Doppler ultrasound. Furthermore, Ganz et al. [42] reported a value of 383–766 ml/min by thermodilution, and Vänttinen [43] reported a value of 239 ml/min using electromagnetic flowmetry. These values are in the same range in those of the present review, despite differences in the method of measurement. Blood flow may also be influenced by the subject's position during measurement and local blood flow per body weight, as well as thigh muscle mass [44].

5.3. Blood flow in the lower abdomen

There is lack of comparative BF_{Ab} data measured by other valid methods (gold standard) such as the thermodilution technique or the cardiovascular magnetic resonance method. However, ultrasound Doppler is also an acceptable valid measure for determining blood velocity/flow in the conduit artery.

Including the results of previous reports [12], the range of BF_{Ab} over the three different days was 1153–4401 ml/min in the 60 participants. Furthermore, the mean value of BF_{Ab} was 2630 ± 649 ml/min in 18 of the participants (age range, 20–38 years) in the previous reports [11].

Based on the general anatomical features shown in Figure 1, the BF_{Ab} values are considered to indicate the sum of blood flow to the coeliac artery; mesenteric arteries; the bilateral renal, suprarenal, gonadal, and internal iliac arteries; and some lumbar arteries.

Previous studies [4,45-47] reported average splanchnic blood flow (including that of the coeliac trunk, superior mesenteric, and inferior mesenteric arteries) as approximately 1500 ml/min, corresponding to 20%–30% of cardiac output. The sum of the blood flow values in the two renal arteries is approximately 1000–1200 ml/min, which corresponds to 20% of cardiac output [48]. In addition, blood flow is 1400 ml/min in the liver, gastro-intestine, and spleen (the so-called splanchnic organs), and 1100 ml/min in the kidney [49]. The range of values for the sum of blood flow in the "splanchnic" and the "two renal arteries" reported in previous studies is similar to the BF_{Ab} values obtained using the present method. However, the wide range in BF_{Ab} may also be related to individual physical features such as body surface area and body weight.

Hemodynamics variable		Ao	LFA	RFA	Ab
Blood velocity (cm/sec)	Mean ± SD	26.1 ± 6.5	8.3 ± 2.4	8.1 ± 2.1	–
	Range	13.9 – 41.1	4.9 – 13.4	4.0 – 12.7	–
	95%CI	24.4 – 27.7	7.7 – 8.9	7.6 – 8.7	–
Vessel diameter (mm)	Mean ± SD	15.6 ± 1.2	9.0 ± 0.7	9.1 ± 0.7	–
	Range	12.4 – 18.1	7.9 – 11.6	7.6 – 10.9	–
	95%CI	15.2 – 15.9	8.9 – 9.2	8.9 – 9.2	–
Blood flow (ml/min)	Mean ± SD	2951 ± 767	316 ± 97	313 ± 83	2323 ± 703
	Range	1585 – 5274	178 – 558	168 – 481	1153 – 4401
	95%CI	2757 – 3145	291 – 340	292 – 334	2145 – 2500

Table 3. Mean values and range for the three arterial hemodynamics and lower abdominal blood flow Mean values are shown for three repeated measurements over three different days in 60 participants. All measurements were performed by a single operator. Ao, abdominal aorta; LFA, left femoral artery; RFA, right femoral artery; Ab, lower abdomen; 95%CI, 95% of confidence interval; SD, standard deviation. This material is reproduced from Osada T. et al. [12,16], with permission from IOP Publishing Ltd. and BioMed Central.

6. The physiological aspect of the three arterial blood flows and blood flow in the lower abdomen

6.1. Relationship of blood flows to body surface area and to body weight

Previous studies have shown that cardiac output increases in proportion to body surface area [49,50], which means that cardiac output is regulated throughout life in almost direct proportion to overall metabolic activity. Furthermore, a positive correlation has been demonstrated between cardiac output and abdominal-splanchnic blood volume, using whole-body scintigraphy [51]. BF_{Ab} is expected to be closely related to body surface area, because the splanchnic system receives ~30% of cardiac output.

A significant positive relationship exists between BF_{Ab} and both body surface area and body weight (Figure 4). The formula used to calculate body surface area is widely used in the target population [52]. Furthermore, an increase in BF_{Ab} with increasing body weight may be reasonable, taking into consideration the total weight of the lower abdomen. This relationship is based on the concept that blood flow distribution is associated with a higher flow per weight to the liver and intestine compared with skeletal muscle at rest [53]. An expected additional finding was that peripheral blood flow at each conduit artery also had a positive linear relationship ($p < 0.05$) with body surface area as well as with body weight (Figure 6). This correlation is in agreement with evidence concerning the relationship between cardiac output supply and peripheral arterial blood flow, with cardiac output being closely related to body surface area [49,50].

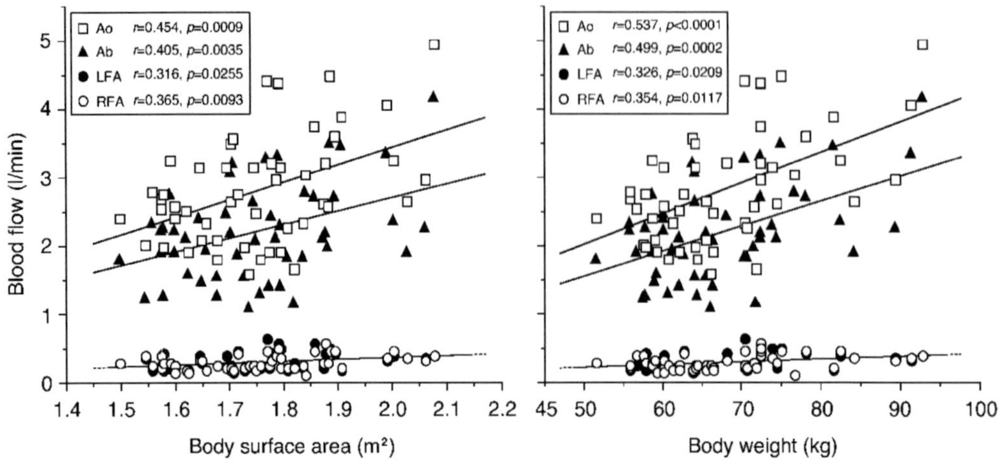

Figure 6. Relationship of blood flows to body surface area and to body weight A significant ($p < 0.05$) positive linear correlation was observed between measured blood flow, and body surface area and body weight for Ao, LFA, RFA, and Ab ($n = 50$). Note overlapping of the circular regression lines for blood flow in LFA and RFA. Ao, abdominal aorta; LFA, left femoral artery; RFA, right femoral artery; Ab, lower abdomen. Figure adapted from Osada T. et al. [13], reproduced with permission from The International Science Literature, Inc.

6.2. Relationship of BF_{Ab} to BF_{Ao}, BF_{LFA}, and BF_{RFA} in estimating blood flow in the lower abdomen

The distribution of BF_{Ab} may be influenced by the magnitude of both cardiac output and limb blood flows. Specifically, it is speculated that alterations in limb blood flow may play an important role in regulating BF_{Ab} via changes in the tone in the vascular bed of abdominal organs during low-intensity exercise when there is little fluctuation in the magnitude of BF_{Ao} [11]. Similarly, it is unclear whether BF_{Ab} or cardiac output at rest has a major impact on limb blood flow in a steady state of neural response.

Day-to-day coefficients of variation in blood flow were relatively high in the femoral arteries compared with BF_{Ao}, even though the absolute BF_{Ao} values were approximately 10 times higher than those of blood flow in both femoral arteries. Accordingly, BF_{Ab} was more strongly related to BF_{Ao} ($r = 0.966$) than to BF_{LFA} ($r = 0.303$) or BF_{RFA} ($r = 0.281$) (Figure 7). Alterations in BF_{Ao} that are closely related to cardiac output (except cerebral and arm blood flows) potentially have the greatest influence on BF_{Ab}, even if blood flow in the femoral arteries has less influence on BF_{Ab}, at least at rest; accordingly, BF_{Ao} potentially has the largest influence on BF_{Ab} as a central hemodynamic factor. Figure 7 shows that precise BF_{Ab} values may be unreliable when there are large variations in both BF_{LFA} and BF_{RFA}. Thus, evaluation of BF_{Ab} may be better expressed by the following formula: BF_{Ab} (l/min) = $0.85 \times BF_{Ao} - 0.19$, if Ao measurement alone is performed (Figure 7).

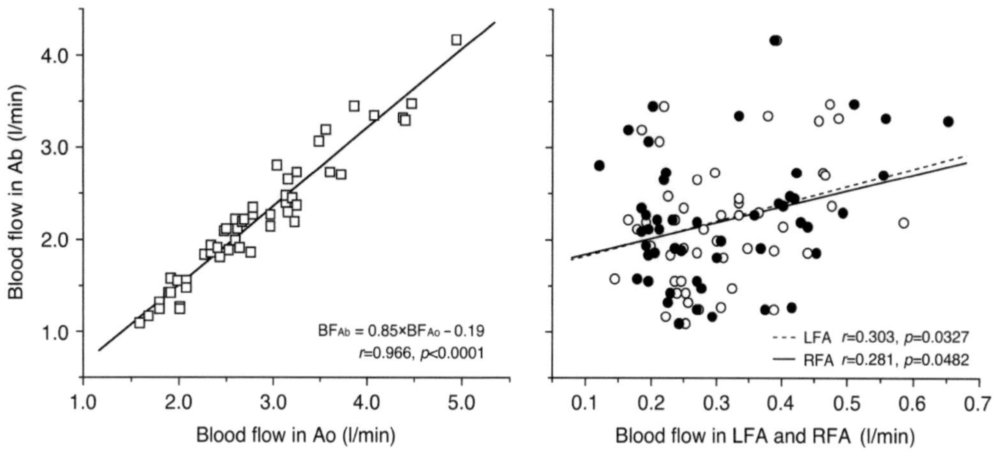

Figure 7. Relationship of blood flow in lower abdomen to the three arteries. BF_{Ab} was more strongly related to BF_{Ao} ($r = 0.966$, $p < 0.0001$) than to BF_{LFA} or BF_{RFA} ($r = 0.303$, $p = 0.0327$ in LFA; $r = 0.281$, $p = 0.0482$ in RFA) ($n = 50$). Ao, abdominal aorta; LFA, left femoral artery; RFA, right femoral artery; Ab, lower abdomen. Blood flow in the Ao, LFA, RFA and Ab is defined as BF_{Ao}, BF_{LFA}, BF_{RFA}, and BF_{Ab} respectively. Figure adapted from Osada T. et al. [13], reproduced with permission from The International Science Literature, Inc.

7. Effect of respiration and posture

Deep thoracic breathing in inspiration produces rapid acceleration of blood flow in veins located near the thorax, such as the hepatic vein, jugular vein, and inferior vena cava [54], while the blood velocity in these veins is reduced just as rapidly at the start of expiration [55]. Mechanical ventilation causing a higher positive end-expiratory pressure-induced increase in lung volume could impede venous return, thereby altering systemic hemodynamics and hepatic venous outflow [56]. In animal experiments, portal vein blood velocity and hepatic arterial blood velocity were shown to decrease with positive end-expiratory pressure as a result of a simple increase in the downstream pressure [57].

Also relevant to the present method are respiratory phase and posture, which are related to alteration in BF_{Ab}, as shown in Figure 8. The difference in BF_{Ab} was approximately 550 ml/min between inspiration and expiration in the sitting position; in the supine position, the difference was 480 ml/min. Blood flow was significantly less in inspiration compared with expiration in Ao, LFA, and RFA, in both the sitting and supine positions. BF_{Ab} was found to be lower in inspiration than in expiration, in both the sitting and supine positions. Respiration-related changes in the hemodynamics of the three conduit arteries potentially lead to alterations in BF_{Ab}. This result may be in partial agreement with the theory that respiratory-induced alteration of BF_{Ab} occurs with impedance of venous return in the splanchnic area.

The change in intra-abdominal pressure during breathing (thoracic-abdominal movement) possibly reflects transient changes in blood velocity in the Ao and femoral arteries. Higher values of venous outflow are found in the hepatic and portal veins in the supine rather than upright position, due to the effect of gravity [54]. In contrast, the reduction of BF_{Ab} in the inspiratory phase is similar between sitting and supine, and thus no postural effect on BF_{Ab} is seen in Figure 8. As the splanchnic circulation is intrinsically susceptible to the adverse effects of hydrostatic force [54,58], redistribution due to postural change between sitting and supine may differ between venous and arterial sites. Respiratory effects should be taken into account in evaluation of BF_{Ab} determined by measurements obtained in the three arteries. The present study demonstrated that changes in blood velocity between expiration and inspiration in the three conduit arteries may potentially indicate alterations in BF_{Ab}, and are only minimally influenced by posture. This phenomenon could be due to mechanical compression of vascular flow perfusion in comprehensive BF_{Ab} or via the vasovagal response. Because respiration and posture effects have an effect when organ perfusion is adequate, it is important not to confuse these effects as a sign of impaired organ perfusion. Evaluation of BF_{Ab} hemodynamics in the three conduit arteries should take respiratory effects into account.

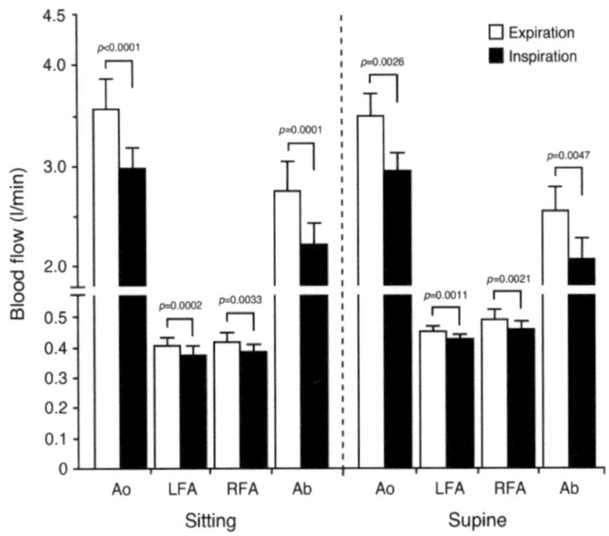

Figure 8. Blood flow in the three arteries and lower abdomen in relation to respiration and posture. Blood flow was significantly less in inspiration compared with expiration in Ao, LFA, and RFA, in both sitting and supine positions. Consequently, blood flow in Ab was lower in inspiration than in expiration, in both sitting and supine positions (n = 10). Values are expressed as the mean ± standard error. Ao, abdominal aorta; LFA, left femoral artery; RFA, right femoral artery; Ab, lower abdomen. Figure adapted from Osada T. et al. [14], reproduced with permission from The International Science Literature, Inc.

8. Redistribution of blood flow in the lower abdomen during/after physical exercise

During exercise, redistribution of blood flow in splanchnic organs is caused by the constriction of the vascular beds that supply oxygen to the working skeletal muscles. Investigations in-

http://dx.doi.org/10.5772/53239

to splanchnic and renal blood flow during stressful conditions, such as exercise, have been carried out in humans [4,5,59,60]. The correlation of splanchnic/renal blood flow and circulatory capacity (oxygen delivery) was validated such that the magnitude in the reduced blood flows was shown to be positive linearly with the increase in percentage of whole maximum oxygen consumption (%$\dot{V}O_{2max}$), as well as heart rate, during whole body high-intensity exercise above 90 beats per minute of heart rate [4,59]. Using the methodology, the magnitude of BF_{Ab} was investigated during low intensity exercise namely one-legged knee extensor exercise (Figure 9). Reduction in the BF_{Ab} also occurred at a low-intensity exercise below heart rate of 90 beats per minute and was closely related to the relative oxygen demand (Figure 9) [11].

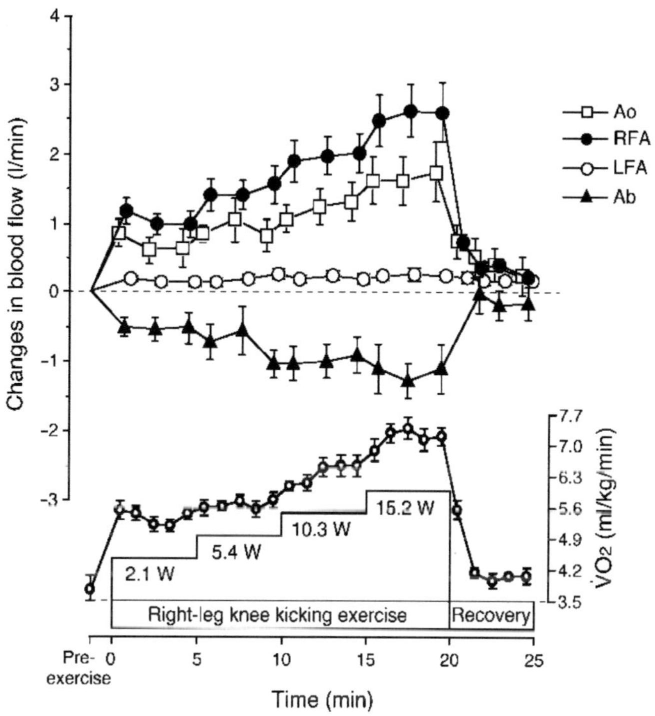

Figure 9. Changes in blood flow in the three target arteries and in lower abdomen and oxygen consumption. The blood flow in the lower abdomen decreased during right leg knee kicking exercise (low-intensity exercise as one-legged knee extensor/flexor exercise) (n = 18). Values are expressed as the mean ± standard error. Ao, abdominal aorta; LFA, left femoral artery; RFA, right femoral artery; Ab, lower abdomen. Figure adapted from Osada T. et al. [11], reproduced with permission from The American Physiological Society.

Furthermore, there is a lack of information on the magnitude in blood flow of splanchnic area in relation to recovery after exercise with various exercise intensities. In the previous study, the magnitude in the mesenteric artery blood flow after running exercise as measured by Doppler ultrasound returned to basal condition according to an exponential curve showing significant reduction until 10 min of recovery [5]. Splanchnic blood flow may not be quickly returning to basal condition immediately after the end of exercise. Consecutively, it is considered that the increase in blood flow to the skeletal muscle (mainly leg) may be partly compensated by the splanchnic organ blood flow not only during but also after exercise. In fact, the mirror image of this effect has been observed in hepatic blood flow and leg blood flow during cycling exercise from 70% to 90%$\dot{V}O_{2max}$ of exercise intensity [61]. This response potentially indicates the shift of blood flow from liver to leg. To consider the redistribution in the lower abdominal blood flow after exercise, blood flow was measured in the Ao and RFA, respectively, after the end of cycling exercise at three levels of exercise intensity (30%, 50% and 85% of maximum oxygen consumption) (Figure 10). The persistence of reduced lower abdominal blood flow after the end of exercise contributes to hyperaemic blood flow in the leg during recovery (after the end of cycling exercise) in proportion to relative exercise intensity and heart rate during recovery.

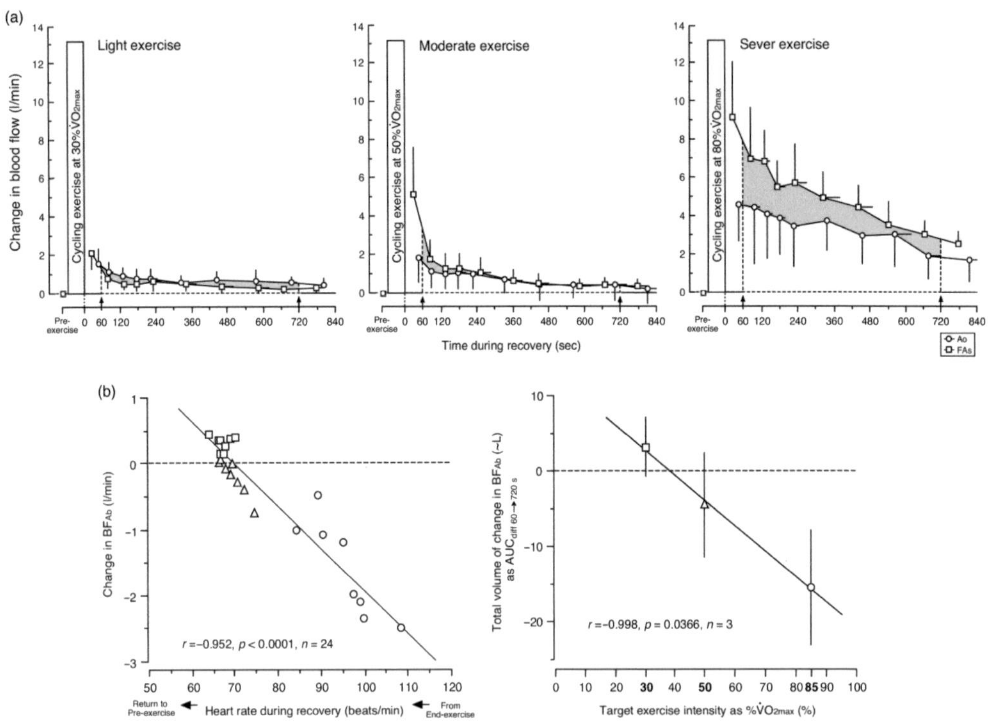

Figure 10. The changes in blood flow for abdominal aorta, femoral arteries and lower abdomen after 6-min cycling exercise, and relationship to heart rate and work load (relative maximum pulmonary oxygen consumption). (a) The change in blood flow was defined as the value compared with blood flow at pre-exercise. The area with gray colour is defined as the difference in area under the curve (AUC_{diff}) between change in BF_{Ao} and those in BF_{FAs} corresponding to contribution of BF_{Ab} (≈ change in BF_{Ab}) shift to persistent hyperaemia in the legs during recovery. The arrows (↑) indicate the AUC_{diff} measurement between 60 and 720 s for the results in b). (b) Heart rate as well as target exercise intensity (%$\dot{V}O_{2max}$) during recovery shows a negative linear relationship with the volume for the reduction in BF_{Ab}.The values expressed in figures are the average data for the 11 subjects at 30%$\dot{V}O_{2max}$, 11 subjects at 50%$\dot{V}O_{2max}$, and 6 subjects at 85%$\dot{V}O_{2max}$. BF, blood flow, BF_{Ao}, BF in the upper abdominal aorta (Ao) above the celiac artery bifurcation; BF_{FAs}, 2-folds of BF in the right femoral artery (RFA); BF_{Ab}, BF in the lower abdomen; %$\dot{V}O_{2max}$, percentage of maximum oxygen consumption. The values are expressed as mean ± SD. Figure adapted from Osada T. et al. [15], reproduced with permission from John Wiley & Sons Ltd.

9. Response in post-prandial state

Many previous studies have demonstrated an increase in the blood flow in the splanchnic area (stomach and small intestine) after digestion. A 38% increase in celiac blood flow rapidly following a liquid food, and a return to normal within 30-60 minutes has been demonstrated [62]. Blood flow in the superior mesenteric artery increased by more than 100% after a solid food and by 63% after a liquid food [63]. The peak systolic and diastolic blood flow increased significantly in coeliac and superior mesenteric arteries after a 710 kcal liquid food. Maximum change in blood flow in the coeliac artery was observed at 40 min and then returned to base value at 60 min, whereas superior mesenteric artery hyperaemia persisted beyond 60 min [64].

Using our method, the increase in BF_{Ab} is also observed after the intake of 1000 kcal solid food (Figure 11). It may be that the food induced functional hyperaemia in the splanchnic area, coeliac and superior mesenteric arteries in lower abdomen. This method may be potentially useful for the evaluation of the comprehensive lower abdominal blood flow vasodilatation in functional hyperaemia regarding nutritious meal intake.

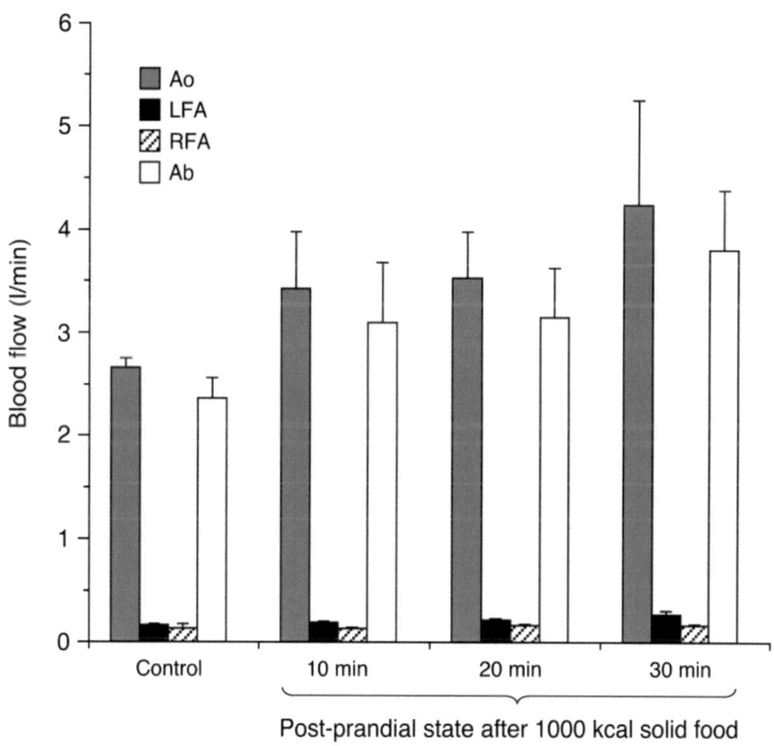

Figure 11. Blood flow in the three arteries and lower abdomen after food intake (post-prandial state). The lower abdominal blood flow increase after 1000 kcal solid food. Unpublished data. *n*=5, Ao, abdominal aorta; LFA, left femoral artery; RFA, right femoral artery; Ab, lower abdomen. Values are expressed as the mean ± standard error.

10. Limitations

The disadvantages of the present methods are that measurement of the three target arteries cannot easily be performed in a short period of time, and that blood flow in the pelvis and other organs (except for the target splanchnic area) cannot be excluded. To avoid over- or underestimation of BF_{Ab}, measurement of the three target arteries should be performed under steady-state conditions at rest, with only minor changes in heart rate and blood pressure.

11. Potential clinical usefulness and application

Evaluation of BF_{Ab} as a quantitative assessment, encompassing physiologic flow, is a potentially useful indicator of 1) reserve blood volume and 2) blood flow in redistribution in the lower abdominal circulation in cardiovascular and hepato-gastrointestinal disease, shock, multiple organ failure, and stressful conditions such as following physical exercise and in the postprandial period. The advantage of the present method is that it enables evaluation of comprehensive BF_{Ab} without interference from intestinal bowel gas, because the three target conduit arteries can be detected relatively easily. It may also be useful for examining pathological hemodynamics, which may influence the abdominal circulation under the conditions of 1) extraordinary hemodynamics associated with abdominal aneurysm; 2) collateral circulation in abdominal-iliac peripheral arterial disease, as well as comparison with the post-operative state; and 3) intestinal neurological dysfunction associated with spinal disorder, in cerebrovascular disease, and in orthostatic hypotension with vasovagal syncope.

Although Doppler methods are less commonly used for quantifying flow in the three target arteries compared with other techniques, the measurement procedure used in the present method is potentially clinically viable. However, because it can be time-consuming to perform routine hemodynamic measurements for the three conduit arteries, measurement may be limited to the region of the femoral arteries around the inguinal ligament close to the genital area, which may not be an acceptable method for general use. It is possible that Doppler ultrasound evaluation of BF_{Ab} using a single vessel (Ao) may enable the necessary information to be obtained (Figure 7). Also of note, because BF_{Ab} values are potentially related to many factors, including mean arterial blood pressure and/or cardiac index, it has potential use as a surrogate parameter for central venous saturation in the clinical setting.

12. Conclusions

The advantage in the described procedure for the determination of splanchnic hemodynamics is that it may potentially enable evaluation of the whole lower abdominal blood flows, assessed by non-invasive measurement using cardiovascular ultrasound. In contrast, it has the disadvantage that measurement of the three target arteries during steady heart rate and blood pressure can be time-consuming, and in measuring blood flow in the target splanchnic area, blood flow of pelvic and other organs cannot be excluded. Respiration and posture related to alterations in BF_{Ab} should be taken into account when measuring the three arteries. Determination of BF_{Ab} by evaluating three-conduit arterial hemodynamics using the technique described in this review may provide a valid measurement that encompasses the comprehensive physiologic arterial blood inflow to multiple abdominal organ systems.

Acknowledgements

The author would like to express gratitude to the deceased Professor Hisao Iwane, as a previous supervisor; Professor Takafumi Hamaoka, as previous co-supervisor at Ritsumeikan University; Dr. Ayumi Sakamoto, as the director of the Tokyo Therapeutic Institute; Mr. Yukihiro Yamamoto of GE Healthcare Japan for his kind support in the initial studies; colleagues Dr. Norio Murase and Dr. Ryotaro Kime; and Professor Toshihito Katsumura, as the present departmental supervisor; and Mr. Eric Sell for his kind assistance. I would also like to thank all of the participants in the studies. This chapter was mainly modified from a recent review article [16] and previous published data reported in original dedicated research.

Author details

Takuya Osada

Department of Sports Medicine for Health Promotion, Tokyo Medical University, Tokyo, Japan

References

[1] Bradley SE, Childs AW, Combes B, Cournand A, Wade OL, Wheeler HO. The effect of exercise on the splanchnic blood flow and splanchnic blood volume in normal man. Clinical Science (London) 1956;15(3) 457-463.

[2] Bradley SE. Variations in hepatic blood flow in man during health and disease. New England Journal of Medicine 1949;240(12) 456-461.

[3] Parks DA, Jacobson ED. Physiology of the splanchnic circulation. Archives of Internal Medicine 1985;145(7) 1278-1281.

[4] Rowell LB. Human cardiovascular adjustments to exercise and thermal stress. Physiological Reviews 1974;54(1) 75-159.

[5] Qamar MI, Read AE. Effects of exercise on mesenteric blood flow in man. Gut 1987;28(5) 583-587.

[6] Christensen NJ, Galbo H. Sympathetic nervous activity during exercise. Annual Review of Physiology 1983;45 139-153.

[7] Alvarez D, Vazquez H, Bai JC, Mastai R, Flores D, Boerr L. Superior mesenteric artery blood flow in celiac disease. Digestive Disease and Sciences 1993;38(7) 1175-1182.

[8] Danse EM, Van Beers BE, Jamart J, Hoang P, Laterre PF, Thys FC, Kartheuser A, Pringot J. Prognosis of ischemic colitis: comparison of color Doppler sonography with early clinical and laboratory findings. American Journal of Roentgenology 2000;175(4) 1151-1154.

[9] Groszmann RJ. Hyperdynamic circulation of liver disease 40 years later. pathophysiology and clinical consequences. Hepatology 1994;20(5) 1359-1363.

[10] Waaler BA, Hisdal J, Eriksen M. Circulatory responses to a meal in patients with a newly transplanted heart. Acta Physiologica Scandinavica 2002;174(2) 101-108.

[11] Osada T, Katsumura T, Hamaoka T, Inoue S, Esaki K, Sakamoto A, Murase N, Kajiyama J, Shimomitsu T, Iwane H. Reduced blood flow in abdominal viscera measured by Doppler ultrasound during one-legged knee extension. Journal of Applied Physiology 1999;86(2) 709-719.

[12] Osada T, Murase N, Kime R, Shiroishi K, Shimomura K, Nagata H, Katsumura T. Arterial blood flow of all abdominal-pelvic organs using Doppler ultrasound: range, variability, and physiological impact. Physiological Measurement 2007;28(10) 1303-1316.

[13] Osada T, Nagata H, Murase N, Shimomura K, Kime R, Shiroishi K, Nakagawa N, Katsumura T. Hemodynamics relationships among upper abdominal aorta and femoral arteries: basis for measurement of arterial blood flow to abdominal-pelvic organs. Medical Science Monitor 2009;15(7) CR332-CR340.

[14] Osada T, Nagata H, Murase N, Kime R, Katsumura T. Determination of comprehensive arterial blood inflow in abdominal-pelvic organs: impact of respiration and posture on organ perfusion. Medical Science Monitor 2011;17(2) CR57-CR66.

[15] Osada T, Iwane H, Katsumura T, Murase N, Higuchi H, Sakamoto A, Hamaoka T, Shimomitsu T. Relationship between reduced lower abdominal blood flows and heart rate in recovery following cycling exercise. Acta Physiologica 2012;204(3) 344-353.

[16] Osada T. Physiological aspects of the determination of comprehensive arterial inflows in the lower abdomen assessed by Doppler ultrasound. Cardiovascular Ultrasound 2012;10: 13.

[17] Rådegran G. Ultrasound Doppler estimates of femoral artery blood flow during dynamic knee extensor exercise in humans. Journal of Applied Physiology 1997;83(4) 1383-1388.

[18] Osada T, Rådegran G. Femoral artery inflow in relation to external and total work rate at different knee extensor contraction rates. Journal of Applied Physiology 2002;92(3) 1325-1330.

[19] Osada T. Muscle contraction-induced limb blood flow variability during dynamic knee extensor. Medicine and Science in Sports and Exercise 2004;36(7) 1149-1158.

[20] Osada T, Rådegran G. Femoral artery blood flow and its relationship to spontaneous fluctuations in rhythmic thigh muscle workload. Clinical Physiology and Functional Imaging 2009;29(4) 277-292.

[21] Osada T, Rådegran G. Determination of limb hemodynamics during rhythmical muscle contractions assessed by Doppler ultrasound. In: Erondu OF. (ed.) Medical Imaging. Rijeka: InTech; 2011. p297-308.

[22] Gill RW. Measurement of blood flow by ultrasound: accuracy and sources of error. Ultrasound in Medicine and Biology 1985;11(4) 625-641.

[23] Holland CK, Brown JM, Scoutt LM, Taylor KJ. Lower extremity volumetric arterial blood flow in normal subjects. Ultrasound in Medicine and Biology 1998;24(8) 1079-1086.

[24] Osada T, Rådegran G. Alterations in the rheological flow profile in conduit femoral artery during rhythmic thigh muscle contractions in humans. Japanese Journal of Physiology 2005;55(1) 19-28.

[25] Osada T, Rådegran G. Alterations in the blood velocity profile influence the blood flow response during muscle contractions and relaxations. Journal of Physiological Science 2006;56(3) 195-203.

[26] Moriyasu F, Ban N, Nishida O, Nakamura T, Miyake T, Uchino H, Kanematsu Y, Koizumi S. Clinical application of an ultrasonic duplex system in the quantitative measurement of portal blood flow. Journal of Clinical Ultrasound 1986;14(8) 579-588.

[27] Leyk D, Eßfeld D, Baum K, Stegemann J. Influence of calf muscle contractions on blood flow parameters measured in the arteria femoralis. International Journal of Sports Medicine 1992;13(8) 588-593.

[28] Isnard R, Lechat P, Kalotka H, Chikr H, Fitoussi S, Salloum J, Golmard J-L, Thomas D, Komajda M. Muscular blood flow response to submaximal leg exercise in normal subjects and in patients with heart failure. Journal of Applied Physiology 1996;81(6) 2571-2579.

[29] Osada T, Katsumura T, Murase N, Sako T, Higuchi H, Kime R, Hamaoka T, Shimomitsu T. Post-exercise hyperemia after ischemic and non-ischemic isometric handgrip exercise. Journal of Physiological Anthropology and Applied Human Science 2003;22(6) 299-309.

[30] Fleiss JL. Statistical methods for rates and proportions. 2nd ed. New York: John Wiley & Sons; 1981.

[31] Bland JM, Altman DG. Statistical methods for assessing agreement between two methods of clinical measurement. Lancet 1986;1(8476) 307-310.

[32] Gabriel H, Kindermann W. Ultrasound of the abdomen in endurance athletes. European Journal of Applied Physiology 1996;73(1-2) 191-193.

[33] Nimura, Y, Miyatake K, Kinoshita N, Okamoto M, Kawamura S, Beppu S, Sakakibara H. New approach to noninvasive assessment of blood flow in the major arteries in the abdomen by two-dimensional Doppler echography. In: Lerski RA, Morley P. (eds.) Ultrasound 82. Proceedings of 3rd Meeting of the World Federation for Ultrasound in Medicine and Biology, 5th World Congress of Ultrasound in Medicine and Biology, 26-30 July 1982, Brighton, England. Oxford: Pergamon; 1983.

[34] Callum KG, Gaunt JI, Thomas ML, Browse NL. Physiological studies in arteriomegaly. Cardiovascular Research 1974;8(3) 373-383.

[35] Fitzgerald DE, O'Shaughnessy AM. Cardiac and peripheral arterial responses to isoprenaline challenge. Cardiovascular Research 1984;18(7) 414-418.

[36] Agrifoglio G, Thorburn GD, Edwards EA. Measurement of blood flow in human lower extremity by indicator-dilution method. Surgery Gynecology and Obstetrics 1961;113 641-645.

[37] Folse R. Application of the sudden injection dye dilution principle to the study of the femoral circulation. Surgery Gynecology and Obstetrics 1965;120 1194-1206.

[38] Wahren J, Jorfeldt L. Determination of leg blood flow during exercise in man: an indicator-dilution technique based on femoral venous dye infusion. Clinical Science and Molecular Medicine 1973;45(2) 135-146.

[39] Reagan TR, Miller CW, Strandness DEJr. Transcutaneous measurement of femoral artery flow. Journal of Surgical Research 1971;11(10) 477-482.

[40] Lewis P, Psaila JV, Morgan RH, Davies WT, Woodcock JP. Common femoral artery volume flow in peripheral vascular disease. British Journal of Surgery 1990;77(2) 183-187.

[41] Hussain ST, Smith RE, Wood RFM, Bland M. Observer variability in volumetric blood flow measurements in leg arteries using duplex ultrasound. Ultrasound in Medicine and Biology 1996;22(3) 287-291.

[42] Ganz V, Hlavová A, Froněk A, Linhart J, Přerovský I. Measurement of blood flow in the femoral artery in man at rest and during exercise by local thermodilution. Circulation 1964;30 86-89.

[43] Vänttinen E. Electromagnetic measurement of the arterial blood flow in the femoropopliteal region. Acta Chirurgica Scandinavica 1975;141(5) 353-359.

[44] Rådegran G, Saltin B. Human femoral artery diameter in relation to knee extensor muscle mass, peak blood flow, and oxygen uptake. American Journal of Physiology Heart and Circulatory Physiology 2000;278(1) H162-H167.

[45] Bradley SE. The hepatic circulation. In: Handbook of Physiology. Circulation, Sect. 2, Volume II. Chapter 41, Bethesda, MD: American Physiological Society; 1963. p1387-1438.

[46] Greenway CV, Stark RD. Hepatic vascular bed. Physiological Reviews 1971;51(1) 23-65.

[47] Hultman E. Blood circulation in the liver under physiological and pathological conditions. Scandinavian Journal of Clinical and Laboratory Investigation 1966;18(Suppl 92) 27-41.

[48] Hollenberg NK. The renal circulation. In: Zelis R. (ed.) The Peripheral Circulation. New York: Grune & Stratton; 1975. p131-150.

[49] Ganong WF. The heart as a pump. In: Review of Medical Physiology. Chapter 29. 21st ed. New York: Lange Medical Books/McGraw-Hill Company; 1998. p567-578.

[50] Guyton AC, Hall JE. Cardiac output, venous returns, and their regulation. In: Textbook of Medical Physiology. Chapter 20. 9th edition. Pennsylvania Philadelphia: WB Sanders Company; 1996. p241-253.

[51] Kiszka-Kanowitz M, Henriksen JH, Moller S, Bendtsen F. Blood volume distribution in patients with cirrhosis: aspects of the dual-head gamma-camera technique. Journal of Hepatology 2001;35(5) 605-612.

[52] Fujimoto S, Watanabe T, Sakamoto A, Yukawa K, Morimoto K. Studies on the physical surface area of Japanese. Part 18: Calculation formulas in three stages over all age [in Japanese]. Japanese Journal of Hygiene 1968;23(5) 443-450.

[53] Åstrand PO, Rodahl K. Physiological bases of exercise. In Textbook of work physiology. 3rd ed. New York: McGraw-Hill Book Company; 1986.

[54] Hsia TY, Khambadkone S, Redington AN, Migliavacca F, Deanfiels JE, de Leval MR. Effects of respiration and gravity on infradiaphragmatic venous flow in normal and Fontan patients. Circulation 2000;102(19 Suppl III) III-148-153.

[55] Abu-Yousef MM, Mufid M, Woods KT, Brown BP, Barloon TJ. Normal lower limb venous Doppler flow phasicity: Is it cardiac or respiratory? American Journal of Roentgenology 1997;169(6) 1721–1725.

[56] Matuschak GM, Pinsky MR, Rogers RM. Effects of positive end-expiratory pressure on hepatic blood flow and performance. Journal of Applied Physiology 1987;62(4) 1377-1383.

[57] Gioia FR, Harris AP, Traystman RJ, Rogers MC. Organ blood flow during high-frequency ventilation at low and high airway pressure in dogs. Anesthesiology 1986;65(1) 50-55.

[58] Culbertson JW, Wilkins RW, Ingelfinger FJ, Bradley SE. The effect of the upright posture upon hepatic blood flow in normotensive and hypertensive subjects. Journal of Clinical Investigation 1951;30(3) 305-331.

[59] Grimby G. Renal clearances during prolonged supine exercise at different loads. Journal of Applied Physiology 1965;20(6) 1294-1298.

[60] Rehrer NJ, Smets A, Reynaert H, Goes E, De Meirleir K. Effect of exercise on portal blood flow in man. Medicine and Science in Sports and Exercise 2001;33(9) 1533-1537.

[61] Nielsen HB, Febbraio MA, Ott P, Krustrup P, Secher NH. Hepatic lactate uptake versus leg lactate output during exercise in humans. Journal of Applied Physiology 2007;103(4) 1227-1233.

[62] Qamar MI, Read AE, Skidmore R, Evans JM, Williamson RC. Transcutaneous Doppler ultrasonic measurement of coeliac axis blood flow in man. British Journal of Surgery 1985;72(5) 391-393.

[63] Qamar MI, Read AE. Intestinal blood flow. Quarterly Journal of Medicine 1985;56(220) 417-419.

[64] Lilly MP, Harward TR, Flinn WR, Blackburn DR, Astleford PM, Yao JS. Duplex ultrasound measurement of changes in mesenteric flow velocity with pharmacologic and physiologic alteration of intestinal blood flow in man. Journal of Vascular Surgery 1989;9(1) 18-25.

Chapter 13

Plasticity of the Visual Pathway and Neuroimaging

M. Gallegos-Duarte, S. Moguel-Ancheita,
J.D. Mendiola- Santibañez, V. Morales-Tlalpan and
C. Saldaña

Additional information is available at the end of the chapter

http://dx.doi.org/10.5772/53013

1. Introduction

Once the formation of cerebral and ocular structures has been completed, the simple light stimulus is enough to activate the necessary neural circuits that integrate the visual tract. It has been estimated that 50% of the cerebral cortex participates in the integration of the human binocular visual system. This system is practically distributed throughout the brain. Therefore, its study has captured the interest of various scientific fields.

The neuronal plasticity of the visual system is the theme of several current works [1, 2, 3]. Nevertheless, very little is known about the adaptive changes and about neuronal plasticity in children who have congenital strabismus (CS), main subject of the current chapter.

The vision is a brain function highly specialized and complex [4]. The structures that perform it are developed by means of division processes, migration, functional integration and regionalization during the corticogenesis [5]. An incorrect development or a bad functioning of the molecular, cellular or physiological mechanisms can induce an altered vision as in the case of strabismus.

The visual process is the result of the elaboration of images generated in the cortical network. This process comprises from the moment the light stimulus reaches the retina until the evocation of visual memories imbued with an affective component generated by the thalamus.

In a simple way, we will say that the visual system is integrated by the visual via and cortical integrator, but in this chapter we will specifically refer to the last one [6, 7]. The visual via takes the information in one direction in an antero-posterior direction. It extends from the eyes as sensorial receptors, arrives to the optical nerves, whose monocular information influences the chiasma, where the nasal sector of the monocular information will perform a crossing of fibers, remaining the temporal fibers without crossing, from this point, the information shared by both eyes continues through the optic bands to the primary visual cortex or striate cortex to systematize the information and generate hyper-complex images [4, 8]. All the steps described, up to now, are considered to form part of the first afferent visual system.

Once the images that have been previously decoded by the striate cortex, in accordance with its temporal frequency space, perceptual-visual process initiates [1, 9]; for that, the visual information must be included in the intern dialog of the brain by means of the cortical network for the purpose of giving it a sense. For that, the information coming from the striate cortex travels through the anterior portions of the brain to be processed in multiple neuronal centers and circuits that shape the cortical integrator [4, 8].

Although the striate cortex is in charge of capturing a great amount of visual elements, it lacks an adequate working memory, for that situation, it results impossible to process the logic of the hyper complex images and give them a ludic sense, to identify and give sense to the environment, it is necessary to resend the information to the working memory sited in the thalamic cortex that adjoins the temporal lobes [4, 8].

Part of the information coming from the grooved area is directed towards the temporal lobes to give a logic sense to answer the question "what am I seeing?" The temporal cortex shares its proximity with the thalamus and auditory areas, because besides de affective sense (like, dislike, danger, repulsion, attraction, etc.) the temporal area processes the visual information to give it directionality [10, 11].

The temporal lobes cooperate with their counterpart of Magno-cellular elements that conform the occipital-parietal via, this last one is the one in charge of assertively answering the question "where is what I am seeing?" the four pathways: left and right occipital temporal as well as the left and right occipital-parietal, give a meaning to the visual information coming from the striate cortex [2, 9].

These associative areas conduct the information that must transform in complex pre-logic elements such as the early recognition of facial expressions or manual attitudes of others (threaten, friendship, indifference), for example, and they are the base for the realization of some specific visual-motor functions such as reading-writing. Once the limbic system adjacent to the temporal lobes, gives affective sense, motivation, and nuance to the visual information, all the observed can be evaluated in relation with other experiences kept in the memory [4, 8, 12].

The cortical integrator works in parallel in an interactive form, as if it were a close cybernetic negative feedback system; its most elaborated product is the binocular vision. It is to be expected that the correct operation and integration of the neuronal visual network depend on an adequate connectivity among the parts that conform the cortical network. In this context, the visual perception is the result of the process of the information that is generated in the neuronal circuits [1, 13, 14].

http://dx.doi.org/10.5772/53013

From this point, all the information is distributed through the cortical network [1, 9] and this is important to consider before analyzing the studies of neuroimaging, by means of a neurometric study [15], electroencephalography [16, 17], or visual perceptual study [18].

Although the CE does not initially affect the superior functions such as judgment or intellect, frequently patients who have this disease may get confused with letters, they require more time to learn to read, are easily distracted, and in general, the development of their activities take more time respecting the individuals with a normal vision. In fact, the children with strabismus present different grades of visual perceptual deficit, which we believe is related with the alterations in the pathway of neuronal interconnection sited in the striate cortex and the cortico-cortical and interhemispheric zones that participate in the processing of the image [6, 15, 17, 19] as it will be forwardly described in the perceptual-visual analysis (Table 1).

Visual perceptual ability	Before the treatment	After the treatment
Fusion Amplitude	-0.4/-0.7	+3 /-1
Stereopsis	0%	0%
Fixation disparity	H: -1.1 V: -0.4	H:-1.1 V: -0.7
Perception Speed	43%	50%
Main elements	88%	95%
Visual memory	87%	93%
Saccadic Movements	72 %	75 %
Shapes and Sizes	42%	80%
Following movements	95%	97%
Peripheral vision	42%	50%
Spatial vision	82%	85%

Table 1. Percentages before and three months after surgery for correction of congenital strabismus H: horizontal, V: vertical.

The Computerized Visual Perceptual Analysis (CVPA) is used to meet the efficiency of visual perceptual system. The CVPA basically estimates the efficiency of the integrator in the posterior portions of the brain, that is, the development of the occipito-temporal and occipito-parietal pathway.

The SPECT (Single Photon Emission Computed Tomography) estimates the metabolic demand of one determined cerebral region, when measuring the energetic demand of the neuronal groups [20, 21]. In these type of studies it is used as a reporter the analog consume of glucose radioactively marked with Technetium-99, which proportionally increments or diminishes based on the functional demand [22], (Figure 1).

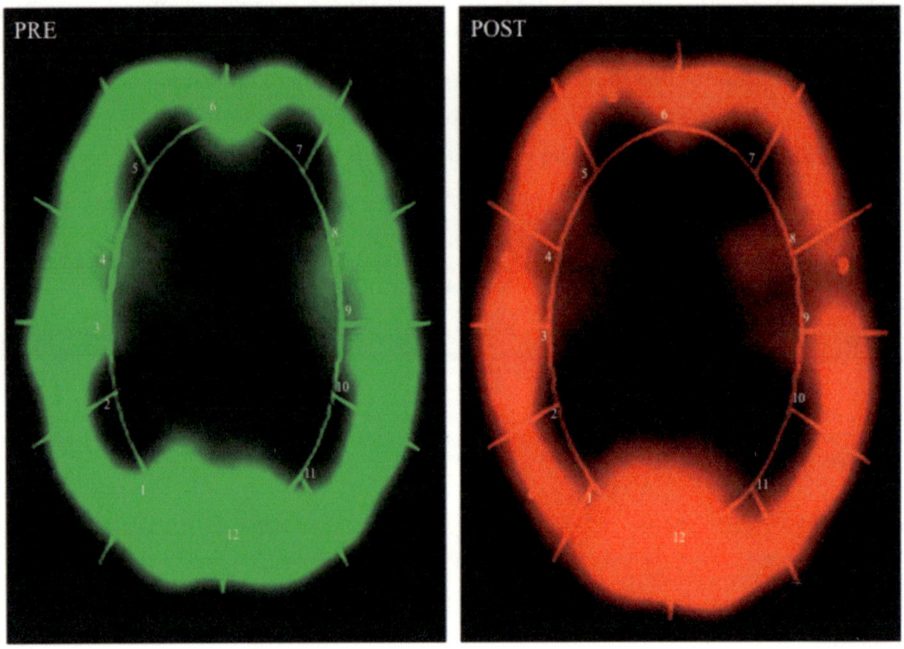

Figure 1. Pictures of the brain SPECT of a girl of 6 years of age. Green shows the status prior to treatment, color red shows the status 4 months after treatment with botulinum toxin. The right hemisphere (left side of the pictures) include zones 1 to 6, from bottom to up and the left hemisphere (right side of the picture) comprises de zones 7 to 12 from bottom to up.

This allows us to get to know the states of normal function, hyperfunction and hypofunction related to the different neuronal groups that work in the specific zones of the brain cortex [20, 21]. In pathologic conditions it is a very useful tool because it indicates us with high precision the normal and affected zones (Figure 2).

The information obtained by means of SPECT has allowed a better understanding of several events referring to the brain behavior and we have used it to determine the behavior and the functional specialization of the visual cortex. The findings that we have found with this methodology have been relevant for the neurology research and specifically to better understand the sickness, and has been helpful to know more about the origin, prognostic, plasticity and improve the life quality in the patients; the neuro adaptive changes that we have found by means of the brain SPECT [23, 24] are next detailed.

The neuronal network generates electric impulses, and this electric activity can be registered by means of the use of the Digitalized Brain Mapping (DBM), (Figure 3), as well as the analysis of the coherence of electroencephalography [25]. These methods provide an objective and noninvasive index of the functional relations that exist between the areas of the brain surface.

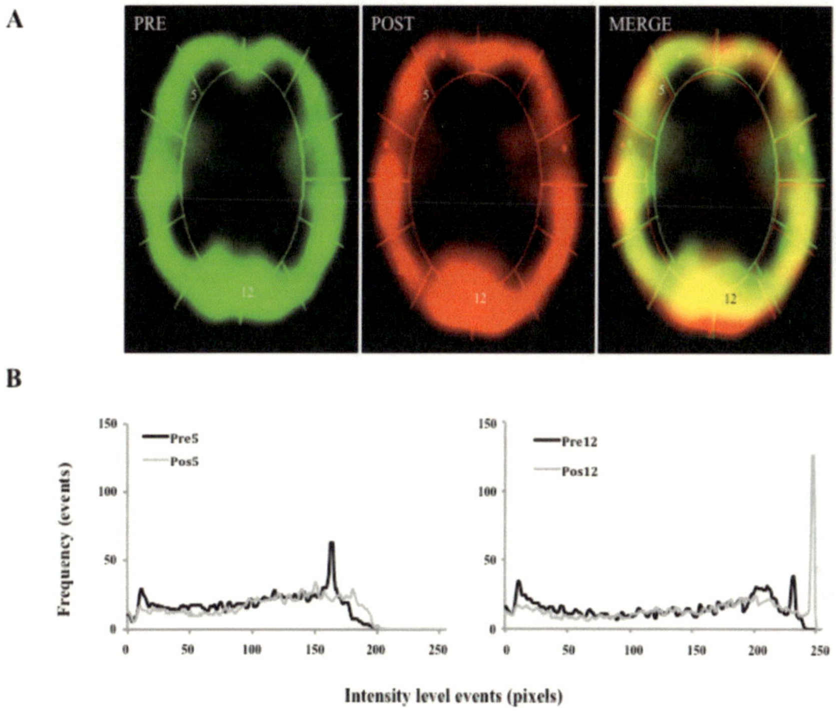

Figure 2. Above, to the right, the picture shows the combination of both studies (MERGE): yellow are those areas that did not suffer many changes, red highlights areas that showed an important metabolic increase (zones 1 and 12), and in shades of green (zones 5 and 9) are those areas that modulated their metabolic activity. At the bottom of the figure, the graphs show uptake of Technetium-99. The black line shows the previous state to the eye alignment by the use of botulinum toxin (Pre), the gray shows the reception levels of the glucose analog 3 months after the treatment (Post). The increase of the uptake after the treatment indicates a greater metabolic activity in V1 and V2. Reception of Technetium 99, the axis "X" shows the intensity level while the axis "Y" indicates the number of times that such intensity is registered

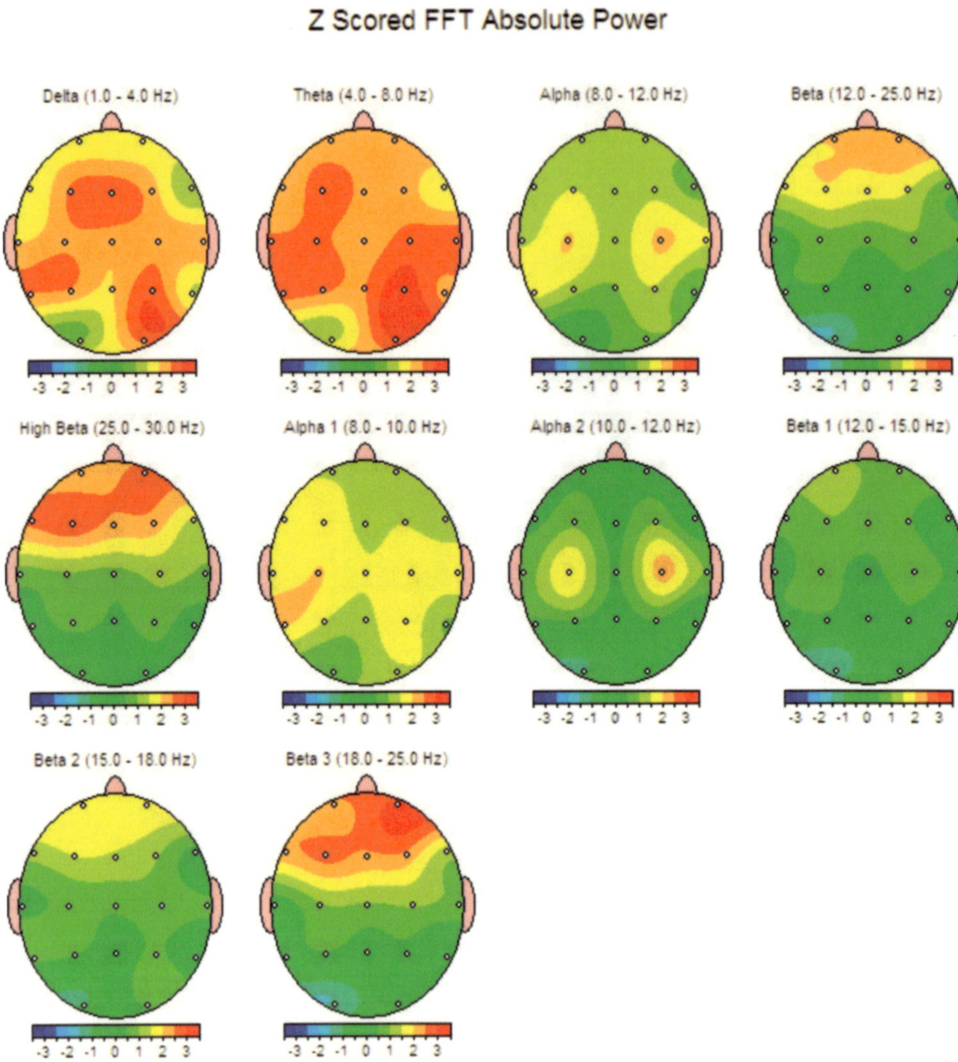

Figure 3. The Brain Mapping shows an increase in the absolute power and hypersimetry in the posterior regions of the brain after the surgery treatment of an 11 years old boy with congenital strabismus. Previous to the treatment he presented slow activity and asymmetry of the background activity in occipital regions.

In a previous study, we reported the results for 193 DBM obtained from children with congenital strabismus [26]. We found that 57% of the patient's studies without treatment presented alterations in the electric behavior that went from mild, such as intertemporal hypo coherence, up to important such as paroxysms and epilepsy, but 6 months after the surgery only 29% of the patients presented alterations in the electric activity (Figure 4). This motivated to perform a more meticulous analysis of the changes of the electric behavior that happen after the surgery by means of Neurometry [15].

http://dx.doi.org/10.5772/53013

Using digitized brain mapping, the authors have discovered morphometric and neurofunctional alterations in the cerebral cortex of patients with essential strabismus, such as intertemporal hypocoherence, cortico-subcortical dysfunction, slowing-down and asymmetry in the frequency, among others (Figures 3 and 4).

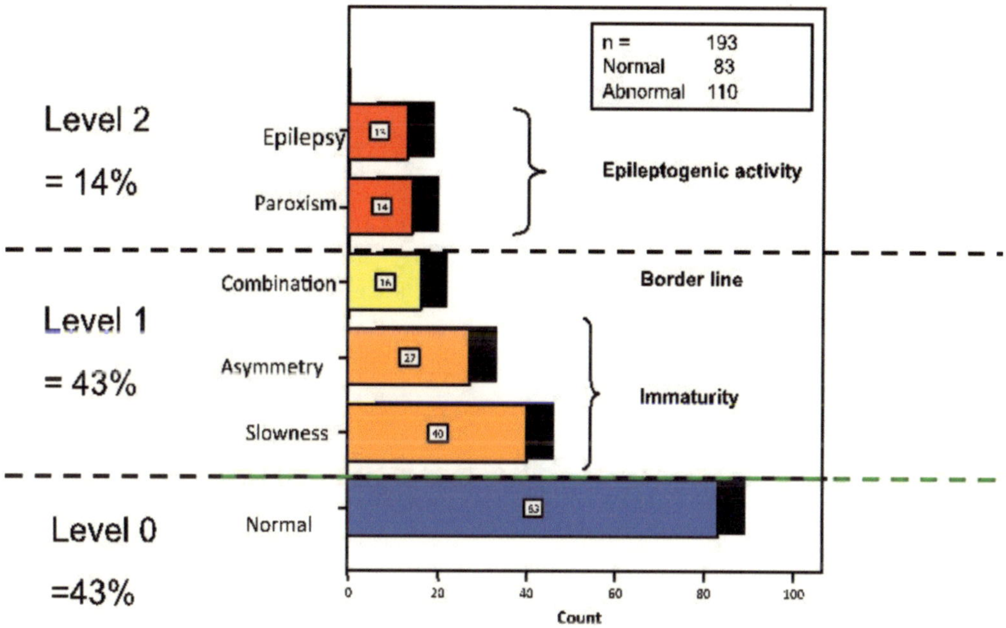

Figure 4. Summary of the reports of the Digitalized Brain Mapping obtained from 193 children with congenital strabismus. The dotted lines separate the sample in 4 levels: 43% were located with a normal electric behavior, 43% in level 1 with low electroencephalographic alterations and 14% presented important alterations

Neurometry allows us to get to know the coherence, which is determined by the activity of the short and large interconnection fibers, intra and interhemispheric, and expresses the synchrony among neuronal groups [15, 27] (Figures 6 and 7). So, meanwhile the hypo coherence expresses the lack of capacity of connection of neuronal groups, the hyper coherence indicates that two or more areas are over connected and work in excessive form. Besides, it allows comparing the obtained results with normative values of the asymptomatic population acquiring a statistical meaning of ±2 standard deviation [26, 15], (Figures 5 and 6).

Z Scored FFT Coherence

Intrahemispheric: LEFT

	DELTA	THETA	ALPHA	BETA
FP1 F3	-0.17	0.78	1.02	1.15
FP1 C3	-1.54	-0.54	-1.76	0.53
FP1 P3	-2.19	-1.58	-1.12	-0.68
FP1 O1	0.42	1.04	1.13	-0.38
FP1 F7	-2.78	-1.79	-0.97	-0.92
FP1 T3	-0.91	-0.19	-0.96	0.18
FP1 T5	-0.11	0.62	0.64	-1.33
F3 C3	-2.29	-1.31	-2.89	-0.52
F3 P3	-2.45	-1.38	-2.25	-1.04
F3 O1	-0.53	-0.66	1.01	-1.40
F3 F7	-1.72	-0.77	-0.78	-0.84
F3 T3	-0.66	0.00	-1.00	-0.13
F3 T5	-1.07	-1.24	-0.13	-1.58
C3 P3	-2.20	-0.89	-1.33	-0.95
C3 O1	-1.65	-2.09	-1.73	-1.65
C3 F7	-1.46	0.03	-0.55	-0.05
C3 T3	-0.13	0.70	0.23	0.28
C3 T5	-2.16	-2.35	-1.49	-1.57
P3 O1	-1.67	-1.98	-0.05	-1.37
P3 F7	-2.09	-0.37	-0.87	-0.40
P3 T3	0.22	1.04	0.50	0.95
P3 T5	-2.02	-1.66	-0.25	-1.35
O1 F7	0.73	0.75	0.68	-2.07
O1 T3	-0.11	-0.56	-0.44	0.30
O1 T5	-1.29	0.07	0.10	0.12
F7 T3	-0.94	0.49	0.26	-0.91
F7 T5	-0.32	-0.72	-0.28	-0.22
T3 T5	-1.14	-0.93	0.09	0.27

Intrahemispheric: RIGHT

	DELTA	THETA	ALPHA	BETA
FP2 F4	-1.03	-1.05	-0.19	0.28
FP2 C4	-2.95	-1.84	-2.84	-0.41
FP2 P4	-2.17	-1.88	-1.31	-1.13
FP2 O2	-0.08	0.31	0.84	-0.60
FP2 F8	-1.99	-2.11	-1.76	-1.48
FP2 T4	-1.39	-1.02	-1.94	-0.26
FP2 T6	-0.85	0.15	0.51	-0.87
F4 C4	-2.85	-1.42	-2.78	-0.53
F4 P4	-2.43	-1.65	-1.84	-1.00
F4 O2	-1.35	-1.12	0.12	-1.49
F4 F8	-1.12	-1.45	-0.83	-0.92
F4 T4	-1.09	-1.07	-1.35	-0.15
F4 T6	-1.27	-1.31	-0.64	-1.30
C4 P4	-2.05	-2.03	-1.27	-1.09
C4 O2	-0.66	-1.37	-1.05	-1.23
C4 F8	-1.51	-1.45	-1.07	-0.58
C4 T4	-0.67	-1.31	-0.07	0.15
C4 T6	-2.31	-2.85	-1.54	-1.85
P4 O2	0.15	-0.04	0.66	0.36
P4 F8	-1.41	-1.42	-1.31	-0.50
P4 T4	0.31	-0.24	0.61	0.62
P4 T6	-1.33	-1.74	0.04	-1.14
O2 F8	-0.11	0.67	-0.19	-1.21
O2 T4	0.44	-0.80	0.40	0.52
O2 T6	-0.58	-0.25	0.74	-0.08
F8 T4	-0.63	0.09	-0.32	0.06
F8 T6	-0.92	-0.68	-1.39	-0.69
T4 T6	-1.23	-1.82	0.13	0.02

Interhemispheric: HOMOLOGOUS PAIRS

	DELTA	THETA	ALPHA	BETA
FP1 FP2	-4.09	-2.77	-1.51	-0.60
C3 C4	-1.47	-1.30	-1.96	-0.92
O1 O2	-0.25	1.51	2.09	2.74
T3 T4	-1.45	0.57	2.26	-0.61

	DELTA	THETA	ALPHA	BETA
F3 F4	-3.54	-3.02	-1.56	-0.80
P3 P4	-0.62	-1.31	-0.15	-1.12
F7 F8	-2.40	-2.47	-2.23	-0.83
T5 T6	0.15	-0.49	0.04	-1.06

Figure 5. Neurometric report before the treatment of the intrahemispheric (up) and interhemispheric (down) coherence analysis of a 7 years old boy with congenital strabismus. The excessive hypocoherence is marked in blue color, the excessive hypercoherence is marked in red. In abbreviation is marked by pairs the zones of interest analyzed (O1= left occipital, T4 = right temporal, as an example).

The Neurometry analysis has enabled us to determine that the following functional relations are altered: occipito-temporal, occipito-parietal and, especially, inter-temporal; the latter includes intra- and inter-hemispheric relations [10, 15, 28]. Similarly, we have employed the brain SPECT technique to define those areas with functional deficits [29, 30].

n a study performed by neurometric analysis we found previous to the surgery treatment of congenital strabismus that 15 of the 16 patients showed everlasting hypocoherence [28]; but after the surgery we found an improvement in this parameter. (Figure 6).

Z Scored FFT Coherence

Intrahemispheric: LEFT

	DELTA	THETA	ALPHA	BETA
FP1 F3	-0.50	0.74	0.83	1.29
FP1 C3	-1.41	-0.29	-1.15	0.07
FP1 P3	-1.86	-0.37	-0.39	-1.12
FP1 O1	-0.88	-1.07	0.40	-1.17
FP1 F7	-1.97	-1.65	-1.01	-0.41
FP1 T3	-0.60	-0.46	-0.72	0.56
FP1 T5	-1.52	-0.84	-0.01	-1.31
F3 C3	-2.48	-0.77	-1.58	-0.78
F3 P3	-1.78	-0.63	-1.43	-1.54
F3 O1	-1.54	-1.45	0.36	-1.41
F3 F7	-1.92	-0.79	-0.78	-0.35
F3 T3	-0.55	-0.13	-0.93	0.32
F3 T5	-1.76	-1.26	-0.35	-0.93
C3 P3	-2.47	-1.58	-2.76	-1.77
C3 O1	-1.70	-1.26	-1.85	-0.91
C3 F7	-1.46	-0.37	-0.27	-0.20
C3 T3	-0.76	-0.01	-0.54	0.63
C3 T5	-2.99	-2.00	-1.69	-1.31
P3 O1	-1.65	-0.39	0.52	-0.06
P3 F7	-1.74	-0.29	-0.66	-0.57
P3 T3	-0.02	0.93	0.66	1.06
P3 T5	-2.37	-0.80	0.29	-0.51
O1 F7	-0.40	-1.11	-0.81	-0.32
O1 T3	0.09	1.43	1.30	2.28
O1 T5	-0.05	1.84	1.58	2.29
F7 T3	-0.88	0.35	0.26	0.39
F7 T5	-1.01	-1.04	-0.62	-0.17
T3 T5	-1.56	-0.33	0.86	0.75

Intrahemispheric: RIGHT

	DELTA	THETA	ALPHA	BETA
FP2 F4	-0.27	-0.08	0.13	0.48
FP2 C4	-1.65	-0.58	-1.60	-0.43
FP2 P4	-1.35	-0.42	-1.24	-0.60
FP2 O2	-0.80	-0.21	1.27	-0.34
FP2 F8	-1.49	-1.67	-1.79	-1.22
FP2 T4	-1.25	-1.12	-2.31	-0.67
FP2 T6	-1.06	-0.13	0.73	-1.16
F4 C4	-2.73	-1.08	-1.69	-1.05
F4 P4	-1.35	-0.38	-1.40	-0.83
F4 O2	-1.66	-0.91	1.02	-0.74
F4 F8	-0.50	-0.59	-0.26	-0.06
F4 T4	-1.33	-1.04	-1.61	-0.64
F4 T6	-1.38	-1.29	-0.39	-1.35
C4 P4	-1.12	-0.33	-0.64	-0.58
C4 O2	-1.43	-1.35	-2.09	-1.42
C4 F8	-1.21	-0.09	0.12	0.33
C4 T4	-1.28	-0.98	-0.40	0.10
C4 T6	-2.55	-2.68	-1.55	-1.33
P4 O2	-1.92	-1.66	-0.79	-1.34
P4 F8	-0.59	0.20	-0.41	0.14
P4 T4	0.76	0.80	1.09	1.18
P4 T6	-2.64	-2.73	-0.49	-1.15
O2 F8	-1.11	-0.14	0.21	-0.71
O2 T4	0.44	-0.66	0.02	-0.01
O2 T6	-1.89	-1.36	-0.01	-0.70
F8 T4	-1.74	-0.67	-0.54	0.08
F8 T6	-1.15	-0.92	-1.44	-0.19
T4 T6	-0.34	-0.38	0.79	1.11

Interhemispheric: HOMOLOGOUS PAIRS

	DELTA	THETA	ALPHA	BETA
FP1 FP2	-3.84	-2.69	-1.88	-1.23
C3 C4	0.03	1.31	-0.85	0.54
O1 O2	-2.47	0.11	0.58	0.85
T3 T4	-1.22	0.83	2.77	0.93

	DELTA	THETA	ALPHA	BETA
F3 F4	-3.17	-2.40	-1.43	-1.10
P3 P4	0.12	-0.19	-0.22	0.12
F7 F8	-1.86	-2.08	-1.89	-0.85
T5 T6	-0.15	-0.45	0.01	-0.61

Figure 6. Neurometric report of the same boy as in figure 9 but 6 months after the surgical treatment. A diminish of the hypocoherence for Delta in frontal regions, an increase of the intertemporal coherences for Alfa and the modulation of the occipito-occipital coherence are observed.

2. Statement of problem

The CS is a neurological disease that manifests as a pathological deviation of the eyes [6, 31]. It represents the maximum perturbation of the binocular visual system and affects 3% of human beings [32, 33]. Due to the sensorial and motor alterations that characterize this disease may be systemized in an accurate manner, and results very simple to correlate the clinic with the neuroimage studies [26].

Given its anatomic and functional repercussions together with its esthetic and social impact, the predominance of CS in humans is patent [34]. In Mexico, where the majority of the population has a mixture of Spanish and Native American origins, this condition is one of the most frequent congenital disabilities [35].

However, one thing is to study the visual tract in healthy subjects and other very different matter is the study of the cerebral cortex of individuals with functional and/or structural asymmetries in their visual system, as happens in patients with essential strabismus. In particular, among our main concerns are the results of surgical and pharmacological manipulations of the extra ocular muscles, which will be addressed in this chapter.

In this manner, strabismus taken as a model of study offers researchers a unique opportunity to gain more insight into the mechanisms the brain uses to compensate the disequilibrium in the cortical network. This network, given the nature of the disease, instead of working in parallel presents peculiarities that should be considered in the study of brain plasticity.

The analysis of the cortical alterations inherent to strabismus has been possible due to neuroimaging techniques. As a result, it has been possible to ascertain, for example, that the fine morphometry in the brain of strabismic children is different from that in healthy children. This is particularly patent in the posterior portions of the brain.

3. Method used

To inquire about the changes that occur in the binocular visual system are analyzed the adaptive changes and brain plasticity before and after the ocular alignment, using the neuroimage studies [36, 37]: SPECT, CVPA, DBM and Neurometry.

To identify these changes, the authors have carried out studies to determine the "before" and "after" in the treatment of strabismus by combining various neuroimaging approaches. As a result, have been identified positive and objective signs of brain plasticity.

To clinically study the perceptual system of the cortical network we use besides the visual acuteness, the CVPA, which examines the 10 basic visual abilities that are detailed in the table 1; these abilities are a reference of the functionality of the visual perceptual system [38].

To get to know the adaptive changes in the perceptual area, we carried out the CVPA on 22 children from 6 to 7 years old before and after the strabismus surgery. These children didn´t received any additional treatment besides the surgery treatment (Table 1).

We have obtained SPECT images previous to the surgery or pharmacological treatment and 4 months after the treatment (Figures 7 and 8). The images were compared to determine the modified area and with that we could localize specifically the metabolic modifications in the several neuronal groups and, afterwards associate them to the neuronal funciton changes in the patients [36].

http://dx.doi.org/10.5772/53013

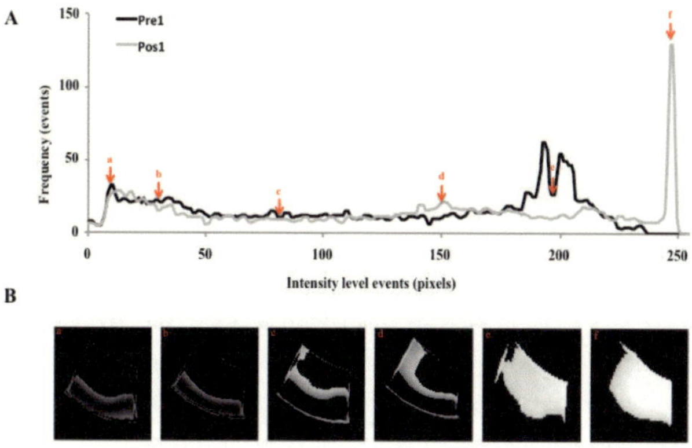

Figure 7. Zone 1 analysis of the SPECT (right occipital) of a 5 years old girl with congenital strabismus. The graphics and photos show the uptake of Technetium-99, the axis "X" shows the intensity level while the "Y" axis indicates the number of times that such intensity is registered. The black line shows the state previous to the strabismus treatment of the first case, and the gray line shows the state after the treatment. This metabolic modulation obeys the neuroadaptative change and the brain plasticity. The pictures show the different zones of interest that that were analyzed (marked in red arrows, has shown in the upper graphic)

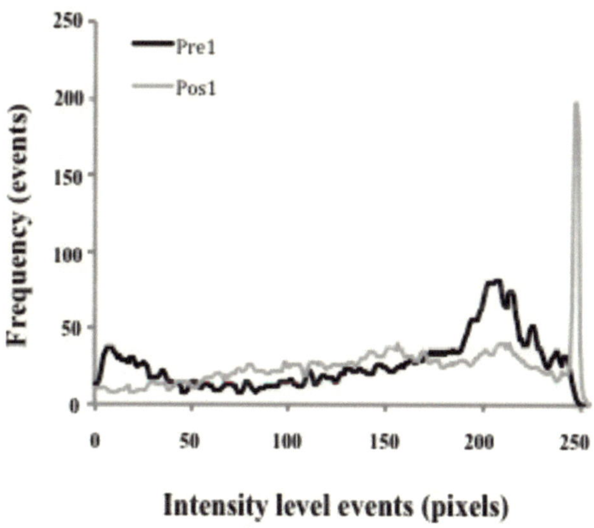

Figure 8. Behavior of the Technetium 99 before and after the treatment with botulinum toxin in a patient of 7 years old with congenital strabismus. The "X" axis shows the intensity level and the "Y" axis shows the number of times that such intensity is registered, the black line shows the previous behavior and the gray line shows the behavior after the treatment. Before the treatment, the zone 1 shows the increase of the density from 183 to 250, after the treatment an important increase is observed in 284, possibly related to the inter-hemispheric connectivity because the patient could obtain a binocular vision

To quantify the neurological adaptative changes related to the CS treatment, it was analyzed and graphed the capturing of the Technetium-99 for the purpose of establishing the grade of hyper and hypo function of the 12 zones of interest. In this communication it is showed the values before and after treatment in the gray scale (Figures 2, 7 and 8).

4. Results

In this study, after the surgery, it was demonstrated a certain recovery in CVPA, some of these changes as is the case of the saccadic movements and the disparity of the fixation were discrete, nevertheless other parameters such as perception of forms and sizes, the magnitude of the fusion or the peripheral vision showed important changes. Up to here, the changes clinically detected by CVPA indicate that there were favorable adaptive changes (Table 1).

From a metabolic point of view, the alterations previous to the strabismus treatment include the presence of hypometabolic regions; these regions show a substantial improvement after the pharmacological treatment with the botulinum toxin (Figures 1, 2, 7 and 8).

The pictures of the brain cortex showed a representative example of the change observed in several patients, in those pictures it is showed the metabolic change in special form, in the same individual before and after the correction of strabismus [4, 36, 37]. The image was divided in 12 sections to locate the prompt changes and to make the analysis easy (Figures 1 and 2).

From a bioelectric perspective, one of the most significant neuro-adaptive changes we have found after the strabismus treatment is an improvement in inter-temporal and inter-parietal coherences (Figure 9 and 10). On the other hand, we have shown the presence of hyper-symmetry and higher efficacy in the cortical input of the primary visual cortex using the Neurometry technique (Figure 11). These findings are in accordance with brain SPECT results (Figures 2 and 8).

When comparing the previous and posterior neurometries to the surgery treatment of 9 patients of strabismus, we found significant changes: improvement in the intertemporal coherences, an occipito-occipital hypersimetry (Figure 11), as well as a diminish in the occipital hyper-coherence, these data suggest that the surgery modifies substantially the connectivity cortico-cotical interhemispheric, as well as an increase in the activity of the striate cortex.

The findings found are congruent with the observed in the brain SPEC, in the sense that after the orientation of the visual axes, it was evident an exponential increase of the metabolism in the cortical areas V1 and V2 responsible of the elaboration of the hyper complex images with the depth sense, and these favorable adaptive changes indicate the presence of neuroplasticity in the binocular visual system in a punctual manner.

http://dx.doi.org/10.5772/53013

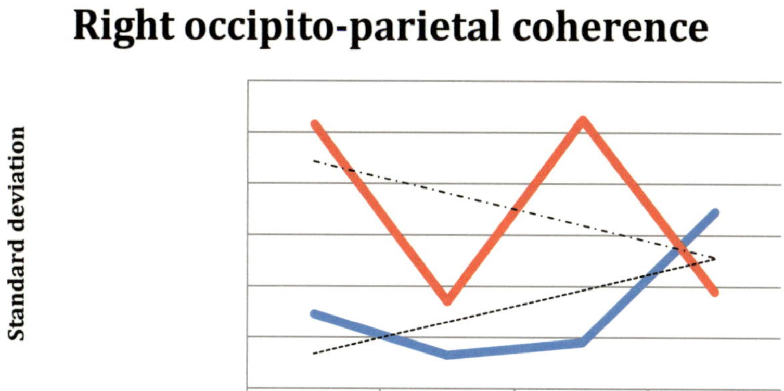

	Delta	Theta	Alpha	Beta
P4-O2 Right pre	-0.71	-0.87	-0.82	-0.31
P4-O2 Right post	0.03	-0.66	0.05	-0.62

Figure 9. Posterior neuroelectric changes to the surgical correction of strabismus in a 5 years old child. A marked hypocoherence in the occipito-parietal via before the treatment is represented with the blue line while the red line shows an improvement for Alfa and Delta after de surgery.

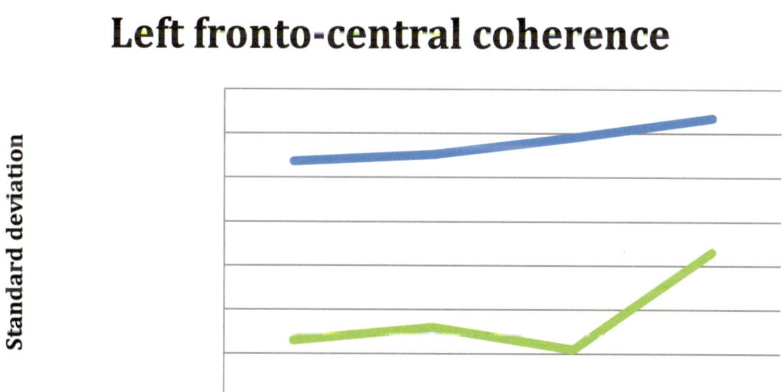

	Delta	Theta	Alpha	Beta
F3-C3 Left pre	1.68	1.76	1.95	2.17
F3-C3 Left post	-0.35	-0.2	-0.45	0.65

Figure 10. Neurometric analysis of a 5 years old child with congenital strabismus. The blue line showed the previous state of hypercoherence and the green line shows the normofuntion 3 months after the treatment.

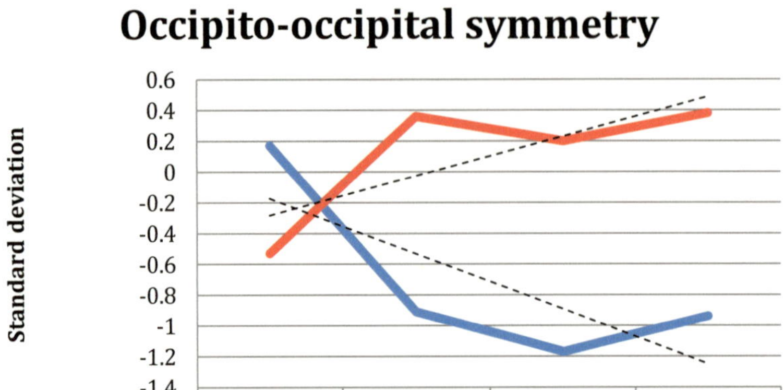

	DELTA	THETA	ALPHA	BETA
01-02 PRE	0.17	-0.91	-1.17	-0.94
01-02 POST	-0.53	0.36	0.2	0.38

Figure 11. Neurometric analysis of a 5 years old boy with congenital strabismus before and 3 months after the strabismus surgery- the blue line shows important occipito-occipital asymmetry before the surgery. The red line shows occipital hypersimetry after the surgery; this hypersimetry is a finding frequently found after the surgical correction of congenital strabismus and indicates an increase in the function of the striate cortex.

5. Discussion

It is highlighted the fact that the human brain has plasticity or capacity to minimize the effects of the injuries through the structural and functional changes [39, 40], and in the best way to evaluate the plasticity, is by means of the clinic situation analysis with respect the previous and posteriors state to the treatment, or more simple, determining a "before" and "after" in the most objective possible mode, and what a better way to do it than by means of a neuro image [36, 37, 41].

To know with more acuteness what happens with the brain plasticity, we have used different functional neuro-image methods such as brain SPECT, the DBM and the Neurometry as we will next see [29, 30, 42].

Although the data obtained through the SPECT are a reflex of the cortical metabolic activity, they don´t measure neither the activity nor the electric connectivity, for such motive it is important to study them by means of other techniques additional to this activity. The combination of both techniques of complementary form allows us to establish with exactness if this events area correlated.

The authors decided to use a combination of three different neuroimaging methods before and after the treatment of strabismus to determine some neuroadaptatives changes in patients with strabismus and have encountered significant neuro-adaptive changes, which we want to share with the reader. In this chapter, we want to share our neuroimaging findings with the international scientific community, as well as our conclusions with regard to this subject.

The idea arose due to evidence that after the correction of the strabismus, the parents reported an improvement in the performance of homework such as reading, playing or writing, without any other different treatment than the surgery or the application of botulinum toxin.

Based on these studies, we have identified metabolic and neurofunctional changes present after the strabismus treatment. This information has shed some light in those neuro-adaptive changes prompted in the cortical integrator as a consequence of the manipulation of the extra-ocular muscles. This evidence has been obtained from neuroimaging techniques.

Regarding this long waited improvement related to strabismus, it is curious that in 1887, George Thomas Stevens had proposed the rehabilitation of an epileptic event and chorea by means of the optical and surgical correction of strabismus. The unusual idea of Stevens to treat in this mode an epileptic event more than one hundred years ago motivated, and not without reason, a scrupulous following for two and a half years to establish a commission of distinguished neurologists pertaining to the incipient neurological society of York. This commission in the middle of a controversial resolution dictated as unjustifiable the offer of the treatment of that doctor [16, 43].

More than once century later, while watching our results, we found three interesting facts related with that controversial proposal of Stevens: a) first of all ,the epilepsy is presented in a relative higer proportion that the general population in children with congenital strabismus, in the same way that some neurological diseases that manifest epilepsy have besides satrabismus [15], b) after the ocular alignement the metabolic and neuroelectrical cortical activity changes positively, c) and finally, the fact that some strabismus manifestations such as the variability or inestability in the deviation angle worsen when a patient with strabismus and epilepsy does not take its medicines but improve when they are under control.

Maybe, Stevens was not so wild as it seem to be on that time; of course that keeping the due distances with what was expected to obtain. We do not suggest that by treating strabismus, the epilepsy is corrected or improved, but now we know that the cortical network can make important adjustments with the purpose to adapt to the new state.

It is now known that patients with congenital strabismus have a greater incidence of presenting depression, suicide, epilepsy, and attention deficit than the general population [4, 6, 15-17]. All indicates that the cortical network is implicated in the origin of strabismus and that the correction of this disease can improve in some way the efficiency of the cortical network.

6. Conclusions

The brain plasticity obeys the brain capacity to diminish the effects of the neuronal damage, being of genetic origin or produced by an injury [44], In spite that the cortical integrator has a specialization level and maximum sophistication, it remains in an invariable state; on the contrary, the studies here shown mark that the plasticity of the visual system to compensate the binocular privation continually present.

The funcitonal observed changes indicate that the simple fact of relocating the eyes in a way that the corresponding areas of the retina are stimulated, allows the cortical network to be in charge of the visual perception.

Effectively, the reactivation of areas relatively silent previous to the correction of the disease indicate that exists a residual capacity of the binocular system to reorganize, improve its connectivity, and the neuroconduction not only through the short and long intra and inter hemispherical interconnection via, but also through zones that comprise great cellular groups and that are capable of reactivating in a relative short time.

The combined use of SPECT, CVPA, DBM and Neurometry allow to best understand the concepts of regional plasticity, distinguishing that at least in the treatment of the strabismus, the occipital symmetry is increased, the metabolism is increased in V1 and V2, diminishes the intertemporal hypocoherence, improves the occipito-temporal coherence and eventually diminished the paroxysms. Clinically diminishes the angular variability, improves the perceptual parameters and in some way we believe that this helps us to contribute to a better visual performance.

As we can see it, the cortical plasticity does not refer simply to repair the damage, but it is a complex strategy of the cortical integrator guided to optimize the resources of the entire network, increasing the efficiency of all the visual system.

Based on all mentioned, we belive that the strabismus instead of being a merely cosmetic problem represents a neurological alteration, and when the treatment is applied involves neuroadaptative changes very favorable for the patient.

Nomenclatures

DBM Digitized brain mapping

SPECT Single Photon Emission Computed Tomography

CVPA Computerized Visual Perceptual Analysis

MERGE combining images computer system

Acknowledgements

The authors wish to thank the Mario Moreno Reyes foundation for the financial support. Jorge D. Mendiola-Santibañez thanks to CONACyT for the financial support, and Carlos Saldaña to PROMEP.

http://dx.doi.org/10.5772/53013

Author details

M. Gallegos-Duarte[1*], S. Moguel-Ancheita[2], J.D. Mendiola- Santibañez[3], V. Morales-Tlalpan[4] and C. Saldaña[1]

*Address all correspondence to: martin_oso@hotmail.com

1 Laboratory of Biophysics of Membranes and Nanotechnology, Department of Biomedical Research, Faculty of Medicine, Universidad Autónoma de Querétaro, Mexico

2 National Medical Center "20 de Noviembre" ISSSTE, Col. del Valle, México

3 Engineering Faculty, Universidad Autónoma de Querétaro, Querétaro, Qro, México

4 Regional Hospital of high specialty of the Bajío, San Carlos La Roncha. León, Guanajuato, México

References

[1] Kusonoki M, Goldberg M.E. The time course of perisaccadic recceptive fields shifts in the lateral intraparietal area of the monkey. J Neurophhysiol 2002; 89:1519-1527.

[2] Ross J, Morrone M.C,Goldberg M.E,Burr D.C.Changes in visual perception at the time of saccades. Trens Neurosci 2001; 24: 113-121.

[3] McCoy PA, Huang HS, Philpot BD. Advances in understanding visual cortex plasticity. Curr Opin Neurobiol 2009;19(3):298-304.

[4] Moguel-Ancheita S, Orozco-Gómez LP. Disfuncionalidad neuronal y psicomotora como retraso en el tratamiento de la ambliopía. Cir Ciruj 2007; 75:481-489.

[5] Bystron I, Blakemore C, Rakic P. Development of the human cerebral cortex: Boulder Committee revisited. Neuroscience. 2008;9: 110-122.

[6] Gallegos-Duarte M, Mendiola-Santibáñez J, Saldaña C. Alteraciones de la sustancia blanca en el estrabismo congénito esencial. Estudio neurofuncional y morfométrico. Acta Estrabológica 2012; 51 (1): 13-40.

[7] Nishitani N, Uutela K, Shibasaki H, Haril R. Cortical visuomotor integration during eye pursuit and eye–finger pursuit. J. Neurosci 1999; 19 (7): 2647–2657.

[8] Wurtz R, Kandel ER. Vías visuales centrales. En: Kandel ER, Schwartz JH, Jessell TM, editores. Principios de neurociencia. 4ta ed. España: McGraw Hill;2000. pp. 524-545.

[9] Merriam E.P, Genovese C.R, Colby C.L. Spatial updating in human parietal cortex. Neuron 2003; 39: 361-373.

[10] Farivar R. Dorsal-ventral integration in object recognition. Brain Res Rev 2009; 61 (2): 144–53.

[11] Bachevalier J, Mishkin M. Visual recognition impairment follows ventromedial but not dorsolateral prefrontal lesions in monkeys. Behav Brain Res 1986; 20: 249–261.

[12] Alvarez P, Squire LR. Memory consolidation and the medial temporal lobe: A simplenetworkmodel. Neurobiology 1994; (91): 7041-7045.

[13] Hall NJ, Colby CL. Remapping for visual stability. Philos Trans R Soc Lond B Biol Sci. 2011; 366 (1564):528-39. Review.

[14] El proceso Cognitivo Cap 2: Publicaciones de la facultad de Medicina de la UNAM. On line: http://www.facmed.unam.mx/publicaciones/otraspub/gea-concurso/Cap2.PDF (accessed 22 mars 2008).

[15] Gallegos-Duarte M, Mendiola-Santibáñez JD, Ortiz-Retana J J; Rubín de Celis B, Vidal-Pineda R, Sigala-Zamora A. Desviación disociada. Un estrabismo de origen cortical. Cir Ciruj 2007; 75 (4): 237-243.

[16] Gallegos-Duarte M, Moguel-Ancheita S. Participación y neuromodulación de la corteza en un caso de estrabismo disociado y epilepsia. Arch Chil Oftalmol. 2006; 63 (2): 199-209.

[17] Gallegos-Duarte M, Moguel-Ancheita S, Rubin de Celis B. Alteraciones en el mapeco-cerebral en la endotropia congénita variable. Rev Mex Oftalmol 2004; 78 (3): 122-126

[18] Visual perceptual learning. Lu ZL, Hua T, Huang CB, Zhou Y, Dosher BA. Neurobiol Learn Mem. 2011; 95 (2):145-51. Review.

[19] Mendiola-Santibáñez JD, Gallegos-Duarte M. Segmentation of the brain and White matter on MRI using morphological connected transformation for the strabismus study. In: Brain Imaging. INTECH Open Access Publishers. p 171-194.

[20] Mullan BP, Oconnor MK, Hung JC, Single photon emission computed tomography brain imaging. Neurosurg Clin N Am 1996; 7(4): 617-651.

[21] Mizoguchi S, Suzuky Y, Kiyosawa M, Mochizuki M, Kacasaki T, Is K, et al. Detection of visual activation of lateral geniculate nucleus by positron emission tomography. Graef Arch Clin Exp Ophthalmol 2003; 241 (1): 8-12.

[22] Ochoa-Madrigal MG, Ortega-Soto H, Valencia-Granados FJ, Cortés-Marmolejo F, Gutiérrez-Trejo MA, Galicia-Tapia et al. Perfusión sanguínea cerebral mediante SPECT en niños con trastorno con déficit de atención con hiperactividad. Neurol Neurocir Psiquiat 2004; 37 (4): 145-155.

[23] Moguel-Ancheita S. Aplicaciones de Toxina botulínica en Estrabismo. Rev Mex Oftalmol 1997; 71(5):194-200.

[24] Moguel-Ancheita S. Tratamiento del Estrabismo con toxina botulínica. Rev Mex Pediatr 2000; 67(4):166-171.

[25] Urretstarazu E, Iriarte J. Análisis matemáticos en el estudio de señales electroencefalográficas. Rev Neurol 2005; 41 (7): 223-434. [35].- Hoyt CS, Good W V. Infantile strabismus: What is it? Where is it? Br J Ophthalmol 1994; 78: 325-6.

[26] Gallegos-Duarte M, Rubio-Chevannier HF, Mendiola-Santibáñez J; Brain Mapping Alterations in Strabismus. Brain Research Journal 2007; 1 (4): 287-337.

[27] Calderón-González PL, Parra-Rodríguez M A, Libre-Rodríguez JJ, Gutiérrez J.V. Análisis espectral de la coherencia cerebral en la enfermedad de Alzheimer. Rev Neurol 2004; 38 (5): 422-427.

[28] Gallegos-Duarte M. Neuroelectic alterations in strabismus. Cir Ciruj 2010; 78 (3): 215-220.

[29] Zeki S, Watson JDG, Lueck CJ, Fristch KJ, Kennard C, Frackowiak RSJ. A direct demonstration of functional specialization in human visual cortex. J Neurosc 1991; 11(3): 641-649.

[30] Marg E. Imaging visual function of the human brain. Am J Optom & Physiol Optics 1988; 65(10): 828-851.

[31] Gallegos-Duarte, M; Estigma y origen de la endotropia congénita. Rev Mex Oftalmol 2005; 79 (1): 10-16.

[32] Engle EC Genetic basis of congenital strabismus. Arch Ophtalmol 2007; 125: 189-195.

[33] A study of heredity as a risk factor in strabismus. Ziakas NG, Woodruff G, Smith LK, Thompson JR. Eye 2002; 16. 519-521.

[34] Michaelides M, Moore AT. The genetics of strabismus. J Med Genet 2004; 41: 641-646.

[35] Hoyt CS, Good WV.: Infantile strabismus: What is it? Where is it? Br J Ophthalmol 1994; 78:325-6.

[36] Moguel-Ancheita S, Orozco-Gómez LP, Gallego-Duarte M, Alvarado I, Montes C. Cambios metabólicos en la corteza cerebral relacionados con el tratamiento de estrabismo. Resultados preliminares con SPECT. Cir Ciruj 2004; 72: 165-17.

[37] Gallegos-Duarte M 2004: Adaptative neurological modifications after medical and surgical treatment of strabismic syndrome with variability in the angle of presentation, may 10, 2004, Spring meeting. French Association of Ophthalmology. Palais du Congrès, Paris, France.

[38] Kavale K. Meta-analysis of the relationship between visual perceptual skills and Reading achievement. J Learn Disabil 1982; (15):1 42-51.

[39] Aguilar-Rebolledo F. ¿Es posible la restauración cerebral? Mecanismos biológicos de la plasticidad neuronal. Plas Rest Neurol 2003; 2 (2): 143-152.

[40] Lobato RD. Historical vignette of Cajal´s work "Degeneration and regeneration of the nervous system" with a reflection of the author. Neurocirugía 2008; 19:456-468.

[41] Pascual-Castroviejo. Plasticidad cerebral. Rev Neurol (Barc) 1996; 24 (135): 1361-1366.

[42] Milner AD, Goodale MA. The visual brain in action. Psyche 1998; 4(12):1-11.

[43] Keane JR. Strabismus surgery for neurological illness. The Stevens commission 1887-1889. Arch Neurol 1989; 46 (3) : 323-4.

[44] Bergado-Rosado JA, Almaguer-Melian W. Mecanismos celulares de la neuroplasticidad. Rev Neurol 2002; 31 (11): 1074-1095.

Chapter 14

Differential Diagnosis for Female Pelvic Masses

Francesco Alessandrino, Carolina Dellafiore,
Esmeralda Eshja, Francesco Alfano, Giorgia Ricci,
Chiara Cassani and Alfredo La Fianza

Additional information is available at the end of the chapter

http://dx.doi.org/10.5772/53139

1. Introduction

The female pelvis is an anatomic region which is quite complex, because it contains some organs and systems accomplishing different and independent functions. The uro-genital system represents the main part of the female pelvis but there are also portions of other organs and systems such as some important blood vessels, gastrointestinal tracts, lymphatics, nerves and parts of the musculoskeletal system. All these structures might house or generate pelvic masses even in para-physiologic conditions, and not necessarily because of current diseases, or congenital alterations, inflammatory illness and tumours.

In order to understand the nature of a pelvic and/or abdominal mass it is necessary to collect as many as possible clinical data. A clinical classification constitutes the first step for finding out the aetiology. The age is indicative for diseases linked to different functional periods of the reproductive system; clinical history must investigate upon possible previous tumours, infectious or metabolic diseases and surgery. When collecting clinical history, pelvic pain which can be divided into acute, chronic and cyclic, must be directly addressed; alterations of body temperature, gastrointestinal symptoms (nausea, vomiting, diarrhoea, constipation, hematemesis, melena), urinary tract symptoms (oliguria, polyuria, stranguria, hematuria, urinary retention, incontinence), taste disturbance; pharmacological treatment in progress (anticoagulants), previous radiotherapy must be addressed.

The are several gynaecological causes responsible for pelvic tumours. These are reported in table 1.

SITE	DISEASE
Ovary:	endometriosis
	organic and functional cysts
	benign and malignant cancers
	metastasis
Fallopian tube:	tubo-ovarian abscesses, pelvic inflammatory disease
	hydrosalpinx
	para-ovarian cysts
	ectopic pregnancy
	neoplasm
Uterus:	uterus body neoplasm
	fibroma
	malformations
	blood-pyometra

Table 1. Gynaecological abdominal-pelvic masses with malignant clinical features.

It has also to be taken into account the possibility that a non gynaecological lesion could be responsible for a mass. In table 2 the principal non-gynaecological causes for pelvic and abdominal swellings are reported.

The role of medical imaging

The best examination in a clinical context is undoubtedly suprapubic and endovaginal ultrasonography. In young patients, especially in those who are in the reproductive age, ultrasonography shows the best accuracy in the differential diagnosis of ovarian and hydrosalpinx cysts, of the ectopic pregnancy, of uterine fibroids [1].

Ultrasonography permits to distinguish correctly between a benign and a malignant adnexal mass and, within these groups of diseases, to give an accurate diagnosis in most of the cases.

Nevertheless ultrasonography isn't free from errors and limitations. Diagnostic errors are probable in the identification of masses which appear solid at US. In these cases is difficult to evaluate the uterine or ovarian or the extra-gynaecologic origin of the lesion. These cases require CT or MRI scan. In particular MRI has proven to be useful in detecting and staging of gynaecological malignancies and in detecting the origin of extra-gynecological pelvic masses [2].

http://dx.doi.org/10.5772/53139

SITE	DISEASE
Gastro-intestinal tract	appendicular abscess
	neoplasms
	diverticulitis, peridiverticular abscess
	Crohn's disease, segmental ileitis
	impaction
	mesenteric cysts
Urinary tract	pelvic kidney
	bladder globe
	urachus cyst
	bladder tumours
Miscellany	lymphadenopathy
	peritoneal carcinomatosis
	musculo-skeletal tumours
	organ ectopia (migrant spleen)
	pelvic vessel aneurysms
	foreign bodies
	pelvic dysmorphisms
	complications of previous surgery
	hematomas
	musculo-skeletal inflammations

Table 2. Abdominal-pelvic extra gynaecological masses with malignant clinical features

2. Intra peritoneal extra gynaecological masses

2.1. Digestive system

They are intra peritoneal masses which originate from the gastrointestinal system, are localized in the pelvis and concern essentially tumours and inflammatory diseases. It is to be taken into account that, especially in adolescents and old patients who have a very long sigma, the loop can be palpated in the pouch of Douglas simulating, when full of faeces, an ovarian neoplasm.

In adolescents this condition can be caused by colon-sigma non-ganglionic diseases (megacolon), where the altered peristalsis implies an abnormal accumulation of faecal material. This condition can also imply the invagination of intestinal traits which is not so infrequent especially in old patients. Among the digestive system diseases, which very frequently can simulate a gynaecological neoplasm, we count inflammatory diseases (acute and chronic) and tumours.

2.2. Inflammatory diseases

An acute, but mainly chronic, inflammation could cause the clinical evidence of an abdominal-pelvic mass and the reasons are the following:

- formation of adhesions in intestinal loops, causing wall thickening and rigidity, sub mucosa and mesentery bleeding and oedema, inflammatory reaction of peritoneum and adjacent omentum.
- bowel perforation and formation of peri-visceral phlegmon; in some cases the wall breaking causes the bleeding of an important vessel and shows the symptoms of haemorrhagic or peritonitic acute abdomen.

These anatomic-pathological aspects correspond to different CT scan findings, classified by Hinchey and his team in 4 stages, depending on the inflammation extension [3]:

- Stage 0: inflammatory thickening of the intestinal wall, with oedema of the mucosa, luminal-stenosis, the inflammation being still circumscribed within the bowel wall.
- Stage I-II-III: abscesses, unique or multiple, showing sometimes air-fluid level images connectible to liquid necrosis; generally these abscesses are adherent to the intestinal wall, or to the peritoneal folds. Such a picture corresponds to the condition of the diffusion of the inflammation beyond the visceral wall.
- Stage IV involves intestinal perforation and faecal invasion of the peritoneum (Figure 1).

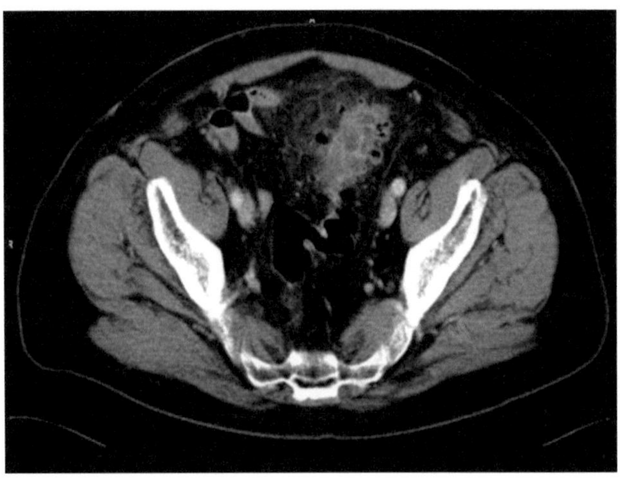

Figure 1. Contrast enhanced CT scan, during a portal phase showing an inflamed sigma, with perforated diverticulum in the medial side of the sigma.

http://dx.doi.org/10.5772/53139

The intestinal inflammation (whether circumscribed or widespread) might cause fistulas with adjacent anatomical regions and/or the most declivous portions of the pelvis such as the vagina and the rectum. The fistula is often the first symptom of the intestinal wall inflammation.

Besides, in patients with generalized sepsis, CT scan is useful for correctly positioning of drainage pipes into the abscesses in order to clean them up by saline and antibiotic washes [4].

2.3. Neoplasms

Sigma-rectum tumours determine swellings of the left adnexal site, but they may also occupy the whole pelvis or the central portion of it. These tumours might appear as solid masses stenosing the intestinal trait where they originate from, or, rarely, masses with mainly extra luminal development.

Not infrequently, the tumoural mass associate with an intestinal inflammatory disease. Nonetheless, the mesenteric vessel congestion and the presence of small perivisceral liquid collections, appear to be the CT scan signs which are most related to diverticulitis and, to a lesser degree, tumours.

When the neoplasm does not involve the pelvic organs the CT scan diagnosis is simple and easy, showing the reproductive system integrity. Thought not infrequently, an intestinal primitive neoplasm may strictly stick to, and infiltrate the uterus; there might also be observed adnexal neoplastic masses which are not in direct continuity with original neoplasm (Figure 2).

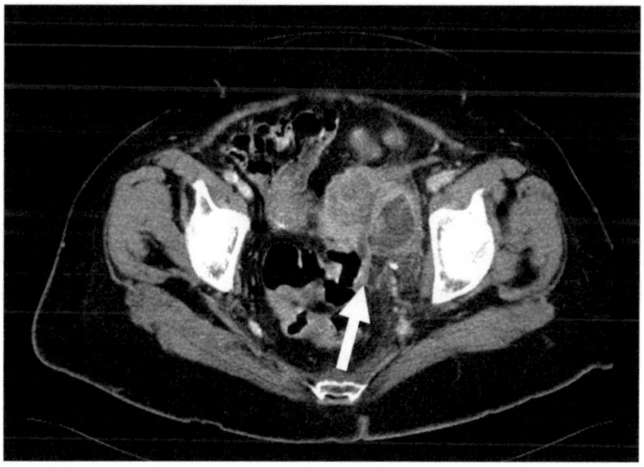

Figure 2. Preoperative axial contrast enhanced CT scan during late phase showing a mass growing in the left ovary (white arrow). An adjacent mass is seen in in the sigmoid colon.

In these cases CT scan is unable to discriminate between a primitive ovarian neoplasm with peritoneal metastasis infiltrating the sigma-rectum, and a primitive intestinal tumour with adnexal metastasis (Krukenberg disease).

2.4. Intra peritoneal foreign bodies

The presence of foreign bodies into the peritoneal cavity represents a not so infrequent finding; they are a consequence of surgical malpractice and that's why they're also known as "gossypiboma". A "textiloma" is a complex made of a non- biodegradable foreign body plus the surrounding reactive tissue [5].

The pelvis can be site of textiloma either because of pelvic or abdominal surgery. In fact the position of the textiloma is affected by the omentum causing the foreign body phagocytosis with consequent fibrinoid-granulomatous reaction and strong adhesions. In this case the textiloma remains into the abdomen. If the surgery implies the removal of the omentum then the textiloma can move to the pelvis. In the case of pelvic surgery, the gossybipoma seems to have greater possibilities of changing its original position and moving either to the pelvic or the abdominal peritoneal cavity.

Recently, in operating rooms, sterile gauze with a radio-opaque marker is being used.

Ultrasonography might be useful in the differential diagnosis of garzomas; they appear as cystic masses, containing the foreign body in their core, with a rather irregular morphology and completely reflecting ultrasonic waves.

At CT scan the finding of a solid mass containing helical, or vortex-like opacities, or the presence of differently dense micro nodules, sometimes calcified, are very suggestive of textiloma. The solid part might be expression of the exudative reaction, while the fibrinoid reaction has a less specific meaning. After c.m. administration a slight peripheral enhancement of the pseudo-capsula. In this case the differential diagnosis with abscesses is very difficult.

At MRI they appear as a solid mass hypointense on T1 and hyperintense on T2, with no specific morphologic features [6].

2.5. Ascites

Very rarely some intraperitoneal liquid collections might be considered as reproductive-system originating tumours. This may happen under particular conditions: patients who underwent previous surgery for abdominal masses; in the cases of intraperitoneal treatment with radioactive drugs where are present so strong adherences causing intraperitoneal fluid flow alterations. Bags of peritoneal effusion may also appear, and they are correctly identified by ultrasonography as liquid masses that can be exchanged as intraperitoneal masses. CT scan results better in defining the liquid bag topography which has low density values (0-10 HU), excluding, more safely, the possibility for the mass to be an intraperitoneal cyst.

2.6. Peritoneal pseudomixoma

It is the accumulation of mucinous material into the peritoneal cavity. It is due to peritoneal metastatic lesions secreting mucin; in most of the cases the principal cause is a mucinous ovarian neoplasia, but less frequently pseudomixomas can be due to malignant mucocele of the appendix and tumours of the stomach, of the colon, of the pancreas and of the breast.

http://dx.doi.org/10.5772/53139

The pseudomixoma typical CT scan appearance is a hypodense, liquid mass localized among the intestinal loops; sometimes, inside the lesions, can be observed images of septa or solid buttons. The HU values range between 15 and 30.

2.7. Mesenteric panniculitis

It's a primitive disease of the mesentery, with intraperitoneal and pelvic metastasis. It is defined as macrophage inflammatory infiltration of the mesenteric fat associated with scar-fibrous component. When this last element prevails, it is defined as liposclerosis. Panniculitis might be also consequent to previous abdominal surgery or radiotherapy.

CT scan is decisive for diagnosis: a fatty mass incorporating some mesenteric vessels without infiltrate them; the mass is homogeneous, circumscribed by a peripheral pseudocapsule well delimited. MRI fat suppression sequences further discriminates the fat components from the liquid ones. These aspects can be unique, affecting portions of the abdominal-pelvic peritoneum with multiple foci.

2.8. Intraperitoneal tumours

Tumours of omentum and intraperitoneal spaces originate from the tissues which constitute these structures: coelomic epithelium, mesothelium, fiber, fat and muscle connective tissue, lymphatic and blood vessels, nerves, embryonic residues. Usually, lesions in these sites are due to primitive abdominal tumours, especially intestinal and ovarian. Therefore, given an intraperitoneal neoplastic mass, it has first to be considered as a metastasis unless a primitive tumoural lesion is found elsewhere.

Peritoneal tumours can be cystic (dermoids, lymphangiomas, benign and borderline serous, micropapillary cystadenomas) and solid (serous, micropapillary cystoadenocarcinoma, malignant mesothelioma, small round cell desmoplastic tumour, fibroma, desmoids tumour, and others). Tumours morphology is often non-specific both at US and CT scans; It might appear either solid or cystic depending on the kind of tissue they are made of. In some casese they cannot be distinguished from mesenteric cysts. The more are the solid component and the complex aspect, the more must be the suspect of the mass being malignant.

3. Extra/retro peritoneal originating extra gynaecologic masses

3.1. Urinary system

In pre-ultrasound age was the most frequent pelvic mass the pelvic kidney originating from urinary system, an extremely easy ultrasound diagnosis even in the gynaecologic area. It is also possible that a pelvic supernumerary kidney leads to the same error.

Occasionally, great kidney-originating masses spreading to the pelvic retro peritoneum can simulate reproductive-system tumours; the same goes for huge cysts, or gigantic hydronephrosis. CT scan and MRI can, instead, easily establish the urinary-system origin of the retroperitoneal lesions.

Other causes for urinary-system originating extra-gynaecologic masses are malformations resulting from Müller ducts alterations associated to Wolff ducts malformations. The most frequent are represented by uterus didelfus with blind hemi-vagina. In the latter the mass is constituted of blood and mucus blocking the vagina. There might also originate some pockets of pelvic endometriosis, which are expression of abdominal reflux of vital endometrium. Finally, even an atresic hemi-horn, with or without communicating endometrium, can be a pelvic mass.

A bladder globe might resemble a pelvic mass in patients who underwent radical hysterectomy surgery or radiotherapy which damaged the bladder innervation and caused large stagnation. The bladder can also be site of extrinsic-diffusion tumours, or huge pseudo-diverticula resembling adnexal masses.

The urachus may be a site of inflammatory processes. Cysts are caused by persistence, of the intermediate tract of the urachus, after birth which doesn't communicate with either the bladder or the navel and therefore may house a very slow-growing liquid collection. It appears macroscopically as a spherical, cystic formation with muscular-fibres and urothelium-constituted walls containing clear, citric liquid and urea. It might be an occasional finding during an ultrasonography or a CT exam. The middle position, the front site (between the Linea Alba and the parietal peritoneum) and the round appearance can easily suggest the origin. These cysts, if inflamed, might be confused with pelvic inflammations.

3.2. Alterations of the sacral canal

By these terms are meant malformations of the sacral canal which is the inferior portion of the vertebral canal. In the sacral canal are contained the spinal meninges, the final portion of the cauda equina and the epidural space between the meninges and the bone walls; often such malformations associate with alterations of kidney, bladder and urinary system-growth. The malformation that is most simulating an adnexal pelvic mass is the anterior, sacral meningocele. This is constituted of meningeal herniation through anterior defects of the sacrum-coccyx. They can be either unique or associated with more complex malformations of the terminal thread, as in the caudal regression syndrome, in the generalized mesenchymal dysplasia (neurofibromatosis type 1 or Marfan syndrome).

The mass appears as a simple cyst, homogeneous and anechoic at US.

CT scan, but mainly MRI can precisely detect the origin of the lesion. It is possible to study the alterations of the sacrum, anterior defects, and the whole morphology of the sacrum-coccyx using sagittal reconstruction with CT. The mass is like a simple cyst, with no enhancement and without capsule.

The main signal characteristic is T2 hyperintensity at MRI. Finally, both CT and MRI is able to perfectly detect the neck of the meningocele (Figure 3).

http://dx.doi.org/10.5772/53139

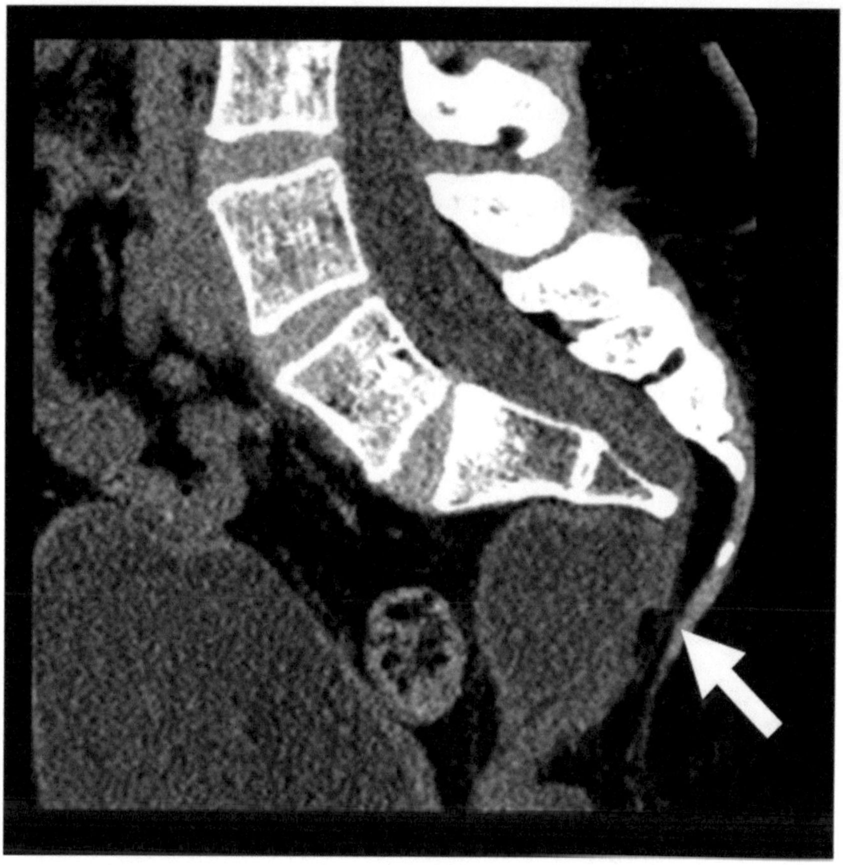

Figure 3. MPR sagittal reconstruction of a CT scan showing an anterior sacral meningocele direcly connected to the medullar canal.

3.3. Pelvic, retroperitoneal tumours

From pelvic retroperitoneum can originate benign or malignant tumours, whose histology might cover all the tissues normally present in the retroperitoneum, mesenchyme: sarcomas, leiomyosarcomas, fibrosarcomas; adipose tissue: lipomas, liposarcomas; nervous system: benign and malignant schwannomas, paragangliomas, neurogenic tumors; hemangiomas: mature and immature teratomas.

The evaluation of these masses is difficult by US. The most preferred techniques are still CT and MRI.

CT imaging appearance is that of a solid mass, only rarely homogeneous in density; it is so mainly as far as neurologic benign tumours (benign schwannomas) or masses rich in well-differentiated striated muscle component (neurofibromas) are concerned. Malignant masses are inhomogeneous, infiltrating the retroperitoneal structures.. Edged and regular contours, the footprint of the surrounding structures without infiltration suggest the benignity.

The masses rich in fatty component, given their retroperitoneal origin, are usually histologically malignant and aggressive; these masses must be distinguished from all pelvic intraperitoneal lipomas. Factors of malignity are represented by the inhomogeneity, the infiltrative character of the edges and the presence of a rich, solid tissue component.

Neurofibromas are solid, neurogenic benign tumours which show enhancement in CT. Both CT and MRI are the first-choice techniques of investigation in the suspect of a pelvic, retroperitoneal mass; this is due to their ability in the topographic localization of the mass and the good ability in the tissue characterization. Probably MRI reaches higher results in the diagnostic accuracy (easy characterization of lipomas, liposarcomas and mature teratomas). If a definitive diagnosis can't be reached by CT or MRI, then guided needle biopsy can be useful. In figure 4 a MRI scan of a schwannoma is presented.

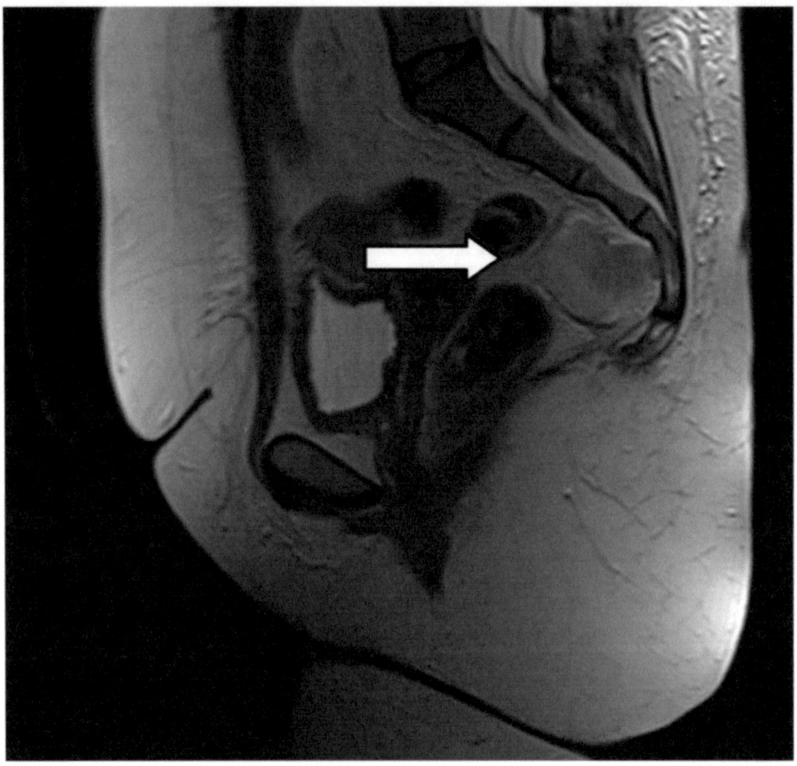

Figure 4. MRI T2-weighted sagittal scan showing a retroperitoneal oval-shaped solid lesion (white arrow) in straight contact with the anterior part of the sacrum, which turned out to be a schwannoma.

They must be considered, finally, other rare, non-gynecological causes for pelvic masses, represented by neoplasias originating from different tissues of the pelvis. We can therefore report some cases of anterior abdominal wall muscles fibromas, pelvic sarcomas, aneurysmal dilatation of the iliac vessels.

http://dx.doi.org/10.5772/53139

4. Tumoural markers

It has been proved that serum Ca^{125} are helpful in the diagnostic evaluation of pelvic masses, particularly in adnexal masses.

An increase (ranging from 80 to 90%) of Ca^{125} serum levels are associated with ovarian, epithelial, malignant, non-mucinous tumours. Besides, Ca^{125} is related to the volume of the tumour mass. Ca^{125} represents the gold standard tumoural markers for ovarian cancer in two different clinical conditions: as a diagnostic tool for evaluating the risk of malignancy of an adnexal mass and as a monitoring tool in the evaluation of the disease state, in patients already treated for adnexal cancer [7,8].

Ca^{125} serum levels equal or below 35 U/ml are normal. Ca^{125} serum levels greater then 50-65 U/ml (in the 80-90% of postmenopausal patients) is associated with a malignancy. Classifying patients with increased Ca^{125} and a pelvic mass by age, permits a rise in positive predictive value of the association of 80% in patients older then 50 and only 50% in younger ones.

On the other hand this marker increases (in 60-70% of the cases) also in advanced endometrial adenocarcinoma and/or in recurrence.

Other gynaecological malignant solid tumours can increase Ca^{125} serum levels (60% in pancreatic cancer, 20-25% in breast, lung and colon tumours). Other non tumoral conditions can be associated with increased levels of Ca^{125} such as endometriosis, peritonitis, tubo-ovarian abscess, diverticulitis, adenomyosis, uterine fibroids, ascites.

Best specificity and sensitivity results have been reached by integrating different diagnostic techniques like markers and ultrasonography and clinical history to create risk index [9].

5. Gynaecological masses: Assessment of malignity/benignity criteria based upon morphologic and multiparametric ultrasonography

Female pelvic masses are mainly caused by gynaecological diseases. For classificatory purposes it's important to know whether the disease originates from the uterus or from the ovaries. This is often difficult to establish, that's why we tend to use another classification based on malignity/benignity criteria. In this case, the main goal of the radiologist is to characterize the mass from a histological point of view, using different imaging techniques.

The imaging main parameters are:

- size and shape;
- vascularisation;
- associated signs.

As far as size is concerned we can say that the bigger the ovarian mass, the higher is the probability that that mass is malignant.

As far as shape is concerned it must be considered the presence of septa, solid components (papillary excrescences) and mass echogenicity.

The presence of septa highly increases the probability of malignity. This finding becomes more relevant when associated with the thickness of the septa.

The presence of papillary excrescences or solid lesions inside or outside a cystic mass is highly suggesting of malignity.

Ultrasonography permits distinguishing between cystic or solid masses. A certain mass is defined as cystic when the content echogenicity is liquid, with back wall shadowing. On the contrary, a completely solid mass is characterized by more or less homogeneous, multiple internal echoes, giving it a parenchimal-like appearance. Generally speaking it can be said that the higher the echogenicity of a mass the higher the risk of malignity.

In table 3 the most important echographic morphological criteria for the definition of malignancy scores are reported.

Simple ovarian cyst, very likely to be benign:	diameter of less than 5 cm
	thin, smooth walls
	anechoic content
	lack of septa or less than 3, thin septa
	no liquid into the Douglas space
	no solid intracystic vegetations
Complex ovarian cyst likely to be malignant:	diameter greater than 5 cm
	smooth, thick walls
	hypoechoic or solid, homogeneous content
	more than 3 thin septa
	a bit of liquid in the Douglas space
	no solid, intracystic vegetations
Malignant ovarian cyst:	diameter greater than 5 cm
	thick, irregular, nodular walls
	many thick septa
	intracystic, solid component
	intraperitoneal carcinomatosis

Table 3. Echographic morphological criteria for the definition of malignancy scores.

http://dx.doi.org/10.5772/53139

Morphological scores for the prediction of malignancy of the masses have been made up by ultrasonography.

Historically the parameters evaluated were size (currently it is considered an adnexal mass a lesion with a diameter greater than 4 cm), echogenicity (considering the masses as solid, simple cystic, complex cystic), presence and shape of septa (single or multiple, whether or not associated with vegetating solid components adhering to them), and persistence over time of the tumour.

Since 1974, Kobayashi reported a 70% diagnostic accuracy of ultrasound in the differentiation of ovarian cancer from other pelvic tumours. The presence of papillae, nodules and thickened septa within cysts were elements suggestive of malignant adnexal disease [10]. In 1979 De Land showed how the risk of malignancy increased linearly with the increase of the solid component within the mass [11]. More recently, Hermann, in 1987, classified the pelvic masses into three categories in relation to the morphological complexity: simple cystic forms, complex forms and solid forms [12].

In 1989 Grandberg went another step further, precisely defining others parameters. He defined: the number of the intracystic papillae, the solid, intracystic component percentage and the presence of septa, reporting the malignancy risk percentage for each of those parameters [13].

In 1990 Jacobs tried to introduce a multifactorial score for the diagnosis of malignancy. He did it considering: the gynecological examination, the trans-abdominal ultrasound and the determination of serum Ca^{125}. It was devised an echographic-morphological score assigning the value 1 to each parameter: multiloculated cyst, presence of solid spots, evidence of metastasis, presence of ascites, bilateral adnexal lesions. All these parameters were included in an analysis that showed how statistically significant were the age, the postmenopausal status, the ultrasound score, the Ca^{125} value and the clinical impression. This score has been defined as RMI (risk of malignancy index) [14]. In 1992 Kuriak linked flow metric data obtained by Colour Doppler to the morphologic score proposing a multiparametric score [15].

Recently, in 2011 a new scoring sistem was proposed called Pelvic Masses Score (PMS). It takes into account the Sassone score, the base 10 logarithm of the Ca^{125} level, the central/septal vascular distribution, the menopausal state and the resistance index [15, 16,17].

Currently, morphological scores have been extensively used in clinical practice mainly because they allowed a better morphologic characterization of pelvic masses.

The vascularisation of a pelvic mass is the second element for a diagnosis of malignancy. Once again, ultrasonography represents the first step in the evaluation of this data. The echo color Doppler examination of a pelvic mass has to be performed when there are masses which are strongly suspected to be malignant. Clearly benign masses don't need such examination. Nevertheless the echo color Doppler examination may be very useful in the interpretation of a mass which isn't clearly benign [15].

The pathogenic factor that justifies the use of colour Doppler in the differential diagnosis of a pelvic mass nature, is represented by the fact that the tumour's new vessels lack a muscular coat, and that causes low resistance to blood flow, generating low Pulsatility Index and Resistive Index values and absence of diastolic notch.

Besides it has to be considered that the flowmeter samples must be multiples and collected from different parts of the mass, that is, not only from the periphery but, more importantly, from the core of the mass. In fact, we believe that many malignant tumours tend to start the new vessel production from the centre of the mass, while peripheral lesion vessels may result from preexisting vessels. A peripheral vascularization of the mass is basically benign, often deriving from ipsilateral uterine artery. Intralesional vascularisation and the presence of vessel in the solid component of the mass or in the septa or papillae, are elements that strongly suggest malignancy. The vascular confluence represents another indication of malignancy [18].

6. Ovarian benign and malignant tumours: Anatomical and pathological classification

Malignant ovarian tumours represent the fifth death cause among US female population; the sixth neoplasia for frequency, the second, most frequent female tumour after endometrial ones and the first death cause as far as gynaecologic tumours are concerned [19].

This illness is more frequent in peri-or post-menopausal women, but there are characteristic histological types for each age group. In adolescents and in women who are younger than 20, half of the tumours comes from germ cells; in post menopausal age they have a most frequent epithelial origin.

The causes for the occurrence of ovarian cancer are not defined; epidemiological studies show that the most affected people by ovarian cancer are represented by peri or post-menopausal, middle or upper class, with no children or just one and with problems in getting pregnant women.

The majority of ovarian tumors begins without well-defined symptoms; as a matter of fact early stages are mostly incidental findings representing just a 20%. In most of the cases they are diagnosed when they are at an advanced stage, that is when the cancer has spread outside the pelvis. The most common symptoms are given by the effect on neighbouring organs: polyuria, dysuria, constipation, sudden increase in abdominal circumference, amenorrhoea, polymenorrhea.

In table 4 WHO histological classification of the tumours of the ovary is presented.

http://dx.doi.org/10.5772/53139

TYPES	SUBTYPES
Surface epithelial-stromal tumours	Serous tumors
	Mucinous tumors
	Endometrioid tumors (including variants with squamous differentiation)
	Clear cell tumours
	Transitional cell tumours
	Squamous cell tumours
	Mixed epithelial tumours (specify components)
	Undifferentiated and unclassified tumours
Sex cord-stromal tumours	Granulosa-stromal cell tumours
	Sertoli-stromal cell tumours
	Sex cord-stromal tumours of mixed or unclassified cell types
	Steroid cell tumours
Germ cell tumours	Primitive germ cell tumours
	Biphasic or triphasic teratoma
	Monodermal teratoma and somatic-type tumours associated with dermoid cysts
	Germ cell sex cord-stromal tumours
Tumours of the rete ovarii	Adenocarcinoma, adenoma, others
Miscellaneous tumours	Small cell carcinoma, Hepatoid carcinoma, Wilms tumours, others
Tumour-like conditions	Luteoma of pregnancy, Stromal hyperthecosis, Stromal hyperplasia, Fibromatosis, others
Lymphoid and haematopoetic tumours	Malignant lymphoma, Leukemia, Plasmacytoma
Secondary tumours	Gastro-intestinal tract (stomach, colon, pancreas), Breast, Renal cell carcinoma, Melanoma, Others

Table 4. WHO histological classification of tumours of the ovary.

7. FIGO staging

Ovarian tumours spread by contiguity, through the intra peritoneal route, by blood and lymphatic. 9% of cases in advanced stage show intra peritoneal carcinomatosis, and 70% ascites.

In table 5 the ovarian tumour FIGO staging is reported [19].

The adnexal masses invasion by contiguity is the direct infiltration of the adjacent anatomical structures. Hence the bladder can be involved through neoplastic deposits in the vesico-uterine fold. The sigma-rectum can also be involved through the rectovesical pouch. In both cases the tumour infiltration very rarely reaches the mucosa.

The intraperitoneal tumour spreading follows the physiologic routes. The most affected sites are: the rectovesical pouch, the para-colic gutters (especially the right one), and the right sub-diaphragmatic peritoneum.

The omentum, through its phagocytic function, collects cancer cells and constitutes an ovarian cancer typical site for cell proliferation. Lymphatic drainage of the ovary in the pelvis and, in the para aortic zone through the infundibulum pelvic ligament, permits the pelvic and lombo-aortic lymphatic metastatic spreading. Neoplastic emboli, reach the left subclavian vein through the thoracic duct, penetrate into the bloodstream and stop in the lung. Pulmonary involvement happens directly through both ovarian veins and the pelvic venous plexus. Upper abdominal metastases (most of the cases liver and spleen) seem to be related to blood-borne neoplastic emboli originating from the sigmoid and superior haemorrhoidal plexus.

STAGE	DESCRIPTION
I	**Tumour limited to ovaries**
IA	one ovary affected, no ascites, absence of capsular infiltration, absence of neoplastic proliferations on the outer surface of the mass;no malignant cells in ascites or peritoneal washings.
IB	Tumour limited to both ovaries; capsule intact, no tumour on ovarian surface; no malignant cells in ascites or peritoneal washings.
IC	Tumour limited to one or both ovaries with any of the following: capsule ruptured, tumour on ovarian surface, malignant cells in ascites or peritoneal washings
II	**Tumour affecting one or both ovaries with pelvic extension**
IA	Extension and/or implants on uterus and/or tube|s|;no malignant cells in ascites or peritoneal washings
IB	Extension to other pelvic tissues; no malignant cells in ascites or peritoneal washings
IC	Pelvic extension (2a or 2b) with malignant cells in ascites or peritoneal washings
III	**Tumour involves one or both ovaries with microscopically confirmed peritoneal metastasis outside the pelvis and/or regional lymph node metastasis**
IIIA	Microscopic peritoneal metastasis beyond pelvis
IIIB	Macroscopic peritoneal metastasis beyond pelvis 2 cm or less in greatest dimension
IIIC	Peritoneal metastasis beyond pelvis more than 2 cm in greatest dimension and/or regional lymph node* metastasis
IV	**Distant metastasis (excludes peritoneal metastasis)** Note: Liver capsule metastasis is T3/stage III, liver parenchymal metastasis M1/stage IV. Pleural effusion must have positive cytology for M1/stage IV.
NOTES	The classification applies to malignant surface epithelial-stromal tumours including those of borderline malignancy. (Non-epithelial ovarian cancers may also be classified using this scheme). *. Regional lymph nodes are the hypogastric (obturator), common iliac, external iliac, lateral sacral, para-aortic, and inguinal nodes.

Table 5. Ovarian tumours FIGO staging

http://dx.doi.org/10.5772/53139

8. Indications for CT scans and MRI.

The use of CT and of MRI in the preoperative phase of malignant ovarian tumours it's a debated argument even today. A correct diagnosis can be done using only ultrasound, as reported in this chapter. However, it is essential to know the CT and MRI appearance of these tumours mainly because they are easy to compare in investigations performed for other purposes.

In literature there are numerous publications which compare ultrasound, CT and MRI for their ability to distinguish between malignant and benign pelvic masses. The CT reaches a specificity and sensibility of about 92,8 and 88% respectively based on the morphology of the lesions and their vascularization after the injection of Contrast Material [20,21].

In our Institution all MDCT studies were performed using a 64-multislices MDCT system (Somatom Sensation 64, Siemens medical solutions, Forchheim, Germany). MDCT images were obtained from the abdomen and pelvic, covering the area from the diaphragm to the symphysis pubis (craniocaudal). The contrast medium (IOVERSOL 350 mg /ml – Optiray, Covidien Imaging Solutions, Hazelwood, MO) was administered at a dose of 1.5 mL per kg, with a variable flow rate of 3-4 mL per second through the antecubital vein of the right arm.

MRI with paramagnetic contrast Material, on the other hand, not only distinguishes better gynaecological lesions from non-gynaecological ones, but also allows a better tissue characterization of the mass. The CT aspect of an ovarian malignant mass is characteristic though, as ultrasound, it is not able to define the anatomical-pathological variant. The mass can be localized exclusively in the adnexal site or, if size is conspicuous, involve the entire pelvic region. Sometimes, when the whole pelvis is filled with the tumour, it is impossible to make out the adnexal origin. The masses are usually complex with thickened and often nodular walls. Not infrequently there are numerous intralesional septa delimiting different chambers which vary in density and are not communicating with each other. Solid components, usually growing in the liquid section of the mass, are often present at the confluence of the thickened septa. An ovarian cancer very rarely infiltrates the retroperitoneal pelvic structures reaching the bone wall.

Even though it's large and closely adjacent to bladder and bowel, this cancer very rarely fully infiltrates these structures' walls, and if there were infiltrations they'd just involve some peritoneal folds and the rectovesical pouch. The nodular peritoneal dissemination can be correctly evaluated by CT scan in the presence of ascites which facilitates the detection of nodules adhering to the intestinal tract and between the mesenteric sheets. The parenchymal nodules adhering to hepatic peritoneum, gastro-colic, gastro-duodenal and spleno-gastric ligament, are more easily distinguishable. An indirect sign of peritoneal microscopic infiltration is the rigidity of the peritoneal layers taking a radial, rail and fanned aspect. When the omentum is highly involved than it's called "omental cake"finding. The great omentum, which has the function of filtering the free, peritoneal liquid, becomes the site of neoplastic solid metastases, sometimes very large, which often join, forming a neoplastic plaster adherent to the anterior parietal peritoneum [22].

At MRI, the malignant ovarian cancer appears as a big, heterogeneous solid and cystic mass. The solid component shows, in T1, low or intermediate signal intensity, while the intensity is quite high in T2. This aspect, however, can be conditioned by the presence of intra lesional haemorrhagic foci, or areas of necrosis. Also the cystic component of the complex mass can have a different signal behaviour. The malignant cystic, ovarian tumours contain abundant proteinaceous or haemorrhagic material causing a high signal intensity both in T1 and in T2. After intravenous paramagnetic contrast material injection, some thickening of the capsule can also be detected, with the presence of septa or intra-cystic vegetations which can be either associated to the mass solid component or not. By gadolinium administration it is obtained an optimal characterization of the solid components of the complex adnexal mass [23]

Lately, Diffusion weighted Imaging (DWI) as a useful tool to improve the radiological diagnosis of malignant tumors, especially for endometrial and cervical tumours. Concerning ovarian cancer, while initially promising DWI in cystic ovarian tumors proved to be limited, particularly for differentiating benign from malignant lesions [24–25]. In a large retrospective analysis the majority of malignant ovarian tumors, mature cystic teratomas, and endometriomas exhibited abnormal signal intensity on DWI, whereas benign lesions did not. A Few studies addressed the use of DWI for peritoneal dissemination of gynaecological cancer assessment: a high sensitivity (90%) and specificity (95.5%) in evaluation of peritoneal dissemination was proven. Nevertheless, the study population was small [24,25].

Preoperative evaluation of upper abdominal organs by ultrasonography or CT scan is important. At the disease onset, in fact, spleen or liver metastases are frequently found according to the tumour stage [26]. For this reason, staging must always include the study of upper abdominal organs. The intraperitoneal, often multifocal, spread of the ovarian cancer is very frequent and well assessable by both CT and MRI (Figure 5).

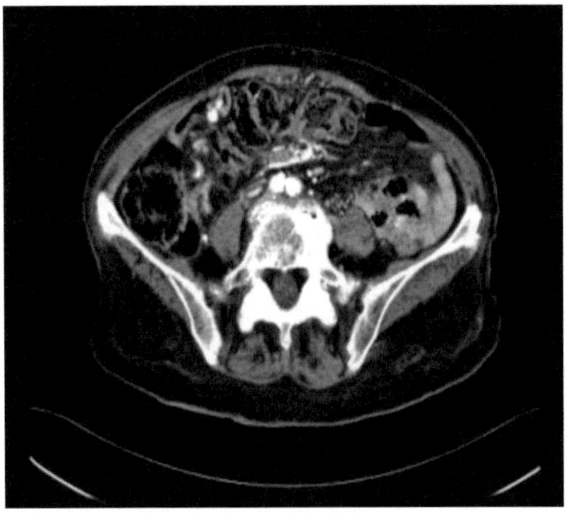

Figure 5. A Contrast Enhanced CT scan showing typical intraperitoneal calcified implants in a serous papillar ovarian cancer (III stage FIGO classification).

The results of preoperative CT and MRI in advanced stages of ovarian cancer can predict the success of the radical surgery. The residual post-surgery tumor must be absent or of a diameter less than 2 cm. This is a very important goal: in these conditions the patients respond better to chemotherapy and have a more favorable prognosis. Through a quantitative score that examines five common anatomic, frequently affected by the disease sites by CT scan, one can select the patients who are eligible to the initial radical treatment. The criteria for the tumor unresectability include the presence of metastases with a diameter greater than 2 cm localized in the following sites: mesenteric root; gastro-splenic ligament; epiploic pouch; hepatic hilum; hepatic, intrasegmental peritoneal reflection; diaphragm and liver dome. Besides other unresectability criteria are: lymphadenopathy greater than 1 cm above the celiac zone; presence of extraperitoneal, presacral disease [26].

9. Adnexal inflammation, tubo-ovarian abscesses and Pelvic Inflammatory Disease (PID)

By the term PID it's meant female genitalia inflammations not only affecting reproductive organs but also the whole pelvic zone, including the pelvic peritoneum. From a pathogenetic point of view PID includes primary and secondary forms, representing In the primary forms, which represent more than 90% of the cases, the inflammation affects initially the lower genital tract (cervico-vaginal tract), spreading subsequently to the uterus, the adnexal glands up to the pelvic peritoneum. In the pathogenesis exogenous factors are involved of such as sexually transmitted germs and instrumental factors; or endogenous factors as in the case of the pathological transformation of cervico-vaginal saprophyte flora. The secondary forms,which are quite rare, are determined from the diffusion to the internal genitalia, through blood, lymphatic or by contiguity, of pathogenic microorganisms from extragenital outbreaks: pyelitis, cysto-pyelitis, cystitis, colitis but especially appendicitis, peri-appendiceal abscess, diverticulitis.

For each pathogenic PID form there have been recognized risk factors. In the case of the primitive exogenous venereal PID they are represented by the young age, frequency and precocity of sexual relationships, number of partners and sex during the menstrual phase.

In the case of primitives exogenous iatrogenic PIDs the most important risk factors are: the use of intrauterine devices (IUD), voluntary termination of pregnancy, endometrial biopsies, hysteroscopy, hysterosalpingography and tubal insufflation. The PID aetiology needs to be continuously updated. It is currently considered to be poly-microbial. We assisted to a reduction of the pathogenic role of Neisseria gonorreae down to 15-20% compared to association of both aerobic and anaerobic germs: streptococci, staphylococci, E.Coli (10-40%); Mycoplasma (10-30%), Chlamydia trachomatis (40-60%). PID includes several pelvic diseases clinically distinguishable into acute and chronic forms. Acute infections are caused by uterine cervical flora that spreads from the mucosal surface to the uterus and fallopian tubes, finally affecting the pelvic and/or abdominal peritoneum. The subacute and chronic form widely varies in extension and severity, including tubal lesions with the formation of pelvic liquid collections and connectival reaction widespread, or by formation of extensive and tenacious adhesions. In order to have an accurate and early PID diagnosis it is essential to the use of imaging techniques. Laparoscopy is essential not only for recognizing the disease but also in order to isolate the pathogenic germs, favouring a targeted therapy.

Based on the laparoscopic findings there are three distinct forms of acute salpingitis, each with different prognostic significance:

- light form: the tubes are hyperemic, edematous, covered with exudate or by deposits of fibrin, but are mobile and with patent ostia;
- moderate form: the signs are more evident and there are doubts about the ostia patency;
- serious form: there is pelvic and peritoneal inflamnation with closed ostia and/or abscess formation.

Ultrasonography was used to confirm the pelvic abscess clinical diagnosis, thanks to its accuracy, sensitivity and specificity. Compared to laparoscophy, endovaginal ultrasonography can recognize almost all of the cases of severe tubal damage, but just 65% of slight tubal damage. Ultrasonography is also very helpful in the follow-up of pelvic inflammation patients, for evaluating the effectiveness of therapy.

On the other hand ultrasonography may be negative both in the acute and in chronic salpingitis. In PID detection of some liquid into the recto-vescical pouch, it may result easy with US, and it may have a higher diagnostic value whenever the liquid presented diffuse or inhomogeneous echogenicity, indicating a blood or purulent collection.

CT scan is not so useful as far as mild and moderate forms are concerned; it's crucial in the recognition and evaluation of the chronic PID.

MRI seems to be very useful in the diagnosis of this disease; it is in fact possible to characterize the inflammation activity, better distinguishing the acute state from the subacute and chronic ones.

The salpingitis initial phase, which is characterized by hyperemia and edema, can be laparoscopically evaluated but not by ultrasound, CT scan and MRI. However, it is a very short lasting phase and is rarely demonstrated even by a early laparoscopy. Salpingitis often follows and is associated with endometritis which can be sonographically demonstrated: the uterus is large, with loss of normal endometrial echogenicity and with irregular, undefined borders; sometimes the cavity may contain hypoechoic material. Even CT scan and MRI don't show, at this stage, any ovarian alterations, while in the presence of endometritis nonspecific uterine abnormalities can be detected: hyper- hypodense endocavitary formations (due to liquid collections) with no enhancement after CM injection.

In the exudative phase, exudate collects in the tubes, covers the fimbrial peritoneum and can spill out of the still open tubal ostium, or, when it's closed, the tubes stretch and become filled with exudate (laparoscopically moderate or severe PID).

By ultrasound, adnexal region appears magnified, with well-defined contours and with a cystic appearance; begins to form a multilobed, often multisepted, sausage-like mass. The

http://dx.doi.org/10.5772/53139

content can be more or less echogenic depending on the blood or exudative component. In some cases of this last condition some pseudo-niches determined by thickening of the tubal mucosa are observable inside the dilated tube.

By CT scan the adnexal region may appear swollen and inhomogeneous; after the CM administration it can be highlighted a marginal rim of intense enhancement delimiting the various ectatic portions of the tube. The pious-sactosalpinge has a more or less folded intestinal-like appearance and by this feature it can be distinguished from other ovarian liquid formations; the density is varying from serous to corpuscular (Figure 6).

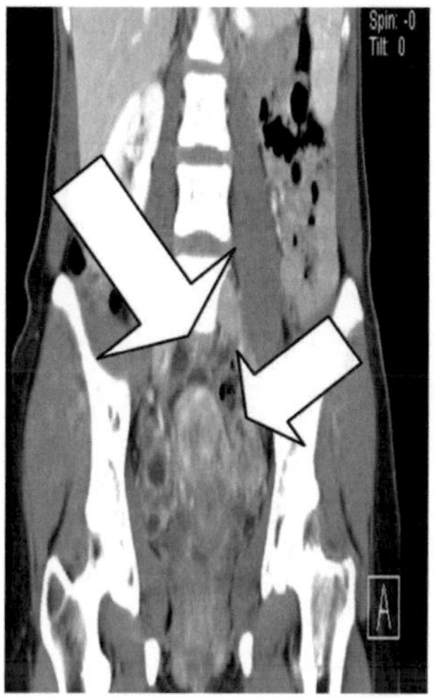

Figure 6. MPR coronal reconstruction of a Contrast Enhanced CT scan during portal phase showing bilateral swelling of the tubes which have an intestinal like appearance in a sactosalpingitis (white arrows).

If an early therapy it hasn't been established, the next step of the inflammation involves the involvement of the ovary. The bag filled with pus extend the the fallopian tubes and ovarian parenchyma making them lose their cleavage planes, wrapped by tenacious adhesions. The tubo-ovarian abscess rupture (3.5%) is a surgical emergency. The tubo-ovarian abscess appears as an adexal or retro-uterine mass, often with internal baffles and sometimes images of gaseous levels. During the appropriate antibiotic treatment the mass becomes better defined and cystic. It can often be found some liquid into the recto-vescical pouch and endo uterine abnormalities can coexist. The echo color Doppler may be helpful in the mass characterization. The hyperaemia and angiogenesis caused by acute inflammation result in an increase of both systolic and diastolic flow velocity, with decreased PI and RI. These altered flow conditions may be reversible during the gradual disappearing of the inflammation. The differential diagnosis must consider the acute salpingitis with sactosalpinx, the tubarian piocele, other conditions of chronic pelvic inflammation without masses.

CT scan, at this stage, detects the adnexal or retro-uterine mass. After CM administration, in the most acute forms, may be evident an intensely enhanced, marginal rim, which is a typical sign of ongoing inflammation. In the acute and sometimes even in chronicle forms the central part of the swelling presents various densities but not contrast enhancement; sometimes there are baffles which delimit internal chambers. In chronic forms the mass may present irregular contours, inhomogeneous density and contrast enhancement.

In neglected cases and in those which do not respond to treatment, the inflammation extends to the entire pelvic peritoneum, the bowel, the contralateral ovary, the bladder and the ureters. The anatomical-pathological framework includes peritoneal inflamnation, distant abscesses and, in the chronicle evolution, adhesions between peritoneal organs, inflammatory infiltration of the peritoneum and retroperitoneal tracts.

By ultrasonography, the pelvis appears very irregular showing ill-defined, irregular contoured masses with both solid and liquid component; under these conditions, the uterus and the ovaries can be indistinguishable. It can be associated, in this framework, hydroureteronephrosis.

CT scan easily recognizes the pelvis structural-anatomical upheaval. By CT scan/MRI certain signs are very obvious which, if present, provide an accurate picture of the disease severity. These signs are: fascial and peritoneal thickening; peri-rectal, peri-vescical, intestinal, pre-sacral, pre-vescical and latero-pelvic fat's increase in density and inhomogeneities; involvement of extra-genital structures; masses that can be dumped to the uterus, may spread to the recto-vescical pouch and to the parametrium. The contours are irregular and hazy [27].

MRI seems to play an important role in the diagnosis of pelvic inflammation as can be used in the initial phase of the disease (the exudative one), or in the tubo-ovarian abscess and pelvic peritonitis. By MRI, the tubo-ovarian abscess appears as a simple or complex cystic mass, with irregular but neat and well defined walls. The cystic component has signal intensity similar or modestly higher than fluid one (low T1 signal and high T2 one); only rarely it may present a high protein content and therefore a blood-like signal (Figure 7).

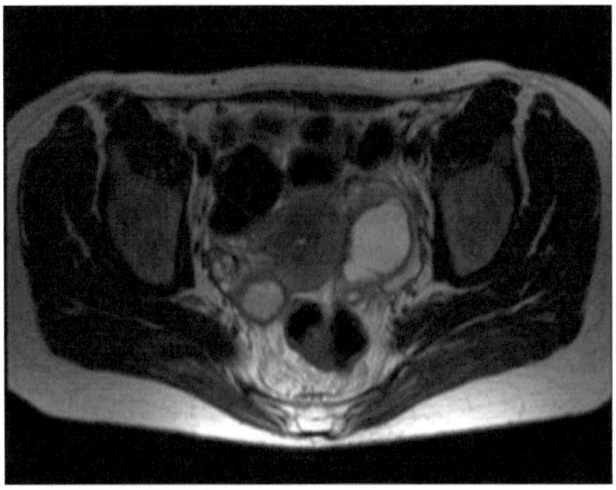

Figure 7. Axial MR scan of a bilateral acute salpingitis. Huge dilatation and bilateral swelling of the tubes can be seen.

http://dx.doi.org/10.5772/53139

10. Metastatic tumours

Ovarian metastatic tumours are quite frequent: they are about 5-10% in the US, and 15-18% in Japan. On Imaging it has to be always considered the possibility of a metastatic tumour whenever a pelvic mass is found. Nevertheless is has been observed that even using all the different imaging methods and machines they can't differentiate with certainty a primary pelvic mass from a secondary one. Both by ultrasonography and CT scan have been described the Krukenberg tumours whose pattern may greatly vary. The common gastric Krukenberg presents a solid, homogeneous, bilateral mass pattern (Figure 8), while the metastasis from colon-rectum have a more often cystic, complex, necrotic pattern.

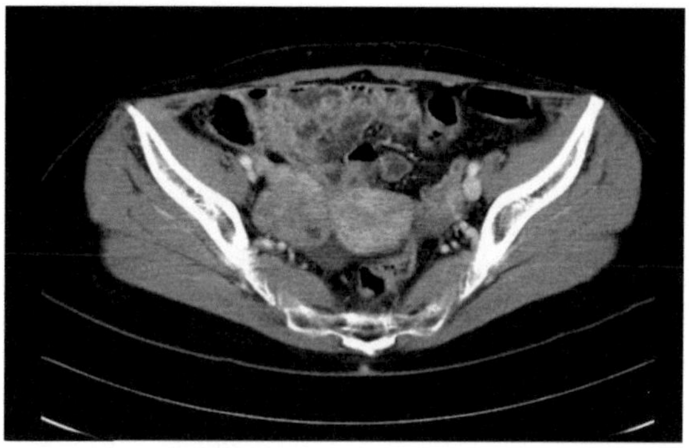

Figure 8. Contrast enhanced CT during portal phase showing two heterogeneously enhanced round masses in a patient suffering from gastric cancer. Histology of the resected masses showed signet-ring cells consistent with Krukenberg metastases.

At US gastric Krukenberg tumours can be bilateral, consisting of complex masses with different percentages of solid and cystic components, frequently associated with ascites. At CT scan Krukenberg tumours are described as mainly solid, with rich peripheral C. E., with cystic component in the cortical or intralesional site masses. The cystic components' walls present a high C.E.

At MRI It is represented by a solid, T2 hypointense, consisting of dense stromal tissue component. It has been than observed that when an apparentely malignant adnexal mass is bilateral, shows well defined but irregular contours, is associated with peritoneal carcinomatosis without ascites, it is 7 times more likely to be a Krunenberg than a primary ovarian tumor.

11. Cystic ovarian teratomas

Mature cystic ovarian teratomas are benign tumours recognisable, using various imaging techniques, by certain characteristics. Already from direct examination of the pelvis, it is possible to obtain very clear images showing teeth-like characteristics, either singular or grouped from a common germinal follicle.

The appearance of dermoid cysts at US is highly variable and depends on the homogeneity and composition of the newly formed tissue. The calcifications inside the mass, characterised by acoustic barriers, are not, however, pathognomonic, as they are also seen in other benign tumours (Brenner) or in malignant adnexal masses. Similar images can be also frequently observed in teratomas and it is possible to recognise not only the Rokitansky protuberance, but also the presence of skin appendages, locks of hair, sebum and glands. The fatty component can also present crude images indicating acoustic barriers, located within a fluid; this is due to varying acoustic impedance of different fat components.

The ultrasound morphology of the mass can be that of a homogenous formation, with elevated echogenicity and a solid appearance; on the other hand it can appear as a cystic formation, either simple or complex depending on the acoustic impedance of the intralesional structures. In some cases, the ultrasound cannot provide a definite diagnosis of teratoma and in others it cannot exclude malignant characteristics.

In CT scans however, the appearance of dermoid cysts is often pathognomonic. CT is the ideal method to evaluate tissue fatty components, leading to a correct diagnosis in case of adnexal fatty mass. Even when other hypodense tissue, like sebum and hair, are present, the fat is recognisable and the, usually, polymorphic appearance in the ultrasound is defined more clearly. CT scans can also correctly identify calcification, better define their morphology and therefore reach a diagnosis. In CT scans it is also very easy to identify fat buoyancy, a pathognomonic sign of dermoid cysts (Figure 9).

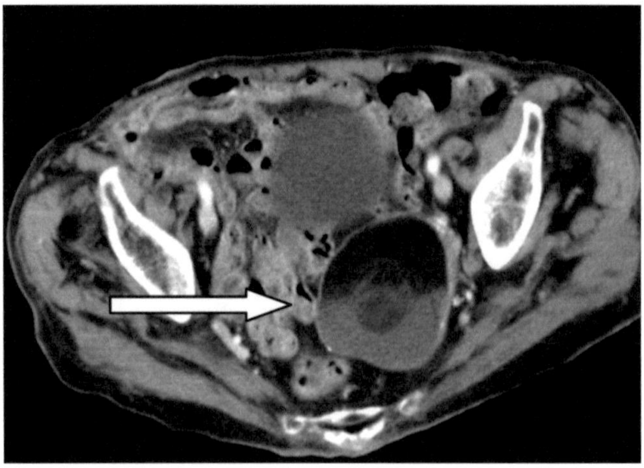

Figure 9. A Contrast Enhanced CT scan showing a huge lesion in the left hemipelvis (white arrow). A fluid –fat level can be seen within the lesion; there is a heterogeneous floating part with soft tissue density. This lesion turned out to be a dermoid cyst.

http://dx.doi.org/10.5772/53139

Even in magnetic resonance imaging (MRI) the diagnosis of dermoid cysts is based on the evidence of fat within the lesion. T1 and T2 weighted images are not enough for this purpose and so fat suppression techniques need to be implemented (Figure 10).

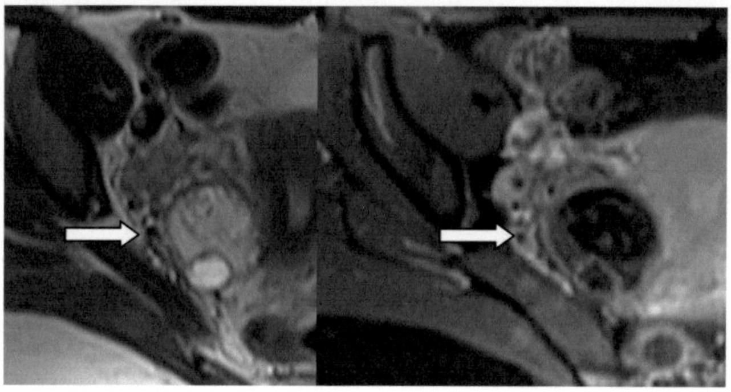

Figure 10. T2-weighted images non-fat saturated (left picture) with fat saturation (right picture) in a MRI scan of a patient with a pelvic mass (white arrow), showing a heterogeneous mass in the left ovary in which there is a signal drop in fat saturated image. The mass proved to be a dermoid cyst.

A differential diagnosis is necessary for endometriotic and mucinous cysts. Diagnostic difficulties may arise when there is a small fat component, or a high levels of hematic content that masks the fatty signals. MRI can correctly evaluate fatty levels and fat buoyancy components, like the Rokitansky nodule; these semiological aspects help differentiate diagnosis. Chemical shift artifacts caused by the presence of fat are also useful in the diagnosis of dermoid cysts. Intravenous administration of gadolinium causes contrast enhancement of the cyst walls and of the Rokitansky nodule [28,29].

Mature teratomas are, in most cases, benign tumours; on occasion, there may be an immature component, with malignant characteristics; this occurs in about 1% of all benign teratomas. The tumour most commonly associated with the teratoma is the squamous-cell carcinoma.

Malignancy signs in a dermoid are indicated by tissue showing clear enhancement. In addition, as the malignant component often infiltrates different dermoid tissues, the capsule, or the extracapsular anatomic structures, it is possible to assess the nature of the cyst by its aggressive morphological appearance. Complications of cystic dermoids are represented by ovarian torsion, or by acute rupture of the mass in the peritoneum.

It is also important to remember that a dysontogenetic pelvic mass may not necessarily originate from the ovary. Sacrococcygeal teratoma and primary retroperitoneal teratomas are more frequent. Sacrococcygeal teratomas are most common dysontogenetic masses in infants; the diagnosis can also be done in uterus, with direct ultrasound visualisation of a presacral mass often associated with polyhydramnios. In many cases the masses are visible externally, developing in the subcutaneous tissue of the intergluteal area;

The masses can have macroscopic appearances, ranging from predominantly cystic, to mixed, to predominantly solid; the last one is most likely to be malignant.

Imaging plays an important role in the diagnosis of these tumours: firstly, through CT ad MRI scans it is possible to differentiate between other abnormalities of the terminal filum such as meningocele and myelomeningocele. It is possible to identify other abnormalities also associated with teratomas in the sacrococcygeal area. Rarely it's possible to observe the growth into the vertebral canal or bone destruction due to teratoma. The association with anal stenosis, vesicoureteral reflux, presacral abscess and skin changes may be indicative of Currarino syndrome.

Acknowledgments

This work has been funded by Covidien AG.

Author details

Francesco Alessandrino[1*], Carolina Dellafiore[1], Esmeralda Eshja[1], Francesco Alfano[1], Giorgia Ricci[1], Chiara Cassani[2] and Alfredo La Fianza[1]

*Address all correspondence to: pragia@hotmail.com

1 Foundation IRCCS, Policlinico San Matteo, Institute of Radiology, University of Pavia,

2 Foundation IRCCS, Policlinico San Matteo, Obstetrics and Gynecology Department, University of Pavia, Italy

References

[1] Liu J, Xu Y, Wang J. Ultrasonography, computed tomography and magnetic resonance imaging for diagnosis of ovarian carcinoma. Eur J Radiol 2007;62:328-334.

[2] Johnson RS. Radiology in the management of the ovarian cancer. Clin Radiol 1993;48:75-82.

[3] Lawrimore T, Rhea JT. Computed tomography evaluation of diverticulitis. J Intensive Care Med. 2004;19(4):194-204.

[4] Neff CC, van Sonnenberg E. CT of diverticulitis: diagnosis and treatment. Radiol Clin North Am 1989;2:743-752.

[5] La Fianza A, Campani R, Dore R, Tateo S. La tomografia Computerizzata nei "garzomi" intraperitoneali. Radiol Med 1991;82.706-710.

[6] Bellin MF, Hornoy B, Richard F, Davy- Miallou C, Fadel Y, Zaim S, Challier E, Grenier Ph. Perirenal textiloma: MR and serial CT appearance. Eur Radiol 1998;8.57-59.

[7] Bast RC, Badgwell D, Lu Z, Marquez R, Rosen D, Liu J, Baggerly KA, Atkinson EN, Skates S, Zhang Z, Lokshin A, Menon U, Jacobs I, Lu K. New tumor markers: Ca125 and beyond. Int J Gynecol Cancer 2005;15(suppl.3):274-281.

[8] Duffy MJ. Tumor Markers in Clinical Practice: A Review Focusing on Common Solid Cancers. Med Princ Pract. 2012 May 15.

[9] Jacobs I, Stabile I, Bridges J, Kemsley P, Reynolds C, Grudzinskas J, Oram D. Multimodal approach to screening for ovarian cancer. Lancet 1988;1(8580):268-71.

[10] Kobayashi M. Illustrated manual of ultrasonography in obstetrics and gynecology. Tokio: Igaku Shoin; 1974.

[11] De Land M, Fried A, Van Nagell JR, Donaldson ES. Ultrasonography in the diagnosis of tumors of the ovary. Surg Gynecol Obstet 1979;148:346-348.

[12] Hermann UJ Jr, Locher GW, Goldhirsch A. Sonographic patterns of ovarian tumors: predictions of malignancy. Obstet Gynecol 1993;69:1225-1228.

[13] Granberg S, Norstrom A, Wikland M. Comparison of endovaginal ultrasound and cytological evaluation of cystic ovarian tumours. J Ultrasound Med 1991;10:9-14.

[14] Jacobs I, Oram D, Fairbanks J, Turner J, Frost C, Grudzinskas JG. A risk of malignancy index incorporating CA 125, ultrasound and menopausal status for the accurate preoperative diagnosis of ovarian cancer. Br J Obstet Gynaecol 1990;97(10):922-9.

[15] Kurjak A, Predanic M. New scoring system for prediction of ovarian malignancy based on transvaginal color-Doppler sonography. J Ultrasound Med 1992;11: 631-638.

[16] Sassone AM, Timor-Tritsch IE, Artner A, Westhoff C, Warren WB. Transvaginal sonographic characterization of ovarian disease. Evaluation of a new scoring system to predict ovarian malignancy. Obstet Gynecol 1991; 78:70-76.

[17] Rossi A, Braghin C, Soldano F, Isola M, Capodicasa V, Londero AP, Forzano L, Marchesoni D. A proposal for a new scoring system to evaluate pelvic masses: Pelvic Masses Score (PMS). Eur J Obstet Gynecol Reprod Biol. 2011;157(1):84-8.

[18] Guerriero S, Alcazar JL, Ajossa S, Galvan R, Laparte C, García-Manero M, Lopez-Garcia G, Melis GB. Transvaginal color Doppler imaging in the detection of ovarian cancer in a large study population. Int J Gynecol Cancer. 2010;20(5):781-6.

[19] Fattaneh A. Tavassoli Peter Devilee, editors. World Health Organization Classification of Tumours. Pathology and Genetics of Tumours of the Breast and Female Genital Organs. Lyon: IARCPress; 2003.

[20] Gatreh-Samani F, Tarzamni MK, Olad-Sahebmadarek E, Dastranj A, Afrough A. Accuracy of 64-multidetector computed tomography in diagnosis of adnexal tumors. J Ovarian Res. 2011;17:4-15.

[21] Tempany CMC, Zou KH, Silverman SG, Brown DL, Kurtz AB, McNeil BJ. Staging of advanced ovarian cancer: comparison of imaging modalities-report from the radiological diagnostic oncology group. Radiology 2000;215:761-767.

[22] Petru E, Schmidt F, Mikosch P, Pickel H, Lahousen M, Tamussino K, Gruendler N, Porsch E. Abdominopelvic Computed Tomography in the preoperative evaluation of suspected ovarian masses. Int J Gynecol Cancer 1992;2: 252-255.

[23] Bazot M, Daraï E, Nassar-Slaba J, Lafont C, Thomassin-Naggara I. Value of magnetic resonance imaging for the diagnosis of ovarian tumors: a review. J Comput Assist Tomogr. 2008;32(5):712-23.

[24] Levy A, Medjhoul A, Caramella C, Zareski E, Berges O, Chargari C, Boulet B, Bidault F, Dromain C, Balleyguier C. Interest of diffusion-weighted echo-planar MR imaging and apparent diffusion coefficient mapping in gynecological malignancies: a review. J Magn Reson Imaging. 2011;33(5):1020-7.

[25] Fujii S, Kakite S, Nishihara K, Kanasaki Y, Harada T, Kigawa J, et al. Diagnostic accuracy of diffusion- weighted imaging in differentiating benign from malignant ovarian lesions. J Magn Reson Imaging 2008;28:1149–1156.

[26] Buchsbaum HJ, Brady MF, Delgado G, Miller A, Hoskins WJ, Manetta A, Sutton G. Surgical staging of carcinoma of the ovaries. Surg Gynecol Obstet 1989;169:226-232.

[27] Rezvani M, M. Shaaban A. Fallopian Tube Disease in the Nonpregnant Patient. RadioGraphics 2011;31:527–548.

[28] Devine C, Szklaruk J, Tamm EP. Magnetic resonance imaging in the characterization of pelvic masses. Semin Ultrasound CT MR. 2005;26(3):172-204.

[29] Imaoka I, Wada, A, Kaji,Y, Hayashi T, Hayashi M, Matsuo M, Sugimura K. Developing an MR Imaging Strategy for Diagnosis of Ovarian Masses. Radiographics. 2006;26(5):1431-48.